NEW LEASE OF LIFE

By Gunnar Espedal

© 2016 Gunnar V Espedal

Published on behalf of Gunnar V Espedal by Forj Marketing

Viktorklinikken, Snekkerveien 22,

4321 Sandnes, Norway

+47 98841615

gunnar.espedal@gmail.com

www.gunnarespedal.com

ISBN-13: 978-0995372603
ISBN-10: 0995372608

Disclaimer: New Lease of Life is intended solely for information and education. Please contact a medical or health professional if you have questions about your health.

"I love what you have written. NEW LEASE OF LIFE is very evocative and poignant and offer many insights and the education in this book should be taught in schools."

(Stephanie Hale, Author, entrepreneur,
Oxford Literary Consultancy)

"New Lease of Life contains vital information concerning the health benefits of alkaline ionized water, ionizing air purification, and so much more. Having been in the air purification and alkaline ionized water purification field for over 25 years, we found the book highly informative and an eye opening look into the importance and beneficial rewards of incorporating pure healthy water and air into our lives."

(Keith Jones, Carey Jones, Author, Vollara Presidential Directors)

"This is the wake-up call the world so desperately needs and has been waiting for, true hard facts, true wisdom, combined with infinite love of life itself. NEW LEASE OF LIFE is the ultimate 'must read'. It is an encyclopedia of vital-to-life information that will change the lives of all who journey through these wonderful pages and in due course of every living creature on this beautiful blue dot we have the God-given privilege to call home.

NEW LEASE OF LIFE is highly informative, warm and sensitive. It draws you in and captivates you completely. You do not want the story to end. You know you are changed and inspired. In essence NEW LEASE OF LIFE is an intelligent work of art that speaks the universal language that all will understand. Our cells turn towards the wisdom and love within its pages as sunflowers turn their faces to the sun; it is an entirely natural process."

(Susannah King. Natural medicine specialist and former secretary of P.M. H. Wilson, UK)

DEDICATION

This book is dedicated to my mother and father who taught me that music and dance, poetry and nature's own beauty are intrinsically and strongly connected to love itself.

This book is also dedicated to my seven colorful children: Louisa Jayne, Camilla Victoria, Viktor Emanuel, Daniel Oliver, Nikoline Florentyna, Magny Simona and Sølve Kristoffer.

I love you with all my heart.

ACKNOWLEDGEMENTS

I am forever grateful for Teta Montaha, now 106 years old, who is a living and thriving example of the advice offered in this book, who danced with me the oriental style of Lebanon and for her granddaughter RoRo, who taught me the pure poetry and emotion, the life enhancing motion of oriental music and belly dance. As an appreciation of the generosity showed to me from the whole Karam family in Beirut, I decided to present the book translated to French for the benefit of the Lebanese people especially, and for this work I am very grateful for the excellent translation of Casimir B. Dassi from Benin. Thank you brother!

A well-deserved thank you to Raymonde Karam Fossan who opened my eyes to her beloved Lebanon, the wonderful cuisine and people. God's cedars and breath taking beauty of the country, so well described by the psalmist: "Well watered are the trees of the Lord, the cedars of Lebanon which He planted" - Psalm 104:6.

A great thank you for helping me out with the typing of the manuscript goes to Lisa Myhren, Ingvild Sara Aarsland, Nikoline Florentyna, Magny Simona and Daniel Oliver. And also, thank you to Ingvild Sara for excellent photographs taken. Thank you also to Martha Dec for producing the beautiful cover for the book.

Thank you to my professional editors Stephanie Hale from Oxford Literary Consultancy and Debbie Brunettin for invaluable suggestions and advice; and Sam Taylor, Olga Rachello for their great work with my website development. On the other side of the world, on a tiny island called Norfolk Island 877 miles east of Australia, God connected me to Sharni-Marie Barney, who is doing a marvelous job with the website, blogs and all the social media presentation, as well as getting this book to print. Without your skills I would have been lost in the tango. Thank you, sister!

A special thank you to my colleague and friend Susannah King for always cheering me on and believing in me!

Thank you to Ralf Iwersen and Carey Jones from Vollara for all your encouragement in the making of this book.

I am indebted and forever grateful to my own brother Odd Birger and his wife Elna for standing by me in the stormy weathers and the walk in the dark valley. Without them this book would not have been completed.

Writing New Lease of Life has been an epic journey, much like a brook flowing and dancing down a hillside to the tune of solids on its way to the sea. Energetically, invigorating and challenging. At the end of the journey, a new circle started with the invention of a unique water generator which transforms and improves the water quality in every way. More of that in book number two... Meanwhile I hope you enjoy this book as much as I enjoyed writing it for you!

PREFACE

A few years ago I received a Christmas present, a book from my oldest son Viktor with the telling title "All the Sad Literary Men." Point taken, it was his way of gently nudging his dad and encouraging him to reach the tipping-point, stop procrastinating and produce the book, long time overdue. "Time to teach the world some of your old wisdom and new discoveries and inventions from your armamentarium, or face being the joke of the family at the annual Christmas party. Show me what you`ve got in your tool-box, dad!"

"Everybody can be great...because everybody can serve", said Dr. Martin Luther King Jr.

Having had the joy and privilege to serve and help people with health problems for almost fifty years as a physiotherapist, counselor, coach, mentor and naturopath as well as inventor/entrepreneur, this book is about the joy of finding the most efficient keys to transform your life completely. I have come from a life with pain, low energy, overweight and so-called incurable ailments to a life without pain, full of energy, creative passion and drive, fit as a fiddle, ready to help and serve others.

In other words: A New Lease of Life!

At an early age I became quite familiar with serious disease and suffering, especially in my teens when our father got cancer and died at 51 years of age. Seeing our dad, hero and Tarzan (Johnny Weissmuller look-alike) gradually withering away, was a shock. Clutching his hand, screaming from my soul for a miracle, whilst holding a book on miracles by a well-known faith healer Katryn Kuhlman, hoping for a divine intervention. Nothing happened, except a seed was sowed. Little did I know that 20 years later I would receive Yeshua as my Saviour and Healer, and receive the gifts of healing and miracles, all by Grace. Terminal cancer patients healed. Blind eyes opened, pain and incurable diseases disappeared, all confirmed by medical doctors. However, in this period evil trolls in the pharmaco family appeared and began many years of persecution and character assassination. But the enjoyment I received from all the happy people who instantly received miraculous healing, was far greater than the lies, harassment and persecution by medical doctors and health government bureaucrats. A crisis as experienced by our dad's passing away also carried within a seed, an opportunity, a stepping stone towards my mission in life. Interesting to note that the Chinese word-sign for crisis and opportunity is exactly the same!

The main area of focus in this book is on vitality of water, air, food, faith, moves, love and humor.

Learning to revitalize and balance these areas in your life is fun, easy and will give you immediate benefits. Just one example is the study of William James, a genius psychologist and philosopher and his 'AS IF' principle. Act the part, be surprised and receive some amazing benefits! There are many other examples of 'TLC', tender, love and care principles, as taught by the great Miss M. Hollis, MBE. Principal, Bradford Hospital School of Physiotherapy.

This book is a playful journey, a proven pathway that has worked successfully for more than 100,000 patients in Norway and abroad. You will learn spiritual truths on health prevention, natural care and cure to modern scientific research on water's ability to receive, communicate and broadcast messages (M. Emotu). You will learn about Pure Energy Norway, a brand new line of frequency water generators that will restructure and purify your water and body giving you a New Lease of Life, and giving you spring water quality every time you turn on the faucet. What fun we have when animals and plants and wild life is seen to be thriving, very rewarding, thanks to a new revolutionary invention!

Change your water and receive significant health benefits straight away. As Teta Montaha, 106 years old from Beirut, Lebanon said: "The greatest health secret is in the water!"

"The greatest wealth is health." – Virgil

Therapeutically Yours,

Gunnar V Espedal

CONTENTS

CHAPTER ONE

One Drop of Water

'And the spirit of God moved upon the face of the waters'. Gen.1.2.

'In one drop of water are found all the secrets of all the oceans; in one aspect of you are found all aspects of existence.' Kahlil Gibran

One fine April morning, I walked down my memory lane in the small village called Eidane, situated by the world-famous and mysterious Lysefjorden, which affords a view across to Norway's most visited tourist attraction, The Pulpit Rock. I sat in the field by the river, reminiscing and singing, 'Those were the days my friend, I thought they'd never end,' a line from the 1968 number one hit song by Welsh singer Mary Hopkins, an original Old Russian romance song, *Dorogoi Dlinnoyu*, (*Along a Long Road*). As the sun illuminated one of the mountains a greyish tinge of purple, the granite mountain came alive, almost vibrating. Energy. A flimsy cloud formation glided past on the blue sky; energy reminding me, as the wise Albert Einstein had mused, that imagination is more important than knowledge. An eagle circled above my head, steadily rising, almost effortlessly.

In the early fifties we arrived in this magical place called Eidane, by the mysterious Lysefjorden, so much praised and loved by my family. That is where we put down our roots, and it was on the farm that our father, the carpenter, artist and nature-loving kind soul, evolved. Every summer we came here and participated in the work at the farm, getting delightfully drunk on the scents and sounds of the season: pink and red roses; gardenias with their beautiful and fragrant flowers; daisies, violets, jasmine; the buzzing of bees and the most annoying horseflies, which unfortunately we could not hear but definitely felt when they stung! At one end of the shimmering lake were the most exquisite bright-coloured water lilies, reminding me of Monet's famous water lily paintings. Enchanting and beautiful as they might be, we were sternly warned never to go swimming there as we might get entangled in the plants. There would be the occasional croaking sound of a toad, mysteriously dead and flat, to wake us in the morning. In fact, all of the animals on the farm—all creatures great and small—talked to us. Henry, our father and Olav, our uncle, together with our cousins, helped out in the fields, shovelling the grass to dry on hayracks. It was tough work, especially for my brother and I, both of us from the city. Sweat would be pouring down our backs. I remember we were very in awe of our cousins, who lived on the farm, walking barefoot on the sharp stubbles of grass. I remember Aunty's last admonishing remark down at the farmhouse: 'Don't forget to drink water in this heat.'

One day, during one of our breaks, we walked further up the hill. And there, all of a sudden, although we couldn't see any sign of a brook, our uncle revealed a water well of fresh, gushing water— coming from some secret place beneath the ground. Amazing!

Wide-eyed, I asked where this extraordinary well came from.

Our father solemnly declared, 'Deep, deep inside the earth, son! From the earth's cathedral!' My little brother and I looked dumbfounded. Getting down on our knees, we gratefully drank the pure, refreshing mountain water. As if by magic, we felt our energy being restored as our cells were rehydrated.

We all felt refreshed after drinking the natural, pristine water from deep down in the earth, an aquifer just as we had imagined it would be, and we resumed our work. For the kids, the days were long and tough, as we worked in the heat. At the end of the day, our uncle Olav would saunter down to the farm and collect two big jugs (called *Norges glass*) of something brown—an unknown liquid to us small, innocent kids. He would put the jugs in the well to cool. It was time to celebrate—both the visit from his youngest brother, Henry, and the help we were providing to his family out in the fields of 'the green, green grass of home' (a line from Welsh singer Tom Jones's hit song, 1966), and for another successful day shovelling, gathering and drying the hay. Two brothers enjoying each other's company and their kids roaming around playing in the fields. Two strong men enjoying homebrewed beer, made from the same gushing well that had so impressed my brother and I, the city kids turned farmers. Two brothers, the oldest and the youngest, quenching their thirst and 'loosening their tongues', as our uncle Olav once expressed it. They reminisced, squinting up at the blue sky, as they were soaking in the healthy vitamin D from the sun. They both agreed that 'happy is the man who has a mouthful of beer'

(Egyptian saying)—especially when brewed by loving, caring hands from pure, mineral-rich healthy water from the earth's cathedral.

In the late afternoon, we sauntered down to the farm to enjoy the wonderful, nutritious and natural whole-food meal prepared by Aunty Helene, a study, strong and portly lady, always smiling. She reminded me of a Russian matryoshka: the commanding, jovial family figurehead of a peasant family. We had completed another blessed summer's day. Our celebrated kingdom of nature at Eidane always magically inspired and rejuvenated us. Gorgeous flowers and myriad colours—vivid reds, elegant whites, warm yellows, rich browns and soft hues of blue.

Natural fertiliser from outdoor loos, buzzing flies and midges—much to the delight of the healthy trout and salmon in the crystal-clear lakes and rivers.

In the early seventies, a noticeable change was observed in our environment as acid rain from the UK and the continent turned many lakes and rivers into hostile environments for fish. This effect was felt greatest in the south and southwest of Norway. My childhood Eldorado was badly affected.

As we all know, rain is slightly acidic, but acidic rain mixed with a whole range of industrial pollutants is different. Airborne pollution such as sulphur dioxide, nitrogen dioxide and associated carbons reacts in the air with sunlight and water to form nitric acid, sulphuric acid and other assorted mineral acids and ammonium salts. In Rome, the rain that lands on the rocks from which it is made is dissolving the famous Pantheon. In India, the Taj Mahal is suffering the same problem.

Both in Norway and Sweden, salmon and trout died as a result of this acid rain. Some improvement was achieved by depositing vast quantities of limestone rocks into the lakes to counteract some of the acidity.

But acid rain is a problem that occurs the world over. In North America, thousands of lakes along the eastern coast are so acidic that fish can no longer survive.

Lysefjorden is located in the Forsand in Ryfylke in south-western Norway. The name means light fjord, possibly derived from the light-coloured steep granite rocks along its edges. The fjord was carved by the action of glaciers in the ice ages and was later flooded by the sea when the glaciers retreated. The geology of Lysefjorden was thoroughly investigated and described by Professor Bjørn G. Andersen in his master's thesis in 1954. The fjord measures twenty-six miles, roughly a marathon, with steep rocks falling 1000 m (3000ft.) into the water. Because of the inhospitable terrain, the fjord is lightly populated; Forsand and Lysebotn being at the opposite end of the fjord. The places of my childhood, such as Eidane, Flørli, Songesand and others, were home to active communities with fishing, farming and small industries. Lysebotn, at the far end, is largely populated by workers from the nearby hydro-electric plants at Lyse and Tjodan, both constructed within inside the mountains. At the Lyse plant, the water falls 650 m into the turbines, producing up to 110,000 kW electricity. At Tjodan the water falls 896m to yield an output of 210.000K.W. The two power plants provide electricity to more than 100.000 people. A spectacular road which rises to almost 900 m (2700ft.) through a series of 27 hairpin bends links Lysebotn with the outside world.

Lysefjorden is an extremely popular tourist attraction, boasting the world-renowned Pulpit Rock (Prekestolen) and Kjerag Mountain, considered the best places in the world for base-jumping. Not only is the fjord long and narrow, but it is in places as deep as the mountains are high. It is only 13 m (43 ft.) deep outside Forsand, where the action of the glaciers has moved stones and gravel from the mountains and a nearby valley, Espedalen, forming a ground moraine in the landscape.

As a little kid, I was awestruck by power of the water each time I visited the hydroelectric power plants in Lysebotn, Måkali and Flørli, and frequently listened to my grandfather's stories of how they had constructed the plant and harnessed the water. Building the pipes and water dam required high physical stamina; in 1934, Kristen Helmikstøl carried 170 kg cement on his back 500 m far up from the water and into the mountains. Together with his brothers Magnus and Thomas and their father Nils Helmikstøl, my great-grandfather, they carried huge weights of cement and timber up the steep mountainside. Kristen was reported in the newspapers to have carried more than the horse! Those people were the Sherpas of Lysefjorden—but a trifle stronger, I might add.

The Pentecostals were quite active during the building process of the power plant and were adamant about keeping liquor-drinking in check. It was believed that they had control over the situation, but one day, calamity broke loose: one of the workers was reported to have fallen into delirium, screaming and behaving like a lunatic. Everybody was visibly shaken by the commotion until another message reached the Pentecostal community. It was not the liquor that had made the poor chap mad, but he had drunk 'herevatn' (herdevann), tempering water to quench his thirst. This is the water that the blacksmith used to harden the steel, and it may well have contained carbon, phosphorus, manganese, sulphur, aluminium, chromium, nickel and iron, or other contaminants. A water far removed from the vital and structured water in the brooks nearby. The poor old chap nevertheless survived and was able to resume his hard work.

Talking of strong, vital and religious people, my grandmother Gunnvor Serina, the sister of the famous strongmen from Helmikstøl, married a Swede, Viktor Lundquist who came to Forsand 1916. They moved to Flørli where Viktor, my grandfather (who was the model portrayed in the well-known statue 'Rallaren'), worked at the hydroelectric plant, before moving to Lysebotn in 1952. Gunnvor worked as cook and matron at the functionary hostel for Lyse Kraftverk. She was a strong woman, often seen carrying 40 kg sacks of flour under each arm as if it were nothing. She was also a wonderful cook of healthy and nutritious Norwegian food, for which she became legendary.

Many years later, after retirement in 1967, she stayed at the home of her daughter Marit and her husband Arne. Because of her diabetes, she often became thirsty at night. One night, Uncle and

Aunty woke up to hollering and screaming from Grandmother's bedroom: 'Arne, Arne, I am dying, I am dying! Come and rescue me!' The whole family shot out of bed, shocked at the incident, only to discover that Grandmother had taken a swig of the bottle of 96% distillation spirit instead of her water bottle, used to disinfect the needles she used for her insulin injection. Grandmother, a very religious Pentecostal woman and teetotal as far as alcohol was concerned, must surely have thought hell and brimstone had fallen upon her.

Later on, once Grandma's burning throat had been soothed by water and she was reassured that she would survive, it became a hilarious family joke. There is nothing like a good laugh for health and longevity. Even Grandma agreed with that saying, and she chuckled when I quipped an old Norwegian saying: 'It is difficult to get rid of old weed!'

The whole story reminded me of the poor chap at Flørli who had quenched his thirst accidentally with 'herdevann', or tempering water, and was thought to be in delirium due to alcohol intoxication.

Nobody would disagree that good old Grandma could be a demanding woman. Sometimes she gathered her religious friends at my aunty and uncle's home. Around a table, always laden with a sumptuous spread of delicious food as Grandma liked to impress people with her cooking skills, they would chat and discuss various topics. Most of her friends were more vocal than Grandma, and perhaps of this fact she would demand immediate attention from Aunty Marit, shouting, 'Phantom pain, phantom pain! Marit, Marit, come and scratch my stump!' Grandma had had to have a below-knee amputation due to complications resulting from her longstanding diabetes. A little wound on her food became infected, resulting in bad circulation and gangrene, and amputation became the only solution for her. When she felt left out, she would shout for help, and many times we were forced to crawl under the table to stretch her amputated limb. Who dare dispute Grandma's phantom pain, argue and oppose the demanding matriarch? Nobody.

Those religious meetings became something of a nightmare for my poor aunty, because it was always the same procedure—every time! Crawling on the floor, scratching Grandma's stump. What a sight!

As a newly qualified physiotherapist at the time, I encouraged Grandma to train. With an enormous push and shove, we managed to get her out of her wheelchair (very reluctantly, I must add). Considerably overweight, she incessantly complained about her prosthesis, which prompted me to design a new strapping, which made her happy for a while. In the end we gave up and until this day, I still do not know who was happiest about the final decision to heave her back into the wheelchair—Grandma, Aunty or me!

Grandma had a big heart, was a legendary cook (see recipes at the end of this book), but also a demanding matriarch.
I was more than happy to drive her to her religious meetings, but used to get quite distressed as she would nudge me from her wheelchair and say, 'Repent and receive Jesus, Gunnar, or else…'

I recall endless letters she wrote to me while I was studying physiotherapy in Bradford, Yorkshire. 'Repent—or else: hell and brimstone. The gnashing of teeth.' She meant well and prayed for me every day. I loved her and, being born on the same date, 20.02, I was able to get underneath that stern and sometimes sour facial expression of hers using humour, teasing and tickling her until she would burst out laughing, tears rolling down her chubby cheeks, wheelchair creaking as her big frame threatened to fall out of the chair.

'Don't forget your fluids, Grandma! See you soon!' would be my well-meaning words of advice each time I left her. She was careful to drink her vital water; due to her diabetes, rehydration was imperative for her well-being. Whether she remembered the poor worker at Flørli who had been wrongly accused of having been deliriously intoxicated, I do not remember. In any case, she never confused her two bottles of clear fluid anymore and remained a teetotaller for the rest of her life, bless her! All her prayers, letters and even admonitions where answered almost twenty-five years later: I received Yeshua as my Saviour, which turned everything upside down. I had never been happier in my life.

Your body has many ways of healing and balancing your life. Knowing yourself is a great stepping stone towards reclaiming your health. Begin today by putting down your final goal. In writing. Become aware of what you put in your body. Is it helping your body to work efficiently—or hindering it? Which lifestyle change can I implement *today*? Remember: The right information put into action will help you take control over your situation.

Victor Hugo's Dark Corridor

A lot of water has passed under the bridge since all this took place. Little did I know how significant and exhilarating the new science and experience of vital water would be, and how many millions of people it would touch, giving them a healthier and better life. Strange to think that it started in Lysefjorden, which the famous French Writer Victor Hugo described dramatically following a visit in 1866:

'Nowhere are these frightful and overwhelmingly compound forces more evident than in this strange fjord up in the north, called Lysefjorden. This is the most dreadful and most fearful fjord arm that exists. Not anywhere is the secret interplay between the elements more complete. Here, in the middle of this wasteland, enters a gloomy street. A no-man's street. A corridor 50 km (*wrong: 42km, dear Hugo*) between 1000-metre-high mountain walls. Where is the wind? Not in the air. Where is the thunder? Not in the sky. The wind is in the sea; the thunder is in the mountains. Sometimes the water is shaken as if under an earthquake. Sometimes thunder can be heard without a cloud in the sky. All of a sudden, a luminous ray shoots out from the mountain wall and retracts like a boomerang, then shoots out again. One mountain attacks another. Bombardment in the walls of the mountains. It is the hate between the cliff's abyss striking yet again.'

In his poetic writing, this is how the great French romantic writer Victor Hugo spoke of Lysefjorden in *Toilers of the Sea*. Maybe Victor Hugo was still depressed following the death by drowning of his daughter Leopoldine Korreles and her husband in 1843, or from living in exile in Guernsey and later Jersey for nineteen years.

Far from the fearful scenery that Victor Hugo described, my brother and I experienced exciting and blissful days with our cousins, swimming and boating in the lake and the fjord. Afterwards, we would climb to the top of the mountain on the opposite side of the famous Pulpit Rock to admire the ice-cream-cone shape of its granite structure. Other days, we rowed across the fjord on botanical excursions to climb Fantajuvet to find rare flowers for our herbarium.

All these stories and many more came flooding back to me when we made a boat trip to Lysefjorden for our daughter Camilla Victoria and Jonathan's wedding. Acting as a guide for our English friends, I pointed out funny and interesting pieces of the fjord's history and peculiarities, to the amusement of our friends. When the boat stopped by a well-known tourist spot next to the steep granite mountain wall, we were offered 'fresh spring water', trickling down the mountain site. Small beakers of water were passed around. Suddenly, a man introduced himself to me: 'I'm a medical doctor; I would not recommend you drink that.' As I heard the distant bells ringing indicating that a flock of sheep were grazing in the vicinity, I got his point. Contaminated by sheep? *Brucella abortus melitensis* (a bacteria) might well be a possibility here—but, in faith, I raised my glass to the other wedding guests and to the soon-to-be-wed couple, Milla and Jono. Fresh water with perhaps a touch of something added, but definitely blessed! Quite honestly, having swum in the River Thames and gulped a few mouthfuls of *that* dubious water, the Lysefjorden water was a no-brainer for me!

The next day, I led my daughter up the aisle at Sola Ruinkirke. Facing the congregation, my back to the beautiful sandy beach at Sola and the North Sea, where my ancestors the fearless Vikings once crossed to Lindisfarne and to England to 'rape, burn and pillage', I read, captivated, from King James, Bible, 1. Corinthians 13 about unconditional love: *'And now abideth faith, hope, charity, these three; but the greatest of these is charity.'*

Viking Heritage

The Sola Ruinkirke, built on the remains of a roman stone church and dating easily from 1100, is a monument that stands on the grounds in commemoration of Erling Skjalgsson (975-1038), a famous Viking leader who lived here and is credited for bringing Christianity to the county of Rogaland. The Christian monks wrote about the fearless Viking sailors of the seas who navigated long distances, using the sunstone, Icelandic Spar, to navigate when the sun was out of sight (ref. the Alderney crystal), and believed to be putting up settlements even in North America as early as the 10th century.

All you Need is Love, Weddings and Singing in the Rain

As I walked out of the church, now overlooking the vastness of the North Sea, I enjoyed the rain as I pondered the water's natural hydrological cycle: Water evaporates from the surface of the ocean. Moist air is lifted, it cools and water vapour condenses to form clouds. Moisture is then transported around the globe until it returns to the surface as precipitation. As I thought about this, I was humming happily and singing Andy Williams' song, *Raindrops Keep Fallin' on my Head*, Hal David and Burt Bacharach's no.1 for the 1969 film *Butch Cassidy and the Sundance Kid* (Academy Award for Best Original Song).

Prancing and dancing around the church grounds in Norwegian national costume, a most happy and proud father, I felt part of the greater wholeness of the magnificent Creation. Have you ever wondered about the fact that the water molecules that land on your head from time to time might have quenched the thirst of an elephant, a dinosaur, Yeshua or Buddha? 'Happiness steps up to greet me!' The line from the hit song caught my imagination as I prepared for the wedding pictures with the rest of my family.

In traditional Agrarian societies, rain was seen as a blessing from above, and drought a signal of divine disfavour. But in the modern-day industry culture, precipitation and clouds are often described using 'lowly' bodily connotations for the phenomenon: in England it 'pisses down'; in Norway, we talk about '*pissvær*'; the French for 'drizzle', '*crachiner*', also implies a spitting; the German '*niesen*', a little sneeze. In the parched Far East, 'Your sky is always filled with clouds' is a symbol of good fortune. In the Western world, prolonged darkness and clouds are associated with S.A.D, seasonal affective disorder and its accompanying symptoms of depression, lethargy and melancholy. A cloud dotted on the in a blue sky is a sign of happiness. But stoically we cheer ourselves up that 'every cloud has a silver living'. The British are best at this, aren't they? Stoicism. In England, at least rain clouds are rarely invoked after protracted periods of drought or on the fifth day of a cricket match against Australia. People are sick of seeing them.

The curative powers of water are not only for the soul, but also for bodily ailments. The mythology of the fountain of external youth is water's most potent power of regeneration is also connected to countering specific maladies. According to the practical wisdom of the ancient Indian Atharva Veda, water has healing powers that drive away diseases and also has a creative capacity. Holy wells and springs embody water's divine life-giving and life-preserving qualities. The human eye is also metaphorically associated with water. This is beautifully described in Henry Thoreau's book Walden, in his description of lakes as a landscape's most wonderful and expressive feature: 'A lake is the earth's eye, looking into which the beholder measures the depth of his own nature.' The trees by the lakeside are its eyelashes; the wooded hills its brows. In the freezing winter, it closes its eyelids to become dormant for three months or more.

The River Thames and Healing Water, Lake Baikal, Pearl of Siberia

Eye disease (ocular ailments) and its connection with water led Peter Ackroyd to describe the River Thames—along with the 26 healing springs found in the vicinity, which resulted in the practice of healing for the eyes being viewed more credibly. Glaucoma is popularly known as 'water of the eyes'. The disease is caused by increased pressure within the eyeball as a result of blockage of fluid. The word shares its etymological roots with Glaucus, one of the Greek sea-gods. 'Glaucus' means bluish-green, the colour of the sea.

The tradition of eye-healing goes back to the time of Augustine's miracles near the river at Crickload, where he enabled the blind to see, as well as to the ophthalmological marvels attributed to the 7th-century princess Frideswide at the well at Binsey near Oxford. This was the well that was transformed in Lewis Caroll's *Alice in Wonderland*— 'Treacle well', where treacle, an old term derived from Latin thermic, meaning *medicine or antidote to poison.*

I find it interesting to think that the London Eye, situated next to the River Thames, is the world's most visited tourist attraction, in the context of eye-healing and the twenty-six healing springs found in the vicinity.

Another modern-day demonstration of the divinity of the water is Lake Baikal, in southern Siberia, the oldest and deepest lake on the planet, which holds one-fifth of the world's fresh water.

Spanning 23,000 cubic kilometres, this is more than all North America's Great Lakes combined. If all our water taps were switched off tomorrow, Baikal's water could keep all six billion of us sated for about forty years. This pristine patch of industrialised Russia, a UNESCO World Heritage Site (1996), holds the greatest secrets in its depths. At the bottom of the lake, where the pressure can puncture three-inch-thick steel, are tiny, transparent fish called golomyanka, made up of thirty-five per cent fat. The Baikal Sea is said to contain more than a thousand epidemic species, including the herpa, the world's only freshwater seal, as well as the legendary giant sturgeon—the Baikal Monster—that preys on them. The lake is known as the Blue Eye or the Pearl of Siberia, and its waters are believed to be life-enhancing. Locals claim that you can add a year to your life when you dip a toe in, five years for a hand, and an extra twenty-five if you risk a swim.

Invertebrates ensure that the lake remains the most translucent in the world. Locals joke that it is 'great for murders', because these tiny creatures rapidly process any organic material found in it. But they have limited power, and poisons from cellulose and paper mills threaten the eco-system. It was Khrushchev, the environmental tyrant, who sanctioned the building of the mills 'to put Baikal to work.' When Putin appeared on TV a few years ago, drawing up a map to show where the oil pipeline would run at least twenty-five miles north of the lake, he seems to have wanted to demonstrate that he wasn't just an old-style Soviet handyman, but was genuinely concerned with the water's apparent life-enhancing qualities.

I crossed the North Sea in the autumn of 1971 on a noble mission to be educated, first and foremost in physiotherapy, exactly 1178 years after Lindisfarne (also called the Holy Island) was attacked by my ancestors, the fearsome Vikings. This was a time of turmoil, strikes, 'The Winter of Discontent', and also described, unfairly I think, as a period of economic decline, during the years of Arthur Scargill and the unions, IRA bombings and much more.

Leeds United and Winger Eddie on the Snow

It was here I bonded with Don Revie's Leeds United, Super Leeds who ruled in UK and Europe. Since much of this book is about water in its entire splendour, I am reminded about one of Don Revie's many statements, this time about the fast-moving Scottish winger Eddie Gray, Frank's older brother whom I met a few times in Bradford where I studied.

'Eddie,' (Gray) said Don (Revie), 'moves along the white chalk lines, light as a feather as if dancing with the ball. Had there been snow on the ground, you'd not see any traces of his feet.'

What is snow but another manifestation of water? Oh, what fun! Those were the happy days of hard work studying and playful ramblings at parties. The word *educate* is derived from the Latin word '*educare*', which means to draw from or be led from ignorance. I might have been a little innocent and green in some fields, but was determined to work smart, hard and diligently.

My work experience thus far had been in a mental hospital, an abattoir, as a construction worker, and at a slate and stone quarry. But my most valuable lesson in life came from loving and caring for our very sick and dying father, who had cancer. When later I was taught the principle of TLC, tender loving care, it resonated naturally with me and has always been a part of every holistic therapy modality I have practised, for which I am grateful for the teaching of M. Hollis, MBE. Lovingly caring for my fellow human beings became interwoven in my heart and mind, the awakening of love and intention engraved in a young man's soul in service to comfort, care, alleviate, uplift and sometimes cure patients.

Sir Titus Salt, Saltaire, Physiotherapy and M. Hollis, MBE

A career as a budding artist, inspired by my father, was stopped in its tracks by my well-meaning uncle, strict teacher and guardian following my father's death, who solemnly declared, 'I strongly advise you not to pursue the arts. It is like throwing your life away and it is not worth your salt!'

I heeded his advice, but finding the prospect of lengthy medicine studies, we opted for physiotherapy. A smart and important stepping-stone it turned out to be.

My appearance raised a few eyebrows, and I was often stopped by Customs, probably because I was wearing and old bluish-grey RAF coat inherited from my uncle, the schoolmaster, and sporting a blue beret. An IRA lookalike, long-haired student.

My residence for the next year became Victoria Road, Salts Hospital in the historical Saltaire Village, a gem of a place that was designated a UNESCO World Heritage Site in 2001, which means that the government has a duty to protect it.

Saltaire got its name from Titus Salt, a very successful weaver of beautiful fabrics that were used to make expensive dresses for the ladies of England. Titus moved the woollen mill from the centre of Bradford to Saltaire by the River Aire, to facilitate access to what is known as the Leeds Liverpool Canal and to the railway. Together with the mill, he built a whole self-contained community. One very important reason for moving the factory outside the city of Bradford was to take his work from the 'dark satanic mills' of Bradford as he described them. 'My workers need more space and fresh air.' Saltaire was a man way ahead of his time, thinking in preventative and holistic terms, and very interested in the health and welfare of the whole community.

The village had shops, bathhouses with running water and a church—another rarity in Bradford. A school, a hospital in Victoria Street (where I took up residency in 1971), a library, a billiard room, a concert hall, and a park in the village named Saltaire, combining his name Salt with that of the River Aire.

I soon became known to my fellow students as the 'All or Non Guy' after the All or Non Law of Physiology, which we became quite familiar with as our strict teaching sank in and the exams rolled on. This law states that the strength by which a nerve or a muscle fibre responds to a stimulus is independent of the strength of the stimulus. It was first described by the American physiologist Henry Pickering Bowditch in 1871—exactly hundred years before I learnt about this principle. All fired up or not at all!

In life's learning process, it is sometimes smart to have a few pegs to hang your facts on—and Mr. Thomasson, our physiology teacher aptly pegged his teaching around a few uplifting, supportive sayings. One of these, from our dearly beloved Norwegian author Henrik Ibsen, is: 'Whatever you do, do it fully and properly, not half-heartedly!'

Acupuncture and Serendipity

My other nickname, 'Cool as a Cucumber' (owing to the fact that I had a knack of keeping my head cool under the stressful circumstances of examination), served me well as I persevered and met the goals that I had set for myself and became one of the award-winning students (J. Brock's Memorial Award). I chose a selection of books on acupuncture as my reward—one of which was the I Ching, the Yellow Emperor of Classical Internal Medicine, which was and still is a classic in the world of acupuncture. Serendipity? I believe so—but I will let you make up your mind once you have come to the end of this book. In any case, I noticed that the audience began to chuckle when the names of the books I had chosen were read out—probably because acupuncture in those days was looked upon as something strange, mystic, weird and very fringe, or at least alternative to mainstream medicine. Little did

I know that medical doctors in Norway would report me to the health authorities for practising acupuncture when I came home, even though I had solid qualifications for this, having studied with Dr. George Bentze and at other acupuncture colleges in Europe. The Norwegian law of 1936 defined acupuncture as surgery, as it uses needles to penetrate the skin, and the health authorities thus branded me a 'quack'. In other words, this was the first 'Bahramdipity troll' of the Serendipity story. Many more were to follow.

What these people failed to understand was that I had already gained experience in the battlefields, where egomaniacal health authorities governed on the basis of fear and obsolete interpretation of laws.

Even my study of osteopathy and my association with the great physician Dr. James Henry Cyriax, the father and Einstein of orthopaedic medicine, was looked upon with great suspicion. I knew full well that if I quoted from his eminent—and now fully accepted—theory and practical management of muscular-scleral disorders, the examination boards would fail me. Dr. James H. Cyriax, whom I met twice in London, became a great inspiration in my work. On one occasion, I had the honour of heading the Norwegian delegation of physiotherapists at a course in orthopaedic medicine. In the evening, we were invited to Dr. Cyriax's private home in Albany Street, near Regent Park, and shared jokes and laughter as he poured wine for these Norwegian Vikings, he himself preferring apple juice.

CHAPTER TWO

The Many Faces of Water—Healing Hands, Faith, Prayers and Miracles

'Kindness is the language the death can hear and the blind can see'. Mark Twain.

Vital Living Water works in so many ways to help your body fight body pollution by getting rid of toxins and contaminants that come from numerous sources: food, air, additives, processed/convenience foods, chemicals, medicines, tobacco, municipal dead water containing heavy metals, et cetera. In addition, revitalised and structured water will provide you with more oxygen, nutrients and energy.

It is worth remembering that the Chinese symbols for *crisis* and *opportunity* are the same: if you are sick and lacking in energy, this can be a welcome opportunity to change—and why not start with the most important element in your body?

Numerous encounters with water seem to have been part of my life, from the hilariously funny to the sad and tragic. Sweet memories about water abound from Yorkshire especially—and, no, I don't mean the famous brown liquid that 'loosens your tongue and refreshes you' as my uncle kept saying to himself. During practical sessions, we were strictly admonished to remember to drink plenty of water—usually in the form of tea with milk and sugar. Since we were in a predominantly hard-water limestone area, calcium and magnesium could sometimes be of concern. But the ingenious folks from the north of England have their own Yorkshire Tea for hard water! Hard water can make quite a bit of difference to the taste of your tea, and the hard-water blend ensures you get a proper brew whenever you stew. Maybe this tea even reaches parts of your body that other teas cannot reach? Borrowed from a well-known beer commercial on TV at the time, we can all agree that vital water, alkaline and restructured water with high redox potential and antioxidant properties are important and something to treasure, be it healing energetic water, real or honest beer and wine.

And yet I see that the industry is largely ignorant about this issue which is so important for the taste and quality of the final product. There is a niche market here, I am sure of that. It would be an omission on my part if I left out a few lines on that great British institution—the pub, or public house.

My first date with a Yorkshire lass was in Ring O'Bells, Saltaire. Trying to get the hang of the broad Yorkshire dialect, which I eventually came to love and became quite good at, was difficult to begin with. My date, who later became my wife, wanted a glass of Dubonnet. As my pronunciation of the said drink failed to bring the desired result—the barman kept saying, 'Jubilee?' which was the name of a beer and not Dubonnet: In the end, much to my embarrassment, having failed to get my tongue properly around the French drink, I had to summon my date to fix the problem; I probably needed something to loosen my tongue!

The public house, what a great institution! The ambiance. The laughter. The icebreakers. The friendliest places to meet—a huge contrast to the places in Norwegian/Scandinavian countries, where very drunk people colour the scene.

Sometimes we would drive quite a distance just to sample a particular pint of Guinness or local beer in the Yorkshire Dales, and forgot about the wisdom in Henry Davis Thoreau's words: 'Water is the only drink for a wise man.'

One night, a crowd of us drove about an hour to reach this rather posh bar. My friend Per and I (who later was best man at my wedding) sauntered up to the bar, both of us commenting in Norwegian about this beautiful-looking lady in a fur coat, saying something like, 'I bet that coat comes from an alley cat!' Whereupon she turned to us, smiled brilliantly and replied in perfect Swedish, 'Hi guys—are you from Norway?'

We were caught with our proverbial pants down—two shamefaced school kids staring down at the floor, searching for a hole to fall into. Anyway, the lady was very courteous and polite, but we both felt we should have been reprimanded—petulant, uneducated and naughty Norwegians that we were! But a good laugh was had by all back at our table with our friends afterwards. A little self-irony goes along way. We ended the evening off on a happy note, hoping not to be punished by the Irish flu or too much under the weather the next morning.

Hydrotherapy and Some Silly Viking Bravado

I cannot recall any healing properties or pleasant experience when I plunged into the ice-covered pond at Manningham Park in Bradford, Yorkshire—the same park where the Yorkshire Ripper operated some years later.

It was a freezing winter's day, and the annual competition between local college and university teams was well underway in the park. A race of self-made floats had to be navigated from start to finish as fast as possible, using oars and sticks. A highly charged and competitive seafaring Viking was placed at the helm of our physio fleet. Undoubtedly my decision to jump into the freezing ice-covered water was in part spurred by the crowd at the side of the pond, led by Miss. M. Hollis, MBE shouting and cheering our team on. Dragging the float forward with a rope in one hand whilst breaking the ice with the other, the intense pain slowly subsided thanks to the icy water, lots of adrenaline pumping through my body and a few drams I'd had before embarking on this overconfident act of bravado. What an introduction to hydrotherapy! But we won!

Exhausted and with a dangerously low body temperature, aching quadriceps muscles, and a crisscross pattern of bleeding wounds from the sharp edges of the ice, I was whisked off in a car, shivering and mentally confused. A hot bath followed. What a contrast! After several hours, I regained my body temperature and strength. The scars on my thighs eventually healed completely. I was something of a hero at the college campus at the time—but with the knowledge of hindsight, that was a bravado stunt never to be repeated again. Reflecting back on this incident, it is true that many of my family members have a natural affinity with and fondness for water—most of them for the pleasantly therapeutic and soothing variety, but some for the scary near-death-experience kind. More on that later.

Curiously enough, our Aunty Torborg apparently knew how to predict the future by deciphering patterns and signs in coffee grounds and tealeaves. Divination and prediction by using tealeaves, tassography, was very popular in England. Potteries, even today, produce teacups for this purpose. Aunty was a kind, fat matryoshka-looking woman, a psychiatric nurse by profession. Much to my mother's shock and consternation, she predicted that I would die by drowning. And this haunted me for many years. I eventually managed to forget this frightening divination, and have a great love for nature and everything connected with water. Shortly after the intoxicating Viking bravado number that came dangerously close to an unhappy ending, I was summoned to the principal's office—Miss M. Hollis, MBE. 'I am proud of you, Mr. Espedal,' she said. I sighed with relief, well aware that all the students had great respect for Miss Hollis; indeed, most were terrified of this energetic, volatile lady.

Even though she had threatened to expel me once because I was sporting a moustache at the time and refused to wear the school uniform and had had the audacity to reply, 'Try me! I won't change,' we became great friends and sometimes she sought my advice on difficult disciplinary questions regarding the students—something that had never happened before. At a reunion twenty-five years later, I was happy to see her again, but sad to hear that she had osteoporosis, had lost some height and was on oestrogen medication. Looking like a petite version of Agatha Christie, she had never heard of my mentor and friend Dr. John R. Lee, who had come to Scandinavia to teach us his new discoveries and had written books on osteoporosis progesterone, the natural way to treat and reverse hormonal imbalance.

Healing Hands

It was Miss Hollis, a formidable teacher in her own right, who first said, 'Mr. Espedal, you've got healing hands.' She proclaimed this during a practical teaching session, but at the time I had never heard such terminology. *Healing hands, hmm…* I looked at my hands, and studied my palms. I didn't see or feel anything extraordinary. But later some of my co-students commented on this phenomenon— except for one female student who quipped, 'Big palm and short sausage-like fingers.' Laugh and the world laughs with you: she later became my wife and we now have two beautiful daughters, Camilla Victoria and Louisa Jayne.

On one of our many excursions into the Yorkshire Dales and moors in a yellow Mini, I pondered on the symbol and significance of ponds, lakes and rivers.

The Strid, The River Wharfe and Bolton Abbey

One of our favourite spots was the River Wharfe and The Ruins of Bolton Abbey, with the stepping stones across the wide part of the river and the narrow, quaint and innocuous-looking country brook called the Bolton Strid or just the Strid. Appearances can be deceptive, and in fact this is part of the tumbling, tumultuous River Strid, which is on the list of 'the most dangerous booby traps in the world.' So what happened to the peaceful meandering? The River Wharfe, the name of which is derived from Celtic and means 'meandering', seems to have been flipped to one side by an unknown force, and at great depths. It simply cannot be measured, as the undercurrents, with its vortex power, are so strong. Unseen caverns and massive underwater pockets hold all of the rest of the river's water. All of this adds up to one simple, terrifying fact: nobody who has ever fallen into the Strid—that harmless-looking brook up there—has lived to tell the tale. It has a one hundred per cent mortality rate, with both suicides and accidents resulting in bodies being trapped in the caverns deep underneath the treacherous stretch of the strip.

In contrast and more peaceful is the old and substantial stone bridge above the Strid where a water pipeline for Bradford Water Works runs its course. The pipe stretches around East Seat and heads off to Grimwith Reservoir. Source: Don Longley. It pleases me to think that I may have sipped some 'Strid Water' whilst studying in Bradford. Have you ever heard that water carries memories? It does indeed—but rest assured that, because of the ingenious design of nature, the same water that has claimed so many lives, the latest being two honeymooners who drowned and were never found, it regenerates through restructuring, dancing and increasing in energy. But that is another story, which I will come back to later.

Stepping Stones and Stumbling Blocks

Close to Bolton Abbey, the twelfth-century priory, fifty-seven stepping stones are beautifully placed across the quiet river, enabling you—provided you are sober—to safely cross the river. Ponds, lakes and rivers are timeless reminders of life's ups and downs. I feel that Henry Thoreau described it so well when he said, 'How perfectly new and fresh the world is seen to be, when we behold a myriad sparkles of brilliant white sunlight on a rippled stream.' Streams and rivers are to our earth as blood is to our body. Trials and tribulations. Grief and sorrow. Joyful gratitude and celebration. All part of the dynamic powers of life. Sometimes we need stepping stones to cross over to a safer and better place, when stumbling blocks seem to hinder us.

Rivers can be seen as consolation and regeneration for body and mind: 'Who hears the rippling of the rivers will not utterly despair of anything.' Rivers have an innate ability for self-cleansing and renewing. Our bodies are the same. We are equipped with the same self-healing system to joyfully cleanse, rejuvenate and regenerate. Crises in life come and go. Recognise that your crisis is only temporary, and that, with a diligent attitude, you can choose to make the seemingly scary stumbling blocks into your personal life-enhancing stepping stones, using the river as a metaphor of life.

The Indigo Dinghy Race—Carpe Diem: A Case of Mindfulness

I mentioned earlier that 'water is the earth's eye, looking into which the beholder measures the depth of his own nature', quoting a saying from Henry Thoreau.

I sat one day in Raymond's car pondering this and enjoying the beautiful scenery as we headed towards the Lake District in Lancashire on a beautiful Sunday for some sailing in Christine's dinghy, immaculately painted in indigo blue. I had been cordially invited to crew with Christine, an active sailor with many years' experience and a keen competitive nature. She reckoned that with me as part of her crew—a Norwegian with traces of Viking heritage in my DNA—we would easily beat all the competitors manoeuvring the boats around the starting line. Bang! The race is on!

Unfortunately, it was my first time ever in a sailing boat. Cruising swiftly along the beautiful lake and approaching the first tackle, Christine shouted a command that would soon become familiar: 'Gunnar, duck! Gunnar, duck!' whereupon I looked around the lake to see if there were any ducks that had escaped my attention. That's the last I remember before the beam hit my head sideways! Stars and stripes danced before my eyes. The consternation and worried look on her face made me realise what a fool I'd been, much

53

to everybody's amusement—including my own after I had recovered. Instead of crunching down in the dinghy and ducking so that the beam with the sail could swing across, I had got the wrong end of the stick and blew it, so to speak. Needless to say, we did not win the boat race.

But I'd say we won the post-race party in the boathouse. A few G&Ts for my skipper Christine and her husband Raymond, and something brownish, Newcastle Brown Ale, for myself, which loosened my tongue and soothed my bruises. Oh, how we laughed at that incident many years later, with my friends always reminding me that 'Norwegians might have been born with skis on their feet, but it's obvious that not all Vikings have sailing skills as part of their DNA!'

Serendipity Favours the Prepared Mind

The above expression is attributed to Horace Walpole from the Persian fairy tale *The Three Princes of Serendipity*. The word is derived from serendipity and is the old name for Sri Lanka—a reference to the ability for making discoveries by accident.

To illustrate this concept, let us look at John Barth's *The Last Voyage of Somebody the Sailor*. You don't reach serendipity by plotting a course for it. You have to set out in good faith for it and lose your bearings... serendipitously. Play is not purely entertainment or something you need to give up when things get serious. The act of playing is itself highly educative and illuminating, and many new discoveries are made when this variability is taken into account. Hence the expression *Homo ludens*, as opposed to *Homo sapiens*.

Some examples of this are Fleming's accidental discovery of penicillin; Louis Pasteur's discovery of the vaccine; Dr. John R. Lee's vital research on progesterone and its role in reversing osteoporosis and many other diseases of the hormonal system. All of these are great examples of a chance observation falling on a receptive eye and an open heart.

Newton's Apple and Other Serendipity Stories

A famous and often cited example of serendipity is Newton's discovery of gravity when an apple fell on his head while he rested under a tree. In the field of observation, 'chance favours only the prepared mind', as L. Pasteur, quoted by Beveridge, said in 1957. However, whether Newton's discovery may have been apocryphal, Becquerel's discovery of radioactivity as a result of his tossing uranium salts into a drawer of photographic material, and many other such events are a unique mix of inspired insight coupled with chance.

The exotic tale of the ancient princes of Sri Lanka, then known as Serendipity, inspired the English novelist Horace Walpole to coin the term *serendipity*. I think it is worth recalling the original story; hopefully it will make you more aware as you travel along the river of your own life, if you can dip down into the water's depths from time to time and come up with one of these gems of a story.

Three godly young princes were travelling the world in the hope of acquiring an education that would enable them take their rightful positions upon their return. On their journey, they met a camel driver who inquired whether they had seen his missing camel. The princes asked whether, by any chance, the camel was blind in one eye, missing a tooth and lame. As a result of these questions, the owner assumed that the three must have stolen his camel, as they knew all these details—and they were subsequently thrown into jail. Soon, the wayward camel was discovered and the princes were brought to the perplexed Emperor of the land. The princes told him that they had known these facts as the grass was eaten on the one side of the road, suggesting that the camel had one eye; the lumps of grass on the ground indicated a missing tooth; and the traces of a dragged hoof revealed the camel's lameness (adapted from *The Peregrinaggio*, 1557).

The moral of this story is that you should not get discouraged if, in your honest endeavour to change and reach out for better health and life quality, you meet Bahram Gur, the Persian King (ca.: 418-38 A.D.), as in the fairy tale *The Three Princes of Serendip:* a powerful individual acting egomaniacally, punishing and persecuting. They may appear on the scene if you dare to challenge their authority, whether they come from the medical or clerical fraternity. With the help of the advice found in this book you will recognise 'the three-headed troll' (as depicted some Norwegian fairy tales)—the Bahrams of the modern-day world—and you will be able to expose them. As with the trolls, they cannot tolerate light, the truth of light—they simply crack up and vanish. The analogy between the Bahram of Persia and some scientific and pontifical Bahram figures is of course a little lame; I will illustrate this aspect later on, as I experienced it first-hand.

As you continue reading this book, I hope you will be able to discover gems of serendipity and synchronicity in your own life. It makes for a much more playful, blessed and joyful ride. Are you ready to cross the river via the stepping stones, to reach the other side—a new, fresh start?

Religious Razzmatazz, an Atheist Journalist and a Religious Bishop

Our clinic expanded into a holistic therapy centre, receiving patients from Norway and abroad. Offering extensive lecturing and post-education training, as well as weekly radio shows for about fifteen years on numerous health issues, we seemed to make quite a stir in the orthodox medical fraternity. So much so that the 'opposition' saw us as a threat and a 'thorn in their sides'.

Holistic therapy in the seventies was looked upon with suspicion and denounced as unscientific and dangerous. However, our patient lists grew thanks to our outstanding results, using natural means and methods: acupuncture, reflexology, crania-sacral therapy, Bowen therapy, electro-medicine and Rife technology, to mention just a few of the modalities we were qualified to practise.

With our practises labelled as quackery by the medical authorities, our family suffered almost twenty years of persecution, harassments, lies and worse. It was a living nightmare. The two elements that kept my sanity and gave me peace of mind were my faith and seeing the many happy patients all around us. Even slanderous, evil newspaper articles could not deter me from reaching out to the sick, who were often misled and manipulated patients who had been blatantly lied to and had so much fear instilled into their poor souls by the cowardly attitudes of medical doctors and the pharmaceutical cartels. They had to be consoled and guided in order to find their footing. I even had patients who had been threatened by their own doctors to stop seeking our advice and alternative health solutions

All this reached a kind of unbelievable crescendo when a major Norwegian newspaper ran a full-page article about the holistic therapy centre that I headed. The journalist, a self-professed atheist, had stirred up the medical authorities, and even the bishop himself, Bjørn Bue, came onto the scene, declaring that I was a charlatan. As a born-again Christian, I knew we were in a spiritual warfare and immediately contacted the bishop who agreed to meet me, and two other experienced Christian warriors.

At our meeting, Brother John immediately took the initiative and went confronted the bishop with a clean tackle worthy of a professional footballer, reminding me of Sir Alex Ferguson's notorious dressing-room 'hairdryer' treatments. Three warriors filled with The Holy Spirit visibly shook this bishop.

The bishop realised that he had been manipulated and hoodwinked by the journalist and prayed to God to be forgiven in his office. He asked if I could forgive him for the injury he had caused my family and me. My heart relieved, I had no problems forgiving the bishop—after all, he was a brother in faith, was he not?

However, when I told him how I met our Yeshua, my Saviour, and how the Holy Spirit revealed to me to receive the full body immersion of *water baptism*, his face immediately changed colour. Now almost red and white, he exploded and spat out; 'You were not led by the Holy Spirit; you were deluded and mislead by another spirit!'

My friends and I were shocked at this outburst, and once outside the bishop's office, I said, 'We knew that the bishop as bishop of a state religious church was very much in favor of baptism of children—the sprinkling of water on the babies' heads—and very much against the baptism that John the Baptist performed in the River Jordan for Yeshua and his disciples.

My friends, John Bjerkestrand and Gunnar Hovden, witnessed the whole ordeal. The promise made by the bishop about an official statement of disclaim to the newspaper now came reluctantly, after some pushing and persuasion from John, my comrade and spiritual warrior. It appeared as a tiny item—nonsensical religious weasel words.

Waterless Canals

As we departed from the bishop's office, I was reminded of the words in the Apocalypse of Peter, who referred to bishops and deacons who arrogantly claimed to be the sole gatekeepers of heaven *waterless canals*.

Confronted with a herd of charging medical puppets whose strings were being pulled, hostile journalists and pontifical writers of all shapes and forms breathing down my neck, I took great consolation in the Holy Scripture: Timothy 3:12 'Yeah, and all that will live godly in Christ Yeshua shall suffer persecution.'

Quietly and humbly I rejoiced. Trials to test one's faith are good; they help us develop maturity and build character. It was a time to value our true friends who stood by us during these stormy years.

Faith, Prayers and Miracles

My sincere prayers went out to those who wrongly accused, misused and persecuted me. The bishop unexpectedly died about one year after this incident.

During this period, we had the opportunity to observe first-hand numerous miraculous healings, either through the use of natural, holistic medicine cures, or prayer and the laying on of hands. The biblical practice of praying for people was not unknown to me as I had seen and heard about this before. The first of many miracles occurred almost exactly five weeks after having received Yeshua as my Saviour and Lord. During a very hectic period with lots of patients at our centre, we received a call from an obviously distressed man. Himself a Christian, he told us his story: 'I have had constant back pain every day for fifteen years. I have been operated on, tried various treatments and have been prayed for, to no avail! Please help me! I am in great pain!'

Even though our day programme was completely full, we moved patients to make room for Mr Sørensen, our Danish brother, who dragged himself to the clinic's door, hobbling on crutches. We needed two people to get him on to the plinth. As he lay before us on his stomach, I heard Gods calling on me to pray for him. I hesitated, as I'd never prayed for anybody before. Then I heard God's command twice with increasing urgency. Still a little hesitant, I placed my hands on his lower back and prayed the Lord's Prayer in my head, as I had neither the courage nor the faith to pray audibly. Before I'd finished, I felt a surge of warmth and trembling going through my hands. 'Was this God's healing?' I wondered. Not telling him what I'd done, I said goodbye and Mr Sørensen left.

Next time he visited, he told us, 'For the first time in fifteen years, I became pain-free and was able to move normally again. I told my wife, who was waiting in the car, that I thought Mr Espedal must have prayed for me, as he laid his hands on me. Did you?'
'Yes, I must confess that's just what I did. And now let me pray and give thanks to our Lord for this glorious miracle.' This time, his skin, which had become wrinkled and scarred following the operation on

his back, was taut and smooth again.

'I think God has given you the gift of healing and performing great miracles for Him,' said Mr Sørensen. These are spiritual gifts of grace as described in the Bible (1. Corinthians 12:11).

Many years later, I met Mr Sørensen again. He told me he'd been well ever since, and now enjoyed long walks through the beautiful countryside of Jæren. Glory to God!

An Amazing Miracle. A Story of Never Ever Giving Up

In the days of harassment and persecution from the medical fraternity and their allies, I received a call from an obviously very anxious and distressed lady. She told me that her husband had incurable cancer and was in a coma with organ failure, according to the doctor's report. She begged me to come to the hospital in a last attempt to pray for a Christian brother and his family who had previously lost one of their sons to cancer. I visited Mr. Steinskog once at the hospital, prayed and laid my hands on him. We did not see any immediate reaction, but as I left the hospital I encouraged his wife to keep praying and to update me daily as I intended to pray and fight for this man´s life. Almost like a medical bulletin from the hospital his wife phoned me several times a day reporting on the ebb and flow of her husband´s condition. One Easter day came the telephone I had been eagerly waiting for:

"He is alive and fully awake, healed and asking for food!"

Joy over joy! After several weeks in coma, he was declared completely free of cancer, healed and well by the medical doctors, much to the surprise of everybody. Straight after he was discharged from the hospital and went home to his farm, where I had the pleasure of visiting him and his family, enjoying his home grown strawberries.

The Dirty Little Secret of our Water

Most people think that ordinary tap water is healthy, but when you examine municipal water, you will discover that it is full of contaminants, toxic compounds, chlorine by-products and heavy metals (mercury, cadmium, led, arsenic, fluoride).

Did you know that the EU has criticised the Norwegian water network? Fifty per cent of the country's water is leaking from the water reservoir to the faucets used in every household, because of old, leaky, rusty water pipes. The fact that these water pipes are placed parallel to the sewage draining system, which is also leaking, means that migrating microbes can move from source one to the other. One of these microbes, Giardia lamblia or Lamblia Intestinalis, which is resistant to chlorine, resulted in 1300 people becoming very sick in Bergen in 2004, 200 of whom developed ME, (myalgic encephalomyelitis or C.F.S, chronic fatigue syndrome). This water scandal could have been prevented. Many scientists have raised concern about the poor quality of Norway's domestic drinking water.

According to the Folkehelseinstituttet, approximately 100,000-300,000 become sick and have to stay at home every year due to poor-quality water. (Ref: Prof. Oddvar Lindholm at the University of Environmental and Biological Science.)

Our drinking water contains dangerous levels of chlorine, trihalomethanes and heavy metals, which accumulate in the body. These include chlorine by-products (C.B.P), together with mercury (Hg), lead (Pb), cadmium (Cd) and aluminium (Al), and chlorine-resistant microbes such as cryptosporidium and Lamblia Intestinalis, as well as many other chemical constituents. This drinking water is far from healthy—and it is the first choice for many of Norway's inhabitants. We should refuse to drink this water, which lacks the necessary ions and minerals, and choose only to drink the very best water: pure, vital, cleansed, ionised, restructured, alkaline water. Is it not about time to reclaim your health, escape the 'sickness industry' and enjoy good health, living a strong and happy life? Your first steppingstone to achieving this goal is vital, restructured water.

Healthy Royal Water and Nobel Prize Winners

Nobel Laureate Albert Szent-Györgyi said, 'Water is the mother and matter of all life. There is no life without water. Vital water hydrates your body at a cellular level. It detoxifies, cleanses, chemically captures (chelates), and brings your cells back to your cells. By stimulating the powerhouses of your cells, the mitochondria, it gives you more energy.

At a therapeutic level, I would say that Royal Living Water reaches and refreshes parts of your body that other waters cannot reach.

If you feel you are venturing into uncharted territory, fear not, because everything will be revealed as you travel this journey with me. These are proven, smart solutions that I have used for my family, friends, patients and myself throughout over forty years of practice. I cannot think of a more natural way than to start the day with vital water, the origin and essence of all life.

According to the Bible, 'In the beginning God created heaven and earth. And the earth was without form, and void, and darkness was upon the face of the deep. And the spirit of God moved upon the face of waters. And God said let there be light and there was light.

(Gen. 1.1-4)

Conclusion

You have the ability to change the stumbling blocks in your life to stepping stones, towards great health and happiness. The rivers have a great capacity for self-cleansing and regeneration—as does our bodies. We are gracefully given the innate tools to fight body pollution and become more energetic. Have a look at your daily routine: Do you need to remove some stumbling stones from your life?

Don't forget to drink plenty of vital, living, restructured water that will rehydrate your body deep inside your cells.

CHAPTER THREE

Escaping the 'Sickness Industry'—Debunking Health Myths

'What we fear doing most is usually is what we most need to do.'
Timothy Ferriss

What you don't know about water, air and food may kill you. A truthful statement.

Our environment is full of pollution. The water you drink, the air you breathe and the food you eat are full of health-damaging elements. Lifestyle diseases are rampant: coronary heart disease, diabetes, cancer, obesity, neurological disorders such as MS, ME, ALS, Alzheimer's, Parkinson's, ADHD, autism, and schizophrenia are all triggered and facilitated by the increasing amounts of pollution. Research indicates that eighty per cent of all lifestyle diseases are caused by these factors.

Your health and well-being are your own responsibility. By realising this and empowering yourself with the correct information, you can take control over your life and escape the sickness industry. Dr. Ivan Illich documented in his book *Medical Nemesis* in the early seventies that the pharmaceutical medical complex was responsible for the third leading cause of death, after cancer and coronary heart disease.

If you jump aboard the happy journey outlined in my book, there is a good chance that the knowledge herein will liberate and set you free.

Prevention of diseases is always the number one priority. Yes, it is possible to live longer and stronger. Both a long and full-quality life is well within reach. Let's use water as an example. Most people take this for granted and assume that the water and health authorities are trustworthy when they claim that our water is of good quality. In Norway, we are led to believe that we have 'the best water in the world'. That is far from the truth.

Due to the long and diligent work of Henri Coandă, the Nobel Laureate and his studies of primitive cultures around the world, we know that the common denominator amongst these people is structured, alkaline, mineral-rich or crystal-clear water. This is the number one reason these people lived a long and healthy life.

Today, we have the technology to recreate the superior physical properties of Hunza water, by processes of filtration, ionisation and restructuring. This water hydrates your body cells eight to ten times faster and more efficiently than ordinary, chemical, 'dead' water. Royal water has gained new properties. With a high negative redox potential and hydroxyl ions, it cleanses, rehydrates and renders cellular environment more alkaline. Municipal water is dead, because it has no energy, opposite ORP (positive polarity) and is an electron thief; it does not flow naturally, since it is forced through contaminated pipes and becomes— yes, dead! Measured by ORP (oxygen reduction potential) and GDV (gas discharge visualisation) and EPI (electro-photonic imaging). As a reference in the field of quantum electro dynamics, you may like to check out the scientific works of Dr. Gerald Pollack, Dr. Vladimar Voelkov and Dr. William Tiller, Konstantin Korotkov and Fritz Albert Popp.

By drinking this type of water, you have taken your first important step in preventing cellular damage and diseases. 'An ounce of prevention is better than a pound of cure', as the researcher, Dr. F. Batmanghelidj, MD once pointed out. Over the last twenty-five years, he has brought the world's attention to water's formidable health and rejuvenating effects through his books: *Your Body's Many Cries for Water, and Obesity, Cancer, Depression: Their Common Cause & Natural Cure.*

Redox Potential: Water's antioxidant power.
Hydroxyl ion: During the ionisation process, the water molecule, H_2O, is split into $H+$ (hydrogen) and $OH-$ (hydroxyl ion).

What about some of the myths? It is often said that 'in the good old days', everything was much better: the word *stressed* was hardly known or used; water and foods were natural, clean and unadulterated. What if the 'consensus truth' out there was in fact more lies and devious marketing strategies to enslave you through your ignorance?

In Norway, we are led to believe that we have the cleanest and best water in the world. Milk and cod liver oil are very healthful and should be consumed on a daily basis—and indeed are major staples in most households. Did your mother urge you to drink milk every day, for your teeth and bones? If calcium in milk is so important for strong bones, how is it that Norwegians are at the top of the world's osteoporosis statistics? A nation of brittle bones, yet big milk drinkers! And strong contenders when it comes to the consumption of soft drinks and coffee—all bone mineral thieves.

The highly praised cod liver and fish oil products, omega-3 fatty acids, are also ingrained in our consciousness as being healthy products, even though they contain residues of chemicals and heavy metals and in fact can do a great deal of damage to your health. A few years ago, a research study was conducted on omega-3 from cod liver oil, examining its effects on bone density and osteoporosis. Shortly afterwards, the study had to be aborted because the participants in the research who were using omega-3 developed more osteoporosis and their bones became more fragile, with loss of bone density. Is it not about time we exposed health myths and got rid of them?

When I first questioned the validity of cod liver oil and fish oil on our regular radio health show thirty years ago, Norway's biggest producer of these products got extremely annoyed and came up with more deceptive marketing tricks. Even today the machinery of propaganda from the industry keeps rolling out advertisements in the media, using our most popular sports personalities as puppets to advocate these unhealthy products. Money is the name of the game—and it seems as if the advertising industry is claiming victory over science. But we have been led to believe all these years that omega-3 essential fatty acids are extremely important for healthy joints and good cardiovascular function, and are a great brain booster and aid in cancer prevention. And now you are saying that it's all wrong? Let's look at the evidence: Professor Brian Peskin's Life-Systems Engineering (Science) work on PEO parent essential oils and why taking fish oil supplements will harm your health is unprecedented. In his first monumental book, *The Hidden Story of Cancer*, he presents PEO, as opposed to fish oil, as the building material and 'oxygen magnets' of cell membranes that will, among other things, prevent cancer. As you may know, a thirty per cent reduction of oxygen to the cells will change the metabolism from aerobic to anaerobic, and cancer will result (Otto Warburg, Nobel Prize Winner).

In his second book, *PEO Solution*, you can read all the scientific facts comparing parent essential oils to adulterated omega-3 fish oil products, backed up by hundreds of confirmed scientific papers which you cannot ignore. If you follow his instructions in this field, take on board, step by step, the new discoveries and technologies related to water and air, and the other lifestyle changes outlined, I can assure you that this goal is well within reach: you will be able to live a full, healthy, harmonious and happy life. In this book, you will see nature's physiological laws revealed as you have probably not seen them before. It is scientific facts, the unbridled truth—not opinions—that form the backbone of this book, gleaned from forty years' experience working in the health field. Are you ready to begin your journey?

Remember, 'A journey of a thousand miles begins with a single step' (Chinese Proverb).

With water being the most important element in our life, the matrix of all living matter, it's about time we took a closer look at it. Hopefully, this new view will empower you to take action and 'escape the sickness industry'—as Elaine Hollingsworth, Director of the Hippocrates Health Centre of Australia, said.

Food for Thought—A Little Zen Wisdom

The following tale was originally told by a Hakawati (storyteller), and is a compilation of Zen wisdom and a lovely anecdote:

There are two fishes swimming along and they happen to meet another, much older, fish swimming in the opposite direction, who nods at them and says, 'Morning boys, how's the water?'

The two fish swim on for a bit and then eventually one looks at the other and says, 'What the heck is water?'

A beautiful story and definitely food for thought! This tale is really about being constantly aware of what is essential and beautiful—in this case, water.

At this point, let me express to you, dear Reader, my gratitude and appreciation for accompanying me on this wonderful journey. But we need to get back to the task at hand: the ugly reality of how the water that we in the Western world take for granted is chemically and energetically toxic and devoid of energy. What follows is a condensed review of the most common toxic elements in our drinking water.

Poisons in our Water

We have all been deceived and lied to regarding our drinking water. The toxic pollution of our planet is reflected in the world's drinking water as well as the oceans. We are faced with an unprecedented loss of species comparable to the great mass extinctions of prehistory. Dr. Alex Rogers, Professor of Conservation Biology at Oxford University, has said that these findings are shocking and worse than the most pessimistic predictions—and our drinking water is no exception, as you will learn shortly. But the consolation here is that the right technology to purify and energise your drinking water exists and is available, for your family's immediate joy and benefit.

Before we talk about the specific pollutants in water and how these affect our health, it is important to trace the sources and how these pollutants came into the water. Water pollution comes predominantly from two sources: point and non-point sources. The former is easy to identify: waste disposal, sewage, industry and radioactivity (Chernobyl, Fukushima). Non-point sources can be more difficult to trace, but these are actually more important: pollution from farming, industry, forestry, mining, and traffic. This happens when rain and melting snow runs over polluted landscapes, picking up toxins on its way to waterways, rivers and lakes.

Over the last decades, we have witnessed an ever-increasing amount of pollution where the ecosystems are destroyed. Herbicides, pesticides, heavy metals, chemical elements, hormone-mimicking material (xenoestrogen) exert a powerful and a negative influence, leading to an overload of the ecosystem. Several species of fish and mammals have changed sex, and children aged as young as four have fully developed breasts caused by poison from pesticides (xenoestrogen).

Our water reservoirs—and therefore our drinking water, including groundwater—are polluted. Many of these pollutants accumulate in the body, which in turn affects neurological functions, and disrupts and weakens the hormone and immune systems.

Rain, coupled with pollution like sulphur dioxide and nitrogen dioxide, and radioactive downfall accelerate the negative cycle of pollution. During heavy rainfall and periods of flood, melting snow and ice, the use of chemicals such as chlorine and its by-products, trihalomethanes, are increased in our water reservoirs.

To assess a drinking-water reservoir, it's important to evaluate the immediate environs, to ascertain whether the area is in danger of being exposed to pollution. In Norway, most of the drinking water originates from surface water. Humus formed by the natural breakdown of plants, soil and animals, forms fulvic acids. When in contact with chlorine, dangerous C.B.P. (chlorine by-products) such as trihalomethanes are formed. This is a known carcinogen.

What happens to your body when you drink polluted water? The acute phase can start within hours or days if the infection is caused by microbes. Both Giardia intestinalis and cryptosporidium are resistant to chlorine disinfection. People with weakened immune systems, patients on steroids, cytotoxic or other medicines are especially vulnerable.

Chronic exposure to chemicals in the water—C.B.P., trihalomethanes, radium, strontium, parasites, heavy metals like lead, mercury, arsenic, cadmic, fluoride, antimony, barium, berry lime, chromium, cupper, cadmium, thallium, aluminium and nitrates—can lead to increased chances of developing cancer, liver and kidneys damage, Alzheimer's, dementia, MS and hormone-related disturbances.

Common Sources of Pollution in our Drinking Water

Microbes

Coliform bacteria are quite common in our environment. When bacteria like these are discovered in our drinking water, it is usually because of leakage due to rusty and damaged pipes. Norway has been informed by the EU to improve its water-pipe system, which is old and leaking. Up to fifty per cent of the water is lost throughout the water-piping system—with ample opportunities for microbial growth. Animal or human faecal matter causes most of the opportunistic infections. Testing for microbes is expensive and time-consuming via traditional laboratory methods, but coliform bacteria is relatively easy to detect. Electro acupuncture—ad modum Dr. Voll—is a reliable alternative test method to detect microbes, and offers real solutions to eradicate any pathological offenders.

Escherichia coli: E. coli is a subgroup of the coliform group of bacteria from faecal matter. Most E. Coli bacteria does not cause any harm and are present in the intestines of man and animal. Some species of E. coli can cause illness. From time to time, we can about 'outbreaks of E. coli', usually through food contamination. (E. coli 0157:H7).

Cryptosporidium: Cryptosporidium is a parasite that stems from animal, man and sewage and can cause cryptosporidiosis, a relatively mild form of intestinal distress, from drinking water infested with this parasite. However, it can be fatal for people with weakened or disturbed immune systems. Infection by this parasite happens in the following way: through eating food or drinking water containing cryptosporidium parvum oocysts (the infective stage of the parasite), or through touch. The symptoms of infection are: diarrhoea, cramps, nausea and fever. Usually two to ten days after being infected, if you have a weakened immune system because of medicine, HIV/AIDS infection, organ transplant or vaccination, you may be at risk. Also, personnel in nurseries, day-care centres and children, and frequent travellers are at increased risk. And of course if you drink infected water, you are obviously at risk of developing an infection.

Most important overall is preventative measures such as personal hygiene, hand-washing, and boiling water, especially when travelling abroad. But even if you follow following this advice, you may still get infected, because both Giardia intestinalis and cryptosporidium are resistant to chlorine disinfection.

Giardia lamblia: Giardia lamblia is a parasite that can spread via sewage and faecal matter from man and animal. One of the most common waterborne microbes, it is found in the intestines of all populations throughout the world. The parasite is transmitted in the same manner as cryptosporidium. The symptoms usually appear one to two weeks after being infected and can last four to six weeks in normal healthy persons. Chronically ill persons affected with Giardia lamblia infection may exhibit ME symptoms, or chronic fatigue syndrome. The same precaution should be noted as for cryptosporidium. But the good news is that it is quite possible to get rid of ME caused by waterborne microbes cryptosporidium, Giardia lamblia or borrelia infection, which can all be treated effectively using electro-medicine applications like Royal Raymond's Rife's Rife technology, Dr. Robert Beeks' protocol or Dr. Clark's method, colloidal silver solution, magnetic day clay and zeolite, to mention just a few.

Contaminants

Radioactivity and nucleotides: Most water reservoirs present the same radioactive pollution. Certain minerals are radioactive and can emit ionising radiation: alpha, beta, gamma and neutron radiation. The Chernobyl accident in 1986 had a big impact in Norway. Besides the old Soviet Union, Norway also received and absorbed most of the radioactive fallout after the accident. Because of the topographical conditions, Switzerland and Austria were badly affected too. After the accident, the wind direction went towards Norway and, combined with heavy rainfall, especially in the middle of Norway in the mountains, it caused extensive damage. The rainwater with the radioactive isotopes penetrated the fields, forests, drinking water and animals. Sheep and reindeer grazing in these areas received these radioactive isotopes in their bodies. Cesium-137, with a halving time of thirty years, is still in the environment today. It is estimated that this accident cost Norway in the region of fifty million Norwegian kroner, (ref. Dagens Næringsliv 17.9.2009).

After the nuclear power accident in Fukushima, Japan, 11.3.2011, measurements of the drinking water in Tokyo have shown dangerous levels of radioactive pollution—more than 210 becquerel pr.kg. This has spread globally to the US and Europe. At present there is still leakage from the Fukushima Daiichi Nuclear Power Plant, and the amount of fallout is considerably greater than that of Chernobyl. Experts tell us that the implications of this accident will stay with us for many years. As you may know, caesium will accumulate in the body via air, water and food. Knowledge on effective ways and means to chelate or detoxify is very important: water technology like alkaline, ionised water, zeolite, herbs, clay, iodine, to mention a few to prevent cancer, is imperative.

Radon: In April 2006 in Simi Valley, California, the soil and water became contaminated by strontium 90, a radioactive element with a long half-life. Radon gas can dissolve in groundwater. Strontium 90 is associated with leukaemia and other types of cancer. Accidents like this one where whole landscapes are damaged have resulted in improved technology such as ionisation, green sand filtration, reversed osmosis, et cetera.

Synthetic organic sources of pollution: Chemicals like ethylene bromide, PCBs, glyphosate (ref. Monsanto's Round-Up), benzene, acrylamide and dioxin are all regarded as very toxic. Dioxin, probably the most toxic product ever produced, consists of up to seventy-five different chlorinated molecules. It has many sources: insecticides, bleach, and combustion to name but a few. Some diseases can be caused by dioxin, including skin diseases, infertility, behavioural and psychological problems, liver damage and cancer.

Volatile Organic Compounds (VOCs): These compounds are found in drinking water and are derived from several sources of pollution: paint, gas, petrol, industrial waste, detergents, et cetera.

Because of its lengthy half-life, VOCs remain in the environment for a long time. The most common forms of VOCs are chloroform, perchloroethylene (PCE), trichloroethylene (TCE) and several derivatives of petroleum. According to a survey published by the United States Geologic Survey (USGS) in 2004, almost all water samples contained VOCs. Even though the effects of VOCs are not immediately seen, long-term exposure to these toxic compounds will cause them to accumulate in your body over time and weaken the immune system. Chloroform is the most common volatile compound from industry (fridges and freezers and also as a result of chlorinating the water). The most common health risk of long-term exposure to VOCs is kidneys, liver and central nervous system diseases such as cancer.

Perchloroethylene and trichloroethylene are VOCs frequently used in industry as solvents. These have known toxic effects, especially in long-term use as they accumulate, causing liver and kidneys failure.

In the US, it is the Environmental Protection Agency (EPA), and in Norway, the Mattilsynet and Folkehelseinstituttet that are in charge of setting limits for these compounds. All clinical experience tells us that the less you are exposed to these chemicals, the better. Simple measurements at home can prevent exposure and the accumulative effects of these toxins.

Several by-products from petroleum belong to the VOCs group and are connected to leukaemia and anaemia. Dichloroethane is a toxic substance that especially damages the liver and the kidneys and is used extensively in the plastics industry. Vinyl chloride used in PVC pipes can damage the hormonal and neurological systems as well as the brain, liver, lungs and lymphatic system. Most of the drinking water in Norway comes from surface water and toxins from VOCs sources are more common in groundwater.

A spokesperson from the EPA's Drinking Water division stated in 1986: 'There are growing concerns about exposure to volatile chemicals in water through inhalation, which suggests that taking a shower is roughly equivalent to drinking two litres of chlorinated water a day. Another concern is chlorine by-products such as trihalomethanes, which can penetrate the skin (DBPs)'.

By-products of disinfection (DBPs): Norway's Water Authority, the *Mattilsynet og Folkehelseinstituttet,* is responsible for providing water for the population that has been disinfected to remove microbes that might otherwise cause infection and spread disease. But in reality it is impossible to remove all faecal matter, of both human and animal origin, in brooks, rivers and lakes. The regulations governing the country's water do not call for any treatment to physically remove chemical by-products that may damage health (BPD). The responsibility of removing chemical by-products such as trihalomethanes, which are carcinogens, from the water falls to individual households. The most common water treatments in the Scandinavian countries are the use of chlorination and UV radiation to prevent microbes, as well as physical measures including chemicals, membrane filtering, coagulation, flocculation and slow filtering.

Norway is among the forerunners when it comes to ultraviolet (UV) treatment of drinking water. In 2003, there were more waterworks using UV than chlorine, which is used mainly small to medium-sized water reservoirs. About half a million citizens benefited from UV-treated water in 2003.

Membrane filtration, coagulation/filtration and slow filtration aim to remove infective material from water, rather than killing microbes using UV, and chlorination. There has been a lot of research and focus on two well-known waterborne parasites, Giardia lamblia and cryptosporidium, the spores of which are not killed by chlorine. These chlorine-resistant parasites exist in the surface water, which is the main source of drinking water in Norway. The world's most major water epidemic caused by a cryptosporidium parvum outbreak occurred in Milwaukee, US in 1993, when more than 400,000 people became ill with digestive and intestinal problems, and more than 100 people died during the outbreak. In 2004, an outbreak of Giardia intestinalis in the drinking reservoir of Svartediket in Bergen caused 1100 people to fall ill, with approximately 200 later developing chronic fatigue syndrome or ME. The reason behind this outbreak lay in the faecal material and high levels of E. coli following heavy rainfall at the end of August 2004.

Water Treatments

As the only water treatment used in this area was chlorination, microbes have escaped this water barrier treatment. There are a number of water treatment options that remove and stop the spread of infection from these two waterborne parasites.

UV radiation: It is well documented that UV radiation is effective in these circumstances.

Membrane filtration: With a nominal opening of 10-nanometers or less, these parasites, viruses and bacteria will be removed.

Ozonation (O3): In sufficient quantities, ozone can be effective, but hazardous and damaging by-products can be formed, especially in coastal regions.

Coagulation—filtration: This method will remove most infective material, but is less effective than UV radiation or membrane filtration.

Health effects of Chlorine By-Products

Most of the trihalomethanes, which are formed from chlorine and humic (fulvic) acid, result in changes in cells' DNA—*mutagenic* being the term used here. Chloroform and bromide chloromethane are characterised as possibly carcinogenic (IARC, LISEPA). The cumulative effect of these increases the risk of developing cancer, especially bladder and colon cancer. Afflictions of the liver, kidneys and nervous system have also been reported.

The concentration of chlorine by-products in Norway is generally lower than the WHO recommended values. In the last year, a lot of attention has been focused on a chlorination product named MX (mutagen X). So far no investigations have been conducted in Norway, but analyses carried out in Finland, the US, UK, Canada, China and Japan show that the highest concentration is 67 nanogram/l.

Inorganic Sources of pollution

This is the largest group of chemicals seeping into the groundwater from polluted soil from industry, forestry, mining, farming, oil and gas drilling, waste disposal, garbage and water-pipe corrosion. Long-term exposure to these toxic substances in water can damage your health and cause several types of cancer.

Arsenic: Arsenic seeps into water from deposits in soil, industry and farming. Arsenic in nature can be released in large amounts during volcanic eruptions and forest fires, or can simply be manmade. Approximately 90% of industrial use of arsenic in the US was for wood preservation, impregnation of fabric or geotextile plant root barriers, soap, metal and medicine.

According to a research study published by the National Academy of Science in 1999, arsenic in drinking water can cause cancer of the bladder, kidneys, liver, lungs and skin. It may also cause damage to the central and the peripheral nervous systems as well as the hormonal system, heart and blood circulation.

Poisons in our Tap Water

Are you slowly being poisoned and drained of energy by the water you drink? The scientific researcher Robert Slovak asked this question some thirty years ago during his investigation into the chemistry of water, when he developed the water technology known as reverse osmosis. Our drinking water is chlorinated, and in this process, health-damaging by-products develop, such as trihalomethanes, which can cause cancer. This happens as due to a chemical reaction between chlorine and humic/fulvic acid as the vegetation breaks down in the water.

Robert Slovak, one of the pioneers in the research into the effect of DBPs (disinfection by-products) warned about the health risks of DBPs, stating that they were 10,000 times more poisonous than chlorine.

There are a host of chemical compounds that have raised concern among researchers in these fields, including fluorine from the aluminium industry, which is a derivate of medicines, pesticides and other products. But clearly DBPs are the worst offender, according to our scientists.

Vital Facts

Most people are unaware of the toxic threat to our health and which filtration systems are most effective for protection. The most common disinfection by-products from chlorine use are trihalomethanes (THMs) and acetic acid (HAA). These are measured in parts per billion and the upper limit has been decided by Mattilsynet og Folkehelseinstituttet. These limits have been persistently lowered, especially in the US, as the dangers and seriousness of these chemicals are becoming more and more evident. Some of these chlorine by-products have a zero limit as the degree of damage is obviously dangerous to our health. But even this zero limit does not guarantee that our drinking water is without these toxic compounds.

How can DBPs damage your health?

Trihalomethanes (THMs) are Cancer Group B carcinogens (shown to cause cancer in laboratory animals). Disinfection by-products (DBPs) are also associated with hormonal fertility problems. Bladder and rectal cancer are increased two-fold.

According to a study published in the scientific journal *Epidemiology* (Jan 1998), smoking and drinking chlorinated water for more than 40 years doubled the risk of developing cancer of the bladder in men, as compared to men who smoked but did not drink chlorinated water.

Another study showed a significant increase in rectal cancer for both sexes who drank chlorinated water. According to a scientific research study published in the *Journal of Environmental Sciences,* swimming in chlorinated water represented an unacceptable health risk. Trihalomethanes from DBPs enter our body via different routes:

- The epidemic layers of the skin let in DBPs during showering or swimming in chlorinated water
- Digestive tract, by drinking water containing DBPs
- DBPs through the skin, through drinking
- Digestive tract during swimming in water containing DBPs
- Inhalation of DBPs from damp/steam when showering or swimming in chlorinated pool

The risk of cancer is greatest from skin exposure. This accounted for 94% of the total cancer risk when exposed to chlorinated water (DBPs).

According to the scientific journal *New Scientist,* a major research study on drinking water in the US revealed that it contained a wide array of chemical substances, including medicine residues, hormone-mimicking substances (xenoestrogen), aspartame, Splenda, cocaine and much more—some of the following may surprise you:

- Atenolol, beta-blockers for coronary disease

- Atrazine, an organic pesticide illegal in the EU. This can cause hormonal disturbances in animals
- Carbamazepine, a medicine used in bipolar disorder
- Estrone, an oestrogen hormone causing sex change in fish
- Gemfibrozil, an anti-cholesterol medicine
- Memprobamate, a sedative used in psychiatry
- Naproxen, an anti-inflammatory medicine as associated with increased risk of asthma
- Phenytoin, an anti-cramp medicine used in epilepsy.
- Sulfamethoxazole, an antibiotic
- TCEP, a reduction substance used in molecular biology
- Trimethoprim, an antibiotic

Killing you softly? Help!

What can I do about this? When faced with these facts, the obvious question is what to do about it. You now know that when you drink, shower or wash yourself with chlorinated water, disinfection by-products (DBPs), or swim in a pool with chlorinated water, you receive a massive dose of toxins. Remember that DBPs are 10,000 times more toxic than chlorine itself!

Help is Near—The Solution is Clear

Fact: 80% of all diseases stem from environmental pollution in water, air and food, according Environmental Protection Agency (EPA). The solution: Filtration, cleansing, ionising and restructuring water; chelation using minerals, vitamins, zeolite, magnetic clay, iodine, chlorella, et cetera.

This new information has led to suggestions that we implement the following steps:

- Install a shower filter to remove DBPs. Remember, the by-products of water chlorination trihalomethanes, et cetera, are 10,000 times more toxic than chlorine on its own—Slovak).
- Hand-wash without chemicals.
- Wash clothes without washing powder or softeners—i.e., no chemicals, but rather oxygen, peroxides, ionisation (active pure technology). This will prevent the growth of bacteria. Furthermore, using only cold water will mean less wear and tear on the textiles and colours don't fade. You save the environment from chemical residues and of course you save a lot of money, never having to heat the water, nor buy washing powder or softeners. Talk about a win-win situation!
- Clean fruit and vegetables with strong alkaline water, Ph10

'We are brought up to a point of choice until we choose correctly ourselves.'—Ancient proverb.

As far as the dangerous chlorine by-products (DBPs) are concerned, most DBPs are absorbed through your skin when you shower, but also through inhaling the steam-creating chloroform. Installation of a simple shower filter with active charcoal removes chlorine by-products.

Take Care of this Problem

Some health-conscious people are of the opinion that distilled water is good for your health. Dr. Paavo Airola wrote about the dangers of distilled water in the early seventies. Distillation is a process you probably know about: water is brought to boiling point; steam rises, condenses and is collected as distilled water during this process.

The documentation indicates, however, that distilled water does not contain any minerals and may be used for a shorter period following a detoxification process, so thus has some merit. But because it contains less vital minerals and electrolytes (sodium, potassium, chloride), as well as zinc and magnesium, this can lead to irregular heart rhythm, arrhythmia and high blood pressure. Cooking in distilled water will result in a reduction of some very important nutritional elements that are vital for all bodily functions.

When you drink distilled water, it will absorb other substances. In contact with air, it will absorb carbon dioxide (CO_2), making the water more acidic (lower pH).

The quantity of distilled water and how long it is consumed will determine the acidity of your body. This, again, can lead to a host of degenerative diseases like osteoporosis, coronary heart disease, diabetes, migraine, asthma, and musculoskeletal problems. Distilled water is around 72-78 dynes per cubic centimetre (a measurement of surface tension). In order for water to penetrate the cells, the surface needs to be lower than 48 dynes. This can be achieved through structuring water using one of several technologies.

Structured water is very different from ordinary, contaminated water. It is ordered pretty much like a crystal. Like ice, it excludes particles and solutes as it forms structures and space—exclusion zones (EZ), according to Professor Gerald Pollack.

The structured water molecules can then easily enter the cells, through the aquaporin channels (Nobel Prize Winner, 2003, Peter Agre).

According to the U.S. Environmental Protection Agency (EPA), distilled water, which is essentially free of minerals, is very aggressive and has a tendency to dissolve substances that come in contact with it. This happens especially when the water connects with carbon dioxide (CO_2) from the air, which makes the water even more acidic and aggressive. Several minerals will dissolve.

The most poisonous forms of mineral water consumed— Coke and all other brands—are made from distilled water. Not forgetting the cheap and unhealthy sugar and artificial sweeteners like aspartame, Splenda and sucralose, these are the most deceptive and health-damaging drinks consumed today. Considerable quantities of calcium, magnesium and other trace minerals are lost and create a serious imbalance in our bodies. Early aging and disease follows. You can't cheat nature and get away with it. This form of water simply damages your health and should carry a health warning label like those have on packets of cigarettes.

Many scientists and health practitioners agree that early aging and diseases are a result of acidity and low pH, which results in too little oxygen for the cells and a gradual breakdown of the cell membranes. Clinical therapists and doctors corroborate this, as they experience first-hand the reversal of so-called lifestyle diseases: cancer, coronary heart disease, diabetes, osteoporosis, asthma, allergy, fibromyalgia et cetera. Toxins from ordinary tap water or bottled water, unhealthy toxic food, pollution from the air and the body itself can create a vicious cycle, culminating in major disruption to the cellular metabolism. This is the backdrop scenario described in the work of Dr. Otto Warburg who received the Nobel Prize in Physiology or Medicine in 1931 for proving that a small reduction in oxygen affects cellular metabolism. Instead of a system fuelled by sufficient oxygen, it becomes to a system of fermentation, using sugar substances as fuel. This is the root cause of cancer. The sad part is that most people are unaware of this scientific documentation. Instead, they are led to believe that the cause of cancer is unknown and that the only chance of survival is early detection and chemotherapy, radiation and surgery. Unknown to most, only three per cent survive after five years of being diagnosed and treated with allopathic medicine. A disgraceful fact that is hidden by a greedy and manipulative pharmaceutical industry.

Oxygen, the Vital Element

All cells have an **absolute requirement for oxygen**, without exception. Deprive a cell of 35 per cent of its oxygen for 48 hours and it may become cancerous. Dr. Warburg discovered that cancer is anaerobic, unable to utilise oxygen, and cannot survive in the presence of high levels of oxygen, as found in an alkaline state.

The following foods can contribute to an acidic body system:

- Sugars including artificial sugars like aspartame, Splenda, sucralose, fructose, MSG (monosodium glutamate, Chinese food). MSG is very often hidden under other names, such as soy, soya lecithin, hydrolyzed vegetable protein, mixed spices, et cetera.
- White flour.
- Milk products.

Stress, either physical or emotional, can contribute to an acidic terrain. Dehydration is often overlooked, but can lead to many problems and diseases. (Ref: *Your body's many cries for Water*, by Dr. F. Batmanghelidj.) It should also be noted that there is a correlation between soft water (distilled water is extremely soft) and a high incidence of coronary heart disease. Cellular structure does not thrive in an acidic environment with a low pH and will do its utmost to counteract this condition by mobilising buffers such as minerals and salts from the skeleton, buffering against the acidity of the cells and their terrain, and producing bicarbonates for the blood.

The more distilled water is consumed; the more minerals are shifted from the skeleton. Even supplementing with minerals is not sufficient to counteract this unhealthy state of affairs. The ideal water should be clean, vital, alkaline, ionised, and restructured with antioxidant properties. It should also contain vital minerals including magnesium, calcium and trace minerals.

Health Myths

Today, health myths abound, and despite the sometimes dangerous side effects, many people still cling to a few products as if their health depended on them.

- Myth 1: Cod liver oil with omega-3 is healthy—Debunked.
- Myth 2: Milk is good for your bone structure—False, debunked.
- Myth 3: Your tap water is healthy—Wrong. It is destroyed and dead and full of dangerous chemicals, with the wrong electrical voltage.
- Myth 4: Fluoride is good for your teeth—Debunked. This toxic element is allowed in many nations' water supplies and even recommended by many dentists.

The Dangers of Fluorides

As this element is often added to drinking water, let us examine the validity of this assumption. Long before any health security tests were carried out, fluoride, a derivate from the aluminium industry, was introduced into the drinking water in some countries. How could a toxic by-product of aluminium be allowed into the US's drinking water?

To understand this, one has to examine the industry's money trail, manipulation of data, and its close connection to the nuclear industry and development of the atomic bomb.

It is well documented that data was manipulated in the Newburgh-Kingston Caries Fluorine Study. Recent declassified documents demonstrated the pro-flour stance by the Public Health Service and The Manhattan Project, during the development of the atomic bomb. It is correct to say that The Manhattan Project sold and recommended fluoride to the American people.

On the other side of the Atlantic Ocean in Copenhagen, Denmark, from 1920-30, a group of world-renowned scientists headed by Niels Bohr were working on the groundwork for nuclear fission. In this environment worked a brilliant and courageous scientist called Kaj Eli Roholm, who paved the way for a proper understanding of the dangers associated with fluoride.

Almost all the world's supply of fluoride came at that time from a large deposit of cryolite in a site in Greenland, which belongs to Denmark. *Cryolite* is a word of Eskimo origin, meaning *ice stone*.

Researchers discovered that aluminium could be more easily extracted by melting the ice stone together with bauxite. These metals where used extensively during the First World War. The factories where these metals were used were heavily polluted and workers became very ill with many diseases such as crippled backs, so-called 'poker back', cancer, osteoporosis, and lung diseases. Kaj Eli Roholm pointed out the cause of these diseases: fluorine intoxication.

Fluoride in our Drinking Water—History and Science

You have probably heard that fluoride is necessary to prevent caries in the teeth and that
fluoride-containing toothpaste and tablets should be used for that reason. The brilliant scientist Kaj Eli Roholm came to the opposite conclusion, however: he says that there is no scientific evidence that fluoride prevents caries (tooth decay), and will in fact damage dental enamel! His warning came 70 years ago. Studies conducted on both humans and sheep confirmed these findings. In Iceland, sheep became ill with bad teeth and crippled deformities, especially with gaddur, when volcanic ashes containing fluoride poisoned the fields in which the sheep grazed. Dental fluorosis (*Colorado Brown Stain* or *Texas Teeth*) is an indication of systemic fluoride poisoning which originates from drinking groundwater polluted by fluoride.

At the time of Kaj Eli Roholm's findings, several new industries were started up based on the properties of fluoride; for example, the production of carbon-based fluoride products and Freon in refrigerators. During the Industrial Revolution, thick clouds of smog hung over Europe. In the early seventies, when I studied physiotherapy in Bradford, Yorkshire, the renovation of the region's black buildings had already started. But whilst most researchers came to the conclusion that sulphur compounds were the main cause of this black pollution, Kaj E. Roholm concluded that it was fluoride, not sulphur, that was the culprit and the real danger in pollution.

The past century's biggest industrial scandal occurred in the Meuse Valley in Belgium where 60 people were killed and several thousand injured in 1930 as a result of fluoride poisoning—not sulphur. Kaj E. Roholm studied the new global aluminium industry and its pollution in Switzerland, Italy and Norway. Commonly observed diseases in these factories were osteoporosis, asthma, headache, nausea, intestinal pain and diarrhoea. The work of A.W. Frostad published in the *Norwegian Medical Publication* (Vol. 56 p.179 in 1936) stated that fluoride intoxication in Norwegian aluminium workers was the main cause of asthma and pulmonary disorders (occupational hazard).

In 1937, Kaj E Roholm published 364 pages of documentation called *Fluoride Intoxication*. Translated into English, it contains 893 scientific references—a monumental works blasting like Danish dynamite, shaking the very foundations of the cryolite, aluminium and fluoride industries worldwide.

With the onset of World War II, the production of fluorine

compounds increased dramatically to meet warfare needs, especially in developing the world's first atomic bomb, under the auspices of research and development project The Manhattan Project. Security requirements kept most information about the use of fluoride and its health hazards a secret during the war and many years afterwards.

Fluoride in our Drinking Water—More Rotten Eggs in the Basket

Based on data, which was deliberately manipulated and hidden, US became the first country to allow fluoride in its drinking water. Sweden was one of the first European countries to fluoridate its water supply in 1952, but this practice was finally prohibited by Sweden's Parliament in 1971. Industries in China and Australia removed some of the arsenic lead and other toxins from the industry and placed it in the water distribution network in greater parts of Australia. The industry saves a lot of money, and citizens are slowly being poisoned, led to believe that it is fluoride in the drinking water that is the cause of the pollution.

Ann Bessington, an independent member of the parliament in Australia, has documented the fact that many toxins, including fluoride and aluminium, pollute the drinking water of the City of Adelaide. The drinking water is destroyed, dead and chemically treated by toxic substances. Fluoride is the main ingredient in rat poison, sarin gas and Prozac (anti-depressant).

As we have seen, fluoridation of drinking water can result in serious damage to health, such as osteoporosis, cancer, and disturbances in brain, liver and kidneys function. The truth about the seriousness of these facts had so far been hidden through corruption and manipulation by the industry and organisations, including health authorities in several countries. The serious and dangerous practice of adding fluoride to drinking water has existed since 1930. Today, it exists in many guises, such as PFC (per fluorinated compounds). Hitler and Stalin used fluoride in concentration camps and gulags to mass-control people, rendering them docile.

About 50 years after the scandal of Newburgh, another source of fluoride's damaging effects is perfluorinated compounds (PFCs). As with fluoride in toothpaste, PFC is present in many household brands, such as Teflon, Gore-Tex and Stainmaster (stain removal agent), and hundreds of others. The truth about the damaging effects of PFCs is hidden or ridiculed by the proponents of this industry—just as with fluoride in 1930.

The truth about fluoride and all its toxic derivatives passes through three different stages, as first described by the German philosopher Arthur Schopenhauer 200 years ago. First, it is ridiculed, before it is strongly antagonised, and finally the truth is accepted as self-evident. When it comes to fluoride in drinking water, I believe we are currently in stage three; hopefully, it is only a question of time before this dangerous practice (i.e., forced intoxication of whole nations and their citizens) ceases. Fluoride is a known neurological toxin, which is biologically active and accumulates in body tissues, interfering with the enzyme systems, damaging the hormonal system and weakening the immune system, leading to neurological diseases. Several hundred scientific studies exist documenting this fact. Twenty-five of these studies show that children achieve a significantly lower IQ when using fluoride.

The chemical industrial giant Du Pont is the leading producer of organic fluorides. Through The Manhattan Project, uranium hexafluoride was used to develop the atomic bomb. After the war, the market was flooded with products based on fluorocarbons: plastic, pharmaceuticals, spray, pesticides, household cleaning materials, et cetera. By the end of the 20th century, millions of tons of CFC and DFC had polluted the atmosphere, our blood and other body systems. In 1966, Theo Colborn, John Peterson Myers and Dianne Dumanoski published the book *Our Stolen Future*. This is an investigation into the disturbances and damage done to the hormone and immune systems throughout our lifetime. The book is one of the clearest warnings in existence today about the health and environment threat that these chemicals represent—but, strangely enough, it contains not a single reference to PFC. Many scientists were quite embarrassed that this class of chemicals had escaped the scrutinising radar of environmental science for almost 60 years. Data on the damaging effects of these chemicals existed, but was not published in the scientific forums until quite recently. The conclusion is that PFC is very durable and lasts a long time in the environment. Fluoride from these sources can be absorbed from carpets, furniture, Teflon, household products, et cetera. Fluoride gradually accumulates in core regions of the brain that govern behaviour, notably the hippocampus and the limbic areas, resulting in hyperactivity or the opposite: apathetic, lethargic behaviour. More than 124 studies carried out on laboratory animals have confirmed these facts.

For over 70 years now, fluoride has been used in household products and water for cooking. Today, one out of ten children is diagnosed with ADD/ADHD, and the numbers are rising rapidly. Alzheimer's, Chronic Fatigue Syndrome, hypothyroidism, arthritis and autism spectrum disorders are all on the rise, and environmental pollution is partly due to fluoride, heavy metals like mercury in dental fillings and vaccination (thimerosal), CFS, PFC. Many environmental organisations are working diligently to implement a ban on fluoride in drinking water. Prof. Paul Connett, a specialist in environmental medicine and member of the Fluoride Action Network, is one of the leading activists in this area.

Fluoride is derived from aluminium, a toxic element for which there are strict rules and regulations on handling and storage. Is it not senseless to allow poisonous fluoride sludge from the aluminium industry into our water, toothpaste and other household products?

The Emperor's Not Wearing Any Clothes!

Dr. John R. Lee, a medical doctor, researcher and author who also became a personal friend when I invited him to Norway and we did a Scandinavian tour to put osteoporosis and natural progesterone firmly on the map. In between lecturing and playing basketball with our kids, he told me many interesting stories, but the one about fluoride has stuck with me. He told me how he had been indoctrinated at medical school to believe that fluoride helps prevent tooth decay. But his thorough and independent investigation into the science of fluoridation, its effectiveness and safety found that 'the Emperor's not wearing any clothes'.

He could not find any evidence of fluoride effectiveness and safety. He even conducted his own very thorough double-blind study in this field. The results were dramatic and clear: regardless of the patients' ailments, they all got worse when drinking fluoridated water, and when drinking non-fluoridated water, their conditions improved, less osteoporosis, hip fractures and cancer. Check out the excellent article by dr. John R. Lee, MD, "The Fluoridation Scam. The selling of Fluoridation in America". There is even a file directory, stop Fluoride Poisoning, which includes EPA whistle-blowers. http://www.net-fluoride/filelist-htm. World famous neurosurgeon Russell Blaylock, MD, says in his book "Health and nutrition secrets to save your life" that only the light of truth can halt this process". (www.blaylockmd.com).

Carefully conducted studies conclusively that fluoride weakens the bone structure, causing an increase of hip fractures in men by 41% and in women 27% (Utah Mormon Study). Fluoride will also damage the brain and the nerve system, especially the developing brain in pregnant women and small children.

Once the majority of our food and water supplies are contaminated along with the soils, everybody will be affected by hazard of fluoride toxicity, (A compounding effect). Drinks packaged in aluminium cans and bottles, i.e.: diet drinks, sodas, fruit juice, bear and energy drinks are the worst. The most toxic brain aluminium fluoride with multiple toxins found in aspartame, sucralose, Splenda, NutraSweet etc., creating the most powerful government approved toxic cocktail imaginable. According to a study done of the University of Oslo, Norway. The measurement of aluminium levels in the drinking water has never been higher than today. And it is steadily increasing.

Below is a list of some toxins, heavy metals and contaminants in our drinking water. The grim reaper has not been idle.

Arsenic: Arsenic is a semimetal in the periodic table and is both odourless and tasteless. It enters drinking water from erosion of natural deposits, runoff from orchards and the electronics industry. Arsenic has been linked to cancer of the bladder, lung, skin, prostate and liver, as well as stomach pain, diarrhoea and paralysis.

Lead: Lead is presented in natural deposits and is a common element used in piping materials. Exposure to lead occurs through breathing in paint fumes and dust containing this heavy metal, but it can also be found in drinking water and can damage your health. Especially vulnerable are babies, young children and pregnant women. Lead can disturb mental development and can later lead to

ADD/ADHD, et cetera. Like other heavy metals, lead has a tendency to be drawn to the central nervous system, kidneys, liver and blood where it reacts and destroys certain enzyme systems. One of the causes of hypertension or high blood pressure is heavy metal toxicity. The latest lead poisoning scandal happened in Flint, Michigan, the hometown of Michael Moore. The authorities ignored the warnings and the poorest kids were hit the hardest and the city was declared to be in a state of emergency before Barack Obama declared it as a federal state of emergency. An outbreak of Legionnaire`s disease in the wake of the poisonous drinking water killed 10 and affecting 77 people.

Chromium: Short-term exposure to chromium can cause skin irritation and sores. Long-term exposure can cause liver, kidneys, blood and nervous system damage. It can also cause cancer.

It is interesting to note that high concentrations of chromium have been measured in the groundwater close to industries and deposits, but also quite a distance from these areas. Chromium can spread via air, soil and water. Chromium 6 is the compound made infamous through the film *Erin Brockovich*, played by Julia Roberts. The company P.G.R.E knew that the carcinogen substance chromium 6 was deliberately put in the drinking water for over 30 years in the small town of Hinkley.

Copper: Copper is a mineral found in natural deposits and mineral ores and is used extensively in piping material. Copper is an essential mineral required by the body in small amounts. Too much copper exposure via food and drinking water can lead to digestive disorders, nausea and vomiting. Patients with Wilson's disease, a genetic disorder in which copper accumulates in the tissues, manifesting in neurological or psychiatric symptoms and liver diseases, are even more vulnerable.

Mercury: Mercury is a liquid heavy metal found in nature together with other elements. Mercury is used in electronic goods such as batteries, light bulbs, et cetera. This accounts for about 50% of its usage. Mercury from industry (coal power stations) can find its way into drinking water through the soil, brooks and rivers. Mercury in the drinking water is inorganic and can easily be converted to the organic methyl-mercury, which is more toxic and can enter the food chain.

Short- or long-term exposure to mercury can lead to kidneys and nerve tissue damage as this neurotoxin is drawn to this part of your body—indeed, the expression 'Mad as a Hatter' is a direct result of mercury poising. Hat-makers in the1800s used mercury in the felting work, which eventually resulted in them suffering chronic occupational mercury poisoning. The direct contact and inhalation of mercury vapour tremors, anxiety, behavioural changes, dementia, et cetera. Lewis Carroll's iconic Mad Hatter character in *Alice in Wonderland* is often linked to the occupational hazards of hat-making.

Mercury is still used in vaccines, and the CDC openly admits this. There is no safe level of mercury. That is a scientific fact.

Today's exposure to mercury can occur in many different ways: exposure to large amounts of water; inhalation—for example, children playing with thermometers. Nausea, vomiting, diarrhoea and kidneys damage can result. Chronic exposure to mercury over longer periods of time can occur through drinking water, and eating fish, especially tuna fish and farmed fish. Before and during pregnancy, it is advisable to abstain from this type of fish because of the content of mercury and other chemical pollutants such as dioxin.

Chronic expose to mercury may result in nervous disorders, kidneys failure, dental problems, infertility, ADD/ADHD, autism, birth defects, prostate problems and cancer. Dental fillings made of amalgam contain mercury, cadmium, thallium and other metals that will weaken your immune system.

But don't despair—there are efficient remedies and methods to remove all these toxins, which you will learn about later (prevention, detoxification, chelating, vitamins, minerals, herbs, vital food and also PURE ENERGY NORWAY for you (Norwegian for *Vital Water and Air*).

Cyanide: Cyanide is a chemical combination of carbon and nitrogen, which are often combined with several other organic and inorganic compounds. The most common is hydrogen cyanide and is mainly used in the production of nylon and other synthetic fibres as well as in pesticides. Cyanide can enter groundwater from industry and waste. Sometimes cyanide is used in road salt in the wintertime. Chlorination of the sewage system can also produce cyanide as a by-product of this process.

Short-term exposure to cyanide can lead to breathing problems, tremors, cramps and other neurological symptoms. Long-term exposure can cause complex symptoms like weight loss, nerve damage and thyroid problems.

Nitrates: When nitrogen and oxygen combine with certain organic and inorganic materials and enter the body from pesticides, nitrates will change to nitrites. Larger amounts of nitrates in drinking water can cause serious disease and death. Children are especially vulnerable. When nitrates are transformed to nitrites, the blood's ability to transport oxygen is diminished. Breathing difficulties and skin changes (bluish) are some of the symptoms. Long-term exposure to nitrates may result in frequent urination (diuresis), internal bleeding in the spleen and liver, and kidneys damage.

Thallium: Thallium is a metal found in natural deposits and mineral ores together with other elements and is used in electronic equipment and sometimes in dental fillings made of amalgam, together with other heavy metals like mercury and cadmium.

The accumulation of thallium in your body through various sources may lead to nervous disorders, damage to liver, kidneys and hormone disturbance. Thallium poisoning through drinking water is rare.

MTBE (Methyl—T- Butyl-ether): MTBE is a group of chemicals added to fuels to increase its oxygen content. In the US, MTBE is added to petrol to reduce the discharge of carbon monoxide and ozone. MTBE has replaced lead to improve the octane effect of petrol. Because of its extensive use, MTBE has been found in ground and surface water in the US. MTBE can reach drinking reservoirs through leakage, and most of the nitrogen material in water can be transformed to nitrates.

The primary inorganic sources of nitrates pollution are potassium nitrate and ammonium nitrates, which are frequently used in farming. Research on laboratory animals has shown that drinking water containing MTBE can cause liver, kidneys and nervous afflictions, ear, nose and throat irritation, nausea, diarrhoea, fatigue and cancer.

Selenium: Selenium is a mineral found in natural deposits together with other elements. Most of the selenium is used in the electronics, glass and pigments industries, metals in pharmaceuticals and in photo laboratories. Selenium is an essential mineral and very important for the body. Soil in Nordic countries lacks sufficient quantities of selenium which is vital for the strength of the immune system and the prevention of coronary heart disease and cancer.

Sedimentation pollution in water

Sediments are loose particles of soil, sand, clay, humus and other elements covering the bottoms of our water reservoirs. They are formed from the degradation of plants, animals and soil. Wind, water and ice can transport sediments across long distances. Sediments in our water systems are polluted pesticides like DDT, chemicals like polychlorinated bisphenols (PCBs). The use of DDT and PCBs were prohibited in the 1970s but these compounds have been discovered in drinking water, especially groundwater.

Is it possible that your own drinking water is polluted by dust particles originating in Asia? A study conducted by Harvard Medical School, published in *Atmospheric Environment*, showed that 41% of the days during which there was poor visibility were the result of dust particles from Asiatic sources. In the same year, it was shown that pollution from North America caused a 33% increase in ozone in the Alps. With the volcanic eruption and its ashes from Iceland, and radioactivity from Fukushima, Japan, the levels of detectable pollution have never been greater. Pollution is spread through primitive organisms to shellfish, fish and animals. Some of these die, become sick and are a threat to people's health.

Recently, the Norwegian farmed fish industry has come under heavy scrutiny because of considerable amounts of heavy metals (e.g., mercury, cadmium), PCBs, POPs (persistent organic pollutants) and DDT—so much so that American and Russian health authorities have warned about this pollution, especially during pregnancy and childhood. The food fed to the fish is sometimes 70% of vegetable origin, with its phytoestrogenic properties, which results in contaminated fish food. Farmed fish live in cramped, unhealthy conditions with insufficient oxygen. The marine landscape is changing because of this pollution, and crabs and other shellfish are exhibiting visible changes; e.g., lack of proper shell, lice et cetera.

There are five main types of pollution in sediments:

- Compounds including nitrogen and ammonium. Too high levels of phosphorus can cause increased growth of algae, leading to less oxygen in the water when the algae die. High levels of ammonium can be poisonous for lower organisms.
- Hydrocarbon in oil and lubrication products.
- DDT and PCBs. Halogen hydrocarbons.
- Polycyclic hydrocarbons (DAH) are a group of organic chemicals including petroleum products.
- Metals like iron, manganese, lead, cadmium, zinc, arsenic, selenium and mercury.

These are toxic compounds for animals and humans alike, depending on the dosage. It is relatively rare to find lead in our drinking reservoirs, but pipe corrosion can release compounds of lead into the drinking water. Older water pipes are very common in Norway and so-called 'lead-free' pipes may contain 8% lead (US).

Lead can also leach from other metal compounds such as chromium and alloys, especially when using hot water. According to our health authorities - EPA in the US,

Folkehelseinstituttet/Mattilsynet in Norway—it is common knowledge that even small amounts of lead represent a health hazard for children and babies and during pregnancy. Baby food mixed with water containing lead or other heavy metals and pollutants can damage and disturb a child's normal development. It is also important to note that baby food very often contains soy, lecithin and hydrolysed vegetable oils that can damage your health. One of the most frequently asked questions under this subject is: 'If lead enters our drinking water after it has left the water reservoir, does the age of our house play a part in the quality of our drinking water?'

The answer is a resounding *Yes*! Drinking water containing lead is more frequently found in older than newer houses. Water pipes in houses built in the 1930s contain higher levels of lead than houses built after this period. There are small variations in housing construction between countries. Only plastic and copper are used in new houses. Experts tell us that the cranes and coupling material used can leach lead (8%). Even though they are technically defined as lead-free, scientific testing proves that newer houses have more lead material leaching into the drinking water. As the house gets older, minerals will be deposited on the insides of the pipes and this may lead to some protection from lead leakage. This tends to occur around five years after the house is built.

Because it is impossible to smell or taste whether drinking water contains lead and other heavy metals, it is safest to test the water for these pollutants, in addition to installing a filtering/cleaning system, reverse osmosis system or ionisation technology. Armed with the knowledge of how to choose the best available solution, which also includes self-administering detoxification and inhalation processes for your body's health and well-being, you can prevent or even reverse diseases coming from your environment. Doctors and therapists worldwide have clinically proven this. 'An ounce of prevention is smarter than a pound of cure,' as the saying goes.

The following is a list of contaminants and heavy metals that should alert you and take measures to avoid them, chelate and detoxify on a regular basis.

Antimony: Antimony is a metal found in deposits and ores mixed with other elements. The most commonly used is antimony trioxide, which is used as a flame retardant, and in batteries, ceramics and glass. Antimony has the same potentials as the poisonous mineral lead. Short-term exposure can cause nausea, vomiting and diarrhoea. Long-term exposure may lead to cancer. This element, which is common in industry, is very mobile, can leach and spread through soil, water and sediments.

Barium: Barium is a silver-white metal, which only exists together with other elements in metal areas and deposits. Barium is used in industry, especially in drilling and in the production of paint, ceramic and rubber, and in medicine as a contrast medium in digestive system assessments. Barium can cause digestive problems, cramps, liver and kidneys failure and arrhythmia (irregular heart rhythm). Barium also comes from cigarette smoking and from chemtrails in air and water. Air particulate samples taken to an EPA-approved lab in Phoenix in 2009 showed a level 1050 times over the toxic limit (http://www.arizonaskywatch.com/charts/our%20charts/air_particulates_2009_a.jpg)

Beryllium: Beryllium is a metal that can be found in naturally occurring deposits and metal ores together with other metal and precious stones. Beryllium is predominantly used in nuclear reactors and in the aviation industry. Exposure to beryllium is most health-damaging through inhalation. Exposure over long periods can cause skeletal diseases and cancer.

Cadmium: Cadmium is a metal found in nature, in deposits and mineral ores. Cadmium is most commonly used in the metal industry as alloys, machinery, enamel, photography, TV and solar batteries, often together with other metals such as nickel. Classified as a heavy metal, cadmium is drawn to the liver, kidneys and nervous system. Short-term exposure may lead to nausea, vomiting, diarrhoea, cramps, epileptic seizure and organ failure. Long-term exposure may damage the liver, kidneys, skeleton and blood system.

Cadmium destroys cell membranes, making it possible for other toxic substances to enter the cells. It leaches from industrial waste and disposal areas that use zinc, lead and copper in the production of nickel-cadmium batteries, paint and electronic equipment. This eventually finds its way into the groundwater where it bio-accumulates together with other heavy metals and is then found in fish and shellfish.

Chromium: Chromium is a metal found in metal deposits areas and is used by industry in the production of stainless-steel cookware, alloys, paint, cement, paper, rubber, impregnation, et cetera. Chromium exists in 2 forms: trivalent chromium, or chromium 3; and hexavalent chromium, or chromium 4. Only a fraction of chromium can be dissolved in water and thus flow into groundwater. Chromium 3 is essential for the body, stabilising blood sugar and normalising the metabolism of fat and protein.

Chromium 4, on the other hand, is highly toxic and can lead to stomach ulcers, skin irritation and sores, cramps, organ failure and death. Fortunately, this happens rarely; however, it is not uncommon to be allergic to both types of chromium. Chromium 4 is very unstable and has a strong tendency to oxidation. The main reason chromium 4 is so toxic is that it can form chromium 5, a known carcinogen, which can attach itself to any tissue and cause cancer.

It is common knowledge that the tar in tobacco can cause cancer. When this became publicly known, the tobacco industry produced light cigarettes with lower tar content. The public was never encouraged to stop smoking. The message that was marketed was 'Smoking is healthy. Keep smoking.' The food industry has followed in the footsteps of the tobacco industry, with so-called 'lite' products being backed by pseudo-science used in marketing to brainwash people. When the question is raised about weight problems, the answer is always the same: 'Less calories, more exercise—and be sure to use our lite products!'

Several studies show that the lite variations came with quite a few health problems. An investigation at the Karolinska Institute in Sweden has show that lite products in fact do not contribute to weight loss; indeed, often the opposite is true. Women drinking milk and cheese containing fat experience less weight gain than their sisters trying to surf on the lite-product wave.

A miraculous bounce back from osteoporosis, asthma and incontinence and the other ailments.

"Thinking themselves wise and learned, fools go aimlessly hither and thither, the blind led by the blind." - Vath Upanishad

Jorunn Anda, an elderly lady hobbled into our clinic, clearly in agony and out of breath, wheezing and told us her long suffering of severe osteoporosis confirmed by bone mineral density measurements (BMD) and was on oestrogen treatment. She also had asthma and was on medication.

"I became almost crippled and could hardly walk", she told the local newspaper journalist. "But after following the advice of physiotherapist and naturopath Gunnar V. Espedal, the osteoporosis vanished, confirmed by the same BMD test and reports from the medical expects. It only took 9 months. I am so happy! As a bonus allergy and asthma has disappeared", exclaimed Jorunn Anda.

A reversal of serious osteoporosis in 9 months was a surprise even for my friend and mentor dr. John R. Lee. On average it takes 2 years to reverse this condition as he documented in Lancet and New England Journal of Medicine.

The reason for the quickest recorded reversal of osteoporosis in the world was due to a unique combination of herbal extract, natural progesterone, minerals and change of food and lifestyle, factors detoxification and a training protocol which you will learn more about in the next chapter.

But before leaving the encouraging story of the Jorunn Anda, she told me a secret: "Mr Espedal, I am very grateful for having been cured of osteoporosis, allergy and asthma, but I have a third problem. Only my husband knows about this. If you can fix this, I don't know what to call you! For the last 30 years I have been incontinent, and have to wear diapers. It is a great problem for me". "Let me try", I said. A simple Bowen procedure of the os coccyx, the tailbone fixed her problem. No more incontinence or diapers.

On the wall in our clinic is a picture of a smiling Mrs J. Anda, holding the journalist's baby, together with a press clipping of her healing story.

You have probably heard the expression, "if a blind man leads a blind, they both fall into the pit" (Mathew 15.13-14). The so called experts in osteoporosis was very much opposed to dr. John R. Lee's work and did not hesitate to attack his work on reversal of osteoporosis which produced 100% great results, i.e.: Reversal and cure! The Norwegian Medical Journal refused to publicize his findings. ¨Abiding in the midst of ignorance¨.

CHAPTER FOUR

Detoxification—An Introduction

'There is a wisdom of the head and a wisdom of the heart.' Charles Dickens.

In this chapter, you will learn how it is possible to detoxify and cleanse your body using different remedies and methods—although the smartest and simplest means of preventing disease is by *avoiding* sources of toxicity or pollution, as opposed to treating the disease.

We all know the expression, 'An ounce of prevention is better than a pound of cure' - or, as the farmers here in Rogaland used to say, 'It is smarter and more efficient to stop and divert the water from brooks than to harness the water masses of a river.' The toxic materials present in water, air and food may prove a little difficult to identify at first—but with a little practice in environmental detective work, and by educating and training yourself, you will soon master the task. First of all, you need to be able to recognise the most dangerous toxins and offenders that can damage your health.

In the fifties, health claims and advertisements tried to indoctrinate people that smoking was a healthy enough habit; and margarine was touted as healthy for your heart and circulation. Now we know better. During the last decades, an overwhelming number of additives have flooded our foods and environment. Scientists claim that 80% of all lifestyle diseases are caused by environmental factors; i.e., toxins, additives and pollutants. We live in a danger zone. By doing something about it, with focused attention and a defined goal, you can achieve better health and vitality instantly. Why wait? As they say in Yorkshire, 'You don't get owt for nowt!'

As we have seen, toxic substances enter our bodies via various routes:

- **Food and drink** via the digestive system, where they are modified by stomach acid, digestive enzymes, bile and various natural bacteria.
- **Respiration**. Toxic substances can be inhaled and act as irritants to the respiratory system. Some particles may be absorbed into the bloodstream.
- **Absorption**. Toxic substances such as VOCs and POPs are absorbed through the skin. Trihalomethanes, by-products of chlorine, easily enter the body via this route, as well as via the lungs and digestive system.

It is therefore very important to prevent this from happening. When heavy metals and other toxic compounds enter the body, detoxification can essentially take place via the following processes:

Elimination: For this method to be effective, the toxic compounds must be dissolved in water, or be connected to a larger molecule (a protein) that can be dissolved. In this way, the toxic compound can be eliminated via the urine or through sweating. In the case of compounds that exist in a gaseous phase, these will be eliminated through expiration.

Conversion: This process occurs when a toxic substance is caught and deposited in specific body tissues. This method entails a greater load for the body's elimination systems. *Example:* Lead is moved to the bone structures, where it competes with calcium and other minerals; or organic compounds such as VOCs in fat cells can deposit it, as these toxic compounds are fat-soluble. Over time, these will accumulate.

The bio-accumulative effect of toxic substances takes place mainly in fatty tissue. Most of the organic substances belong to this group, including polychlorinated bisphenols (PCBs), dioxin and esters. This accumulation tends to occur at an increasing pace because the body does not manage to eliminate these toxic substances fast enough.

Sequestering: This process takes place when toxic substances are deposited in certain tissues. *Example*: Lead is moved to bone tissue where it competes with calcium, or volatile compounds (VOCs) are deposited in fatty tissue.

In summary, the total toxicity load increases. It is therefore imperative to reduce toxicity via filtration, ionisation and other means, to attain water with high redox potential and antioxidant properties, high zeta potential and high hydrogen content. This will improve the detoxification process.

Through the enzyme system of the liver and gall bladder, the body can be stimulated to increase its capacity for elimination. The efficiency of the functioning of these systems is dependent on many factors, including genetics, age, body mass and composition, stress levels, nutritional status, and the methods and remedies chosen to stimulate these processes.

Babies and children are most vulnerable to these toxic substances, since their elimination systems are not properly developed. One aspect here is the ever-increasing amount of additive toxins used in vaccinations: mercury, formaldehyde, polysorbate (also used in car antifreeze products), squalene, aluminium and much more. Other groups that are particularly vulnerable to developing disease as a result of the bio-accumulative effect of toxins and pollutants are pregnant women and the elderly. The body's normal development may be disturbed and can cause birth defects and other ailments, in addition to complications during pregnancy.

A person whose stress levels are high will naturally have a reduced capacity to eliminate toxic compounds due to weakened enzyme and immune systems. Poor nutrition and general poor health will further reduce the body's capacity for this important function.

Calamity might be just around the corner. Many people seem to forget when all is going well and life's a breeze—when a disease hits, seemingly out of nowhere. But in fact a series of small steps breaking the Divine Instruction (as found in the Bible, for instance) have led you to this point: 'Many small streams make a big river,' as the saying goes.

The quickest and most common solution people tend to go for is the 'get-me-out-of-this-predicament-quick solution—i.e., medicine to reduce anxiety, depression, pain, et cetera). This symptomatic, superficial form of treatment is in every way inferior to a holistic approach where the *cause* is treated. The best solution is also free of any side effects: assessment and reliable guidance on further health choices empowers the client, giving him choices and enabling him to take full responsibility for his health. Mastering this aspect of one's life is liberating and exhilarating. The laws of nature and the keys are there for everyone to use, but one step at a time, with good support from a health teacher, coach or therapist. Ignoring these rules is just like violating traffic regulations: it can have a damaging effect on your health.

Winning with Water

Pure Energy Norway is Norwegian for *Vital Water and Air*. It is time to celebrate the *New You*. By taking an active stance, fighting and winning the war on internal body pollution, you are playing alongside your inner body-healing team members, by following the rules of body physiology. You detoxify, avoid certain foods and drinks, exercise, alkalinise and oxygenate through vital water, food, air and oxygen therapies.

Royal, antioxidant, restructured hexagonal water provides you with more oxygen and more energy. Pure Energy Norway! The water that refreshes parts of your body other waters cannot reach. Your body will greatly appreciate the epigenetic modifications that are made, and the positive influences this water has on your body and you will truly be able to feel the difference. We have thousands of testimonials from laypeople, doctors, professional athletes, and fitness enthusiasts, which are backed by solid science from many countries around the world.

What you invest in preventative measures now you will reap later—with interest. Indeed, you will be a winner in so many aspects: you will reduce—and in many cases eradicate completely—the likelihood of your getting cancer, diabetes, osteoporosis, coronary heart disease, allergies, asthma, et cetera.

Good hygienic conditions, clean work surfaces, washing and soaking both fruit and vegetables in alkaline, ionised water with the addition perhaps of a little colloidal silver solution will all kill microbes. Colloidal silver has been recognised for centuries now as being a remarkably effective natural antibiotic. Research has shown that it can even eradicate antibiotic-resistant microbes like MRSA, bird flu and SARS virus (corona).

The following is a list of preventative measures you can start implementing today:

- Drink ionised, alkaline, antioxidant, restructured water in between meals. This provides your body optimal working conditions. This water's high redox potential enables a cellular detoxification process to take place. Increased oxygen going to cells' mitochondria means more vitality and energy. You will learn more about the scientific background to the new water and air purification systems later on. Researchers including Alfred Searle, founder of the global Searle Paramedical Company, who, in the early 1900s, wrote the book *Colloids in Biology and Medicine, 1919*. Colloidal solutions have astonishing results and are rapidly fatal to microbes, without toxic side effects. Dr. Robert Beck at Syracuse Medical University confirmed these findings in the 1970s.

- Make sure to install an air ioniser in your home to provide clean air with plenty of negative ions. This will saturate your body's red corpuscles with oxygen, which will be transported throughout your body.

- Avoid refined foods with their pesticides, additives, xenon-oestrogens, artificial, synthetic, non-vital foods. Go back to basics: prepare dishes from food that comes from the ground, preferably of the organic variety; involve the whole family in the kitchen whenever possible. The kitchen, being the heart and soul of your home, is also an ideal place to educate. The word *educate* comes from the Latin word *educare*—to bring from within; from your heart, your innermost sanctuary, all life originated. Once you have committed to your goals and equipped yourself with the relevant knowledge about health laws and health matters, education flows naturally from within and will resonate accordingly.

- As I mentioned earlier, certain types of fish, such as tuna, shark, eel, swordfish and all farmed fish such as salmon, trout, cod, et cetera, are polluted with contaminants—PCPs, POPs and heavy metals. These should be avoided.

- Avoid smoking, including passive smoking, as cigarette smoke contains the heavy metal cadmium. This has a special affinity to the nervous system and kidneys in particular. Air ionisation with negative ions is a good solution to purify and eliminate toxins and dust from the atmosphere.

- Alcohol: Consume only in very small amounts. Mixed with mineral waters, juice and Coke, it becomes even more acidic and will weaken the detoxification and immune systems as well as the liver.

- Use only natural products for health and well-being in the household. Many creams and lotions are riddled with synthetics, mineral oils and parabens, which can be deposited in the cell structures like fatty tissues, dehydrating and causing premature aging of the skin. Many cosmetic products contain ingredients that are banned from oral use, yet are absorbed through the skin, with all its detrimental effects.

- Take medicine only when absolutely necessary. This may sound obvious, but it is a known fact that medicines cause side effects and are often over-prescribed.

- Avoid neurologically toxic products such as Splenda, sucralose, fructose (as in HFCS—high-fructose corn syrup), aspartame, NutraSweet, amino sweet, canola (rapeseed) oil, soy oil, soy lecithin, palm oil, corn oil, gene-manipulated foods (GMOs), white sugar, common table salt, MSG monosodium glutamate). MSG is often hidden on labels, listed as vegetable seasoning, bouillon, vegetable oil, hydrolyzed oil, et cetera. Chinese food (Chinese food syndrome) often contains MSG.
- Avoid 'lite' products. Who needs lite products? Avoid fat? Not all fat is bad—as examined in the well-known book by Erasmus, *Fat that heals and fat that kills*.

Did you know that Splenda, used in Cola Zero, Pepsi-Max and Coca Cola Light is a modified sugar molecule containing chlorine and is 600 times sweeter than sugar? It is also found in ketchup, soda and yoghurt. Your body cannot detoxify this chlorine compound. It pollutes both your body and the environment.

I don't know about you, but I need a little break, some breathing space from 'swimming in this almost endless chemical soup in which we breathe, drink and live'. Refreshments are in order. So why don't you come with me into our kitchen to enjoy some physical and spiritual nourishment? The kitchen, where a blend of Norwegian and Lebanese dishes are heartily devoured each day. The heart of the home—which reminds me of the great English designer and restaurateur Terence Conran who provided us with this fabulous description of the kitchen some 20 years ago: 'A kitchen provides physical and spiritual nourishment, and for many is now the heart and soul of the family.' I would add to that: 'And from the heart springs all life' (Bible).

The lady of the house offers me a refreshing glass of vital water in an atmosphere with a surplus of negative ions produced from an ioniser. Delicious, nourishing energy; clean, restructured water. Pure Energy Norway —the water that refreshes the parts of the body that other waters cannot reach (restructured and high-zeta potential). I sit and ponder the amazing properties of this water. I sip and let my mind wander. Its features resemble the Hunza water of the Himalayas—the water that has baffled brilliant minds, including Nobel Prize winners in medicine and physiology Henri Coandă and Albert Szent-Györgyi. I am, after all, in a Lebanese-Norwegian home.

Restructured and Vitalised Water, A Right Royal Water!

There is an old Norwegian saying, '*Du kan ikke få i pose og sekk,*' which equates to the English saying, 'You can't have your cake and eat it too.' However, having it both ways, creating a win-win situation, is in fact easy using ionised water with its myriad new physical characteristics. Refreshing, detoxifying, alkalinising and energy-rich water with a great new taste!

This water is the key to increased vitality and a long life inspired the conquistador, Ponce de Leon in the 15th century and

Nobel Prize winners like Albert Szent-Györgyi and Henri Coandă—the latter being particularly fascinated by the fact that the common denominator amongst healthy, long-living cultures around the world—and in particular the Hunza people in North Pakistan, in the Himalayas—was their water. These people enjoyed a long, healthy and vibrant life, often living 120-140 years. Henry Coandă came to the conclusion that the glacial water they drank was the secret to their good health and longevity. Their water came gushing down the mountainsides, which were often covered by glaciers. It had a completely different surface tension and viscosity to the water that most of the civilised world was drinking: a high pH, alkaline water that is restructured and contains an abundance of free hydrogen electrons, high negative redox potential (ORP), and rich in colloidal minerals. The sum of these parts became greater than each individual component—perfect synergy.

The scientists researching this water knew it would be impossible to recreate identical Hunza water with all these properties. But one fact was certain: through technological progress, the characteristics of this vital water could be recreated so closely that you and your family could reap the benefits each and every day.

A 'Happy Health' Invention from the Good Old Days

In the 18th century, Michael Faraday invented an apparatus enabling him to electrolyse and separate hydrogen from oxygen. Russian scientists further developed the method of electrolysis in 1940-50, and Japanese scientists gave us the technology that can be found today in the new brand of ionisation units that has perfected this invention.

How is alkaline, ionised water produced? An electrical current is transmitted via two electrodes of titanium covered in platinum. When water flows through the electrolysis chamber, the water molecules are split into an alkaline and acid water component where hydrogen (H+) ions and hydroxyl ions (OH-) are formed.

In 1996, the Japanese Health Authorities issued an official statement claiming that alkaline, ionised water is considered beneficial for people's health and should be used for medicinal and therapeutic purposes (Japanese Health and Rehabilitation Ministry). In Japan, alkaline, ionised water is used daily in hospitals and clinics to prevent and treat a whole range of ailments. The evidence gathered over 30 years is that this kind of vital water has a profound effect on the body's physiology and chemistry. It is estimated that 30 million Japanese drink alkaline, ionised water daily.

Considerable progress has been made in developing the ultimate electrolysis apparatus, and today's technology is first class. Personally, I prefer plate technology, with a constant and reliable output and correct pH, ability to tolerate warm water (though not recommended), ease of maintenance and durability. Thousands of satisfied customers can vouch for its quality and great results.

Research on the Health Benefits of Antioxidant, Restructured Water

Research in this field has been conducted in many countries, particularly Japan, by the Department of Bioscience and Biotechnology (Hakozaki, Higashi-Ku et al).

In the past decade, global pollution of the environment including our waters has become a major social and health issue. Air pollution also affects water in the soils, rivers and water reservoirs. Chemicals from the pharmaceutical and food industries generate oxidative stress—measurable in the placentas of pregnant women. This can cause various types of diseases in newborns (Obolenskaya et al 2010). Several exotoxins such as heavy metals, MSG, aspartame, and xenon-oestrogen, pesticides, herbicides and derivatives of several medicines are found in drinking water.

It is useful to remind ourselves that the human body consists of approximately 60-80% water.

Leonardo da Vinci said that water is the driving force in nature, and the Nobel laureate Albert Szent-Györgyi stated, 'Water is the mother and matrix of all life.' A good enough reason for you and I to educate and inform ourselves about the necessity to take swift and decisive action on the water issue. Your health and life is your responsibility. Agree?

A useful way to classify water's function is as follows:

- Water molecules themselves. Flowing water affects all of cellular function and the development of organs (Hirokawa, Tauaka, Okada, 2006). Hydration and Brownian movements of water are fundamentally important for protein function (Iwaki, Iwane, Shimokava, Cooke & Janagida, 2009).
- Atoms and molecules derived from water molecules, such as protons ($H+$), hydrogen atoms (active hydrogen, H), hydrogen anions ($H-$), hydrogen molecules ($H2$), oxygen molecules ($O2$) and reactive oxygen species (ROS).
- Molecules dissolved in water, such as mineral ions, mineral nanoparticles, organic and inorganic compounds and gases.

Functional, restructured water is activated water with many specific functions. Some of most researched activation methods are:

- Electrolysis
- Treatment with negative field, paramagnetic field
- Ormus elements (orbitally rearranged monotonic elements). This is a group of substances showing many miraculous properties, such as healing and super conductivity at room temperature. (Para magnetism is the ability of a substance to collect and resonate to the magnetic field of cosmos.)
- Light irritation.
- Ultrasonication.
- Silica microclusters (Dr Patrick Flanagan)
- Hydrogen Stick (Dr. H. Hayashi)

- Crystal Amplifiers (Dr. Marcel Vogel)
- Cymatics: wave phenomenon and vibration by Hans Jenny.
- Electromagnetism, Prills (Dr. Shealy)
- Anchi Crystals (Dr. Konstantin Korotkov. Gas Discharge Visualisation, (GDA) Laminar crystal, Anchi crystal and QMP (Quinton Marine Plasma)
- Structured water. Vortex. V. Schauberger. Clayton Nolte
- Grander water (Johann Grander, Austria)

Pure Energy Norway, a new water generator which purifies and restructures water without batteries and electricity, one hundred percent sustainable and environmentally friendly.

Over the past 80 years, it has been scientifically demonstrated that functional water such as is produced by electrolysis exhibits useful and health-related properties. Electrochemically reduced water (ERW) is produced near a cathode and electrochemically oxidised water (EOW) is produced near an anode. ERW will be further examined here. EOW is also termed electrolyzed acidic water and is functional water exhibiting a sterilising action, which is mainly due to hypochlorous acid, chlorine gas and ozone (Bari, Sabina, Isobe et al, 2003).

The most health-beneficial and well-known water is ERW, also called hexagonal, clustered, electrolyzed, alkaline, ionised, restructured water. ERW has an alkaline pH, is rich in hydrogen molecules and has a negative oxidation-reduction potential (ORP) and reactive oxygen species scavenging activity (ROS) (Shirohata et al 2007). The first studies of this type of water were initiated in 1931. Its application in agriculture was first tried in 1954. In 1960, it was utilised in medical care as healthy and beneficial water. In 1966, The Industry of Health, Labour and Welfare of Japan declared that this water was effective for:

- Chronic diarrhoea
- Indigestion
- Abnormal gastrointestinal disorder
- Fermentation (Candida, yeast infection)
- Antacid. Hyperacidity. Reflux

A double-blind placebo-controlled study on the effects of ionised, alkaline water was conducted from 1996 to 1999 using subjects with abdominal problems and distension, chronic diarrhoea and constipation.

The placebo control was on purified water only. The patients drank at least 0.5 l of ionised, alkaline water of pH 9.5 per day for two weeks. The results showed that ionised alkaline water significantly improved their abdominal complaints, especially chronic diarrhoea—94.1% compared with those who drank purified water (64.7%). Tashiro, Kitahora et al, 2000. The Japanese Society for Functional water was established in 2001 and several active studies have been performed to date. During my years working in our holistic therapy centre, I have first-hand witnessed many truly wonderful healing miracles: clients, who came to see, learn and decided to take action. There is no question in my mind that ionised water (ERW) offers tremendous benefits for the young and old alike. The following example is a very touching one:

> Karen, who is in her fifties, came to our clinic with her doctor's diagnosis showing she had developed advanced osteoarthritis over the last 15 years. This is a very painful condition with a gradual onset and loss of movement, reduced function and muscular tone due to lack of exercise. Also disabled in many other ways, Karen told us she was suffering from an irregular heart rhythm, was menopausal, had oestrogen dominant symptoms (ref. Dr. John R. Lee), lots of stress, sleep disturbance, swollen hands and finger joints, and had to take up to 100 painkillers a month. She permanently lacked energy and had also been prescribed anti-inflammatory agents and several hydrocortisone injections, with considerable side effects.

> Beaming with happiness, she returned to the clinic one day and continued her amazing story: 'After having drunk ionised, alkaline water for three weeks, all my pain has vanished. Look, look, I can bend and stretch my fingers again! No more medicine! Remember, I took about 100 painkillers a month! I was a wreck! Look, my irregular heartbeat is now normal. I sleep soundly at night. As an extra bonus, I have lost 6 kg and am full of energy. All this in four

weeks with restructured antioxidant water! I talk about this miracle to everyone, and my daughter, who is an athlete, started to drink it before and after training. She tells me her training is much easier and the recovery period much faster. She also got rid of her acne, which bothered her quite a bit, after just a few weeks on alkaline antioxidant water. What a joy! We are all rejoicing in our newfound health,' beamed Karen.

One year later, she is still 100% well, still without medication. One of her kidneys had only 5% function before the treatment began; now it works perfectly.

What is the exact mechanism that occurs at the cellular level when we drink alkaline, electrolyzed water? Clinical data suggests that this water improves oxygen to the cells and that ROS (reactive oxygen species) are scavenged and removed (detox). The water also inhibits DNA damage in vitro (Shirahata et al). *In vitro* means 'conducted inside a laboratory' as opposed to *in vivo*, inside the body.

Platinum-coated titanium electrodes are often used in the electrolysis of water, when hydrogen atoms (active hydrogen) and hydrogen molecules emerge from the cathode and its vicinity, and mineral nanoparticles are also formed.

According to health reports worldwide, diabetes mellitus 2 is almost epidemic in its rampant and wide circulation. Type 2 diabetes is associated with oxidative damage due to stress, bad eating habits, being overweight and lack of exercise. Alkaline antioxidant water has been shown to scavenge and remove ROS and rapidly accelerate the secretion of insulin from the pancreas. The water acts on several physiological levels and also alleviates sugar tolerance damage in type 2 diabetes. These positive changes can be seen and measured after drinking the water for just six days.

Timeless Secrets to a Long, Healthy and Happy Life

Our health should be highly valued and treasured. Why is it that so many are sick, tired and chronically ill? Lifestyle diseases are rampant, and obesity, diabetes, cancer, coronary heart diseases, asthma, allergy and depression are almost of epidemic proportions. The reasons for this can be found in many areas: environment, food, air, medicine, stress, lack of nurture and nutritional support, loneliness, lack of knowledge, vision, wisdom, homelessness, toxic thoughts.

Perhaps the time has come to ask yourself whether your health and well-being are your responsibility and yours alone. When I first asked this question in my lectures about 40 years ago, very few listened. One of my main duties is to teach, inform and guide others in disease prevention and treatment. This education is liberating, enabling people to master life's enjoyable journey by empowering them through the keys to achieving full responsibility. I am always mindful of the wisdom of these words: 'It is your *attitude*, not your *aptitude*, that determines your altitude.'

Richard Bach, the author of the bestselling book *Jonathan Livingston Seagull*, tells the story of a seagull and its love for flying: its mastery of this art, and its adventures in achieving this objective. If it is not up to us to take responsibility, stand up, take action and face the challenge—whose responsibility is it, then?

It is too easy to fall into the role of victim and to blame circumstances. The ultimate liberating key is *finding the healer within you—and doing so with tender, loving care.* Honour God, your maker and creator, because you are intelligently beyond anything created in His image, and all of you will sing in harmony. Your very own cells, all 6 trillion cells, will celebrate and exult! Praise the Lord!

By applying these wise choices, you can make epigenetic modifications that will result in a healthier, happier and more whole you. Yes, you can alter your genetic makeup through these wise choices! Isn't that wonderful news?

Many of my patients came to the Viktorklinikken with the notion that they actually expect to have some kind of ailment due to their age or other factors. But according to God's plan, health, joy and longevity are naturally built-in and become a reality if we follow His instructions, as outlined in the Bible. It is natural to 'die old and fulfilled.'

If we receive the full truth of knowledge through love in health issues, we will live a harmonious life, according to His Instruction (Torah). Research shows that less than 5% experience the bliss of dying peacefully, without any disease—simply old and fulfilled. But unless we acknowledge God's knowledge and plan for our lives, it remains a hidden possibility, shrouded in confusion and conflicting information designed to numb and dumb you, rendering you a helpless victim of unfortunate circumstances.

Driving a car requires a certain amount of knowledge and respect of the regulations in place. Driving through orange (wait!) and red lights, is illegal and punishable, and can have serious consequences for yourself and others you may endanger, hurt or even kill. The same applies to your body and your life. *As you sow, so shall you reap* (Galatians 6:7-8).

The consequences of wrong choices will sooner or later manifest themselves in your life. Our lifestyle has changed dramatically over the last years. An imbalanced state of affairs where toxins and acidity accumulate from food, drink, pollution, physical, mental, social and spiritual stress. The most common foods consumed are meat, fish, milk products, refined sugar and salt, low-fat dairy products and sugars, fructose, hydrolysed vegetable oils, white flour, alcohol, coffee, tea and refined foods devoid of nutrients, vitamins and minerals. All of this leads to cellular degeneration. The acid-alkaline balance is disturbed and the body's homeostasis is seriously challenged on a constant basis by poisons such as aspartame, Splenda, sucralose, HFCS (high-fructose corn syrup), MSG (monosodium glutamate). Heavy metals and carcinogens from food, drink, water and air accumulate at ever-increasing amounts and speed. *Example:* Soda has a pH of 2.4-3.3.

It goes without saying that our alkaline buffering systems in the skeleton and organs are highly taxed as they have to fight to neutralise the acidity caused by these imbalances in our food, drink and air.

Even athletes competing at the highest levels ignore these facts. Their intake of food and drink amazes me. *Example*: In Norway, people seem to love readymade frozen pizza, consuming tons of it every year. Coupled with a huge intake of soda, often diet soda (another trick by the industry, leading us to believe it is a healthier alternative), they gobble this stuff before and after training. Personally, I would not give this pizza to my dog. He would sniff at the pizza and immediately reject it, as if saying, 'I just don't eat junk—throw it in the garbage.'

So next time you see athletes competing at international levels, don't be surprised if they are one of the many who ingest horrible foodstuffs and drinks, and perform despite the obvious health-damaging effect this has on their health and performance. If they were armed with the knowledge about today's technology in water, air and oxygen therapy, they would not fall victim to the greedy food and drugs industries, but rather would reap the following benefits:

- Remain injury-free: More oxygen to the cells and membranes, and use of PEOs, (parent essential oils)
- Shorten recovery times through negative ionisation of the water they drink and the air they breathe, using advanced NASA Space Technology

- Perform at a higher level
- Avoid colds, flu and virus infections, which often lead to a disruption in training
- Lay the foundations for a much longer and lucrative career, and a healthy and happy life thereafter

Accumulated acidity comes mainly from four sources: water, air, food and stress. The last element can be the most overwhelming factor as it involves the autonomic nervous system. The stress may be emotional, physical, mental, social or spiritual. Or it may operate on a subconscious level. Many clients are not aware that they carry a high level of stress as part of their everyday life. A stress test in the form of heart-rate variability (HRV) is a useful tool to objectively determine stress levels. HVR is a scientific, objective and 100% reliable test.

Stress management is an important tool in the therapeutic process to take control over increased adrenaline and cortisol levels. Through ionised, alkaline water and negatively ionised air, proper deep, diaphragmatic breathing and relaxation techniques, tapping, trampoline bouncing, oriental belly-dancing and more, this can easily be achieved. In this way the inner terrain will be balanced and a normal pH results from a balanced acid-alkaline environment.

Many people would probably recognise the following scenario: Hectic pace at work, shopping, house-cleaning, kids to pick up from kindergarten, meal preparation, driving kids to various leisure and sports activities, et cetera; eating precooked meals, fast food with poor nutritional value, and drinking juices with HFCS, diet sodas, too many sweets, cravings, bad conscience, et cetera. All of these induce stress, which in turn creates acidity in our bodies, reducing oxygen supply—which weakens the proper functioning of our body's systems, making a good breeding grounds for viruses, bacteria and parasites. Poisons from these microbes weaken the immune system, resulting in inflammation. The pH-balance is further disturbed and more stress ensues. You are in a bad spiral, making yourself vulnerable to illnesses such as diabetes, coronary heart disease, cancer, osteoporosis and even accelerated aging.

Back to my driving metaphor: this can be likened to a driver crossing the continuous line in the middle or the lines on either side of the road, or driving through orange and red lights. Forbidden! Danger!

As Monty Python said: 'Always Look on the Bright Side of Life.' A Short Story of a High Five!

It all comes down to ionised water and air, specific activities including exercise, pure and real food, and a mental attitude of joy and gratitude, mindfulness and awareness of your own self-healing tools and abilities, divinely inspired and given to you by your heavenly Father.

Carpe diem—seize the day and run it with. A 'Don't worry, be happy' and 'Always look on the bright sight of life' attitude is a useful recipe for a healthy life. Joy and gratitude, above all else, triggers your personal sprinkler system of cascading hormones, creating harmonious DNA epigenetic environment. Drs. Masaru Emoto, Len Horowitz and Goldman have all documented this excellently.

Scientific studies show that happy people fall sick less frequently, even when exposed to bacteria and viruses. A state of blissful happiness and love ensures greater resistance to disease. But healthy states cannot be achieved if there is an undercurrent pattern of bitterness, resentment, anger, fear, guilt, and anxiety. These states need to be resolved before moving on to let the body's own healing resources take over and recharge the immune system. The main focus is on the person and the cause, not the symptoms.

Self-help programs involving tapping, kinesiology, relaxation, meditation and exercise such as trampoline and dance may be helpful in this respect. I like to use this sweet little story to illustrate this point: You have probably heard that the greatest joy is achieved through making others happy. Why? Because in doing so, you become happy yourself. Focusing your attention on helping others can bring unexpected and life-changing results. One morning on the way to work, I was riding my bike downhill. A large group of youths was blocking the road as they slowly moved down the hill. It was impossible to get past them. Going at a good speed, in a split second I shouted, 'High five!' whereupon they quickly turned around, smiled, and laughed. The closest reached his hand up to touch my free hand and they parted in a flash to let me through! Remember, I had two choices in this situation: the bad one (which luckily I didn't go for) would have been to shout out something like, 'Move out the way! Think you own the road!?' Anger and hostility would have ensued, without a doubt. Instead, the outcome was ripples of applause, smiling faces all round and a great boost of feel-good hormones, with murmurs of, 'Cool! A cool old dude on his racing bike.' The whole incident became a talking point amongst these young folk as they made way to school.

Opportunities like this will come on a regular basis if you train yourself to be receptive. Look around in joy and imagine these moments coming to greet you or begging to be found—small bright parcels ready to be unpacked.

Small yet significant moments of illumination will also take place every time you drink pure, alkaline, ionised water *consciously, with a grateful mind.* Remind yourself that this noble water rehydrates, cleanses, and revitalises and boosts your energy.

Welcome to the WWW brigade! Winning with Water—positive energy for your cells' mitochondria and DNA. God divinely blesses every drop of this precious water that is received in this manner.

- Win No. 1: Alkaline Water
- Win No. 2: Detox water with high ORP
- Win No. 3: Highest level of rehydration and antioxidant properties

All of these elements work together harmoniously. Drink it with joy, gratefulness and the right intentions. It will never let you down. Treat it with honour and respect. Feel the great taste! Roll it around in your mouth—the physiological change of improvement has already begun, and you can look forward to a joyful journey boosting your immune system. Cheers to living, vital water!

More Messages from Water

Masaru Emoto's book *Messages from Water* contains some stunning pictures of water crystals in various settings, 20,000 times enlarged. To prepare the crystals, the water was first cryogenically frozen. The pictures illustrate in beautiful, intricate detail the crystalline structure and how this differs in pure, vital, energised water as compared to tap water, which is chemically destroyed and dead, and distilled water. Are you ready to do the right thing regarding *your* water?

As you have probably understood by now, this section of the book contains some advanced scientific information in physiology, physics, endocrinology, psychology and histology (our cells). If you don't grasp everything, please do not despair or worry—simply drink alkaline, high redox water (ORP). It is for you, me, and royalty alike. Experience a new spring, a new lease of life!

Hexagonal structures in water are called 'clustered water'. Water that is frozen cryogenically resembles breathtakingly beautiful snowflakes. Dr. Lee Lorenzen is one of the leading experts in water technology. He discovered that these crystals created hexagonal clustered water molecules and were part of the supportive matrix of a healthy DNA. These water molecules play a key role in receiving and broadcasting electromagnetic signals. Fritz-Albert Popp describes this phenomenon in medicine as photon-phonon radiation for intercellular communication. Eminent scientists such as Herbert Froelich and Nobel Laureate Ilya Prigogine have confirmed the importance of this discovery. The main function of the DNA is to receive and send electro-magnetic signals, rather than solely being involved in protein synthesis. Only 3% of DNA's function involves protein synthesis; the rest is about the bioelectrical system.

Throughout our lifetime, with its onslaught of destructive forces from environmental pollution, to diseases, DNA's ability to perform as a coded signalling system is weakened. This is one of the main causes of aging and disease. The hexagonal structures in this reconstructed, hexagonal, antioxidant water, however, vibrate with specific resonating frequencies, maintaining homeostasis in cellular structure through transduction. This is the process where one type of energy is converted to another type of energy. So you drink this water, this high-frequency information will be transmitted; this wave-like information takes place at DNA level and will act like a wake-up signal, normalising your cellular function.

Wonderful news if you ask me! Ready for the new wave? This is the hexagonal water wave that touches the innermost sanctuary of your cells.

Let's look at some more science. An expert in bioelectronics has theorised that the communication between each cell occurs by means of so-called piezoelectrical impulses, which change between phonon/photon transmissions and are influenced by small, external factors, electromagnetic signals. These signals are either manmade or come from nature and can be harmonious or disharmonious. The integrity of your DNA—and hence your state of health—is dependent on the effects of oxygen and water molecules. The opposite is also true: imagine the disharmony created by polluted, chemical and electrically dead water containing poisons—a sure foundation for a weakened internal structure, disease and premature aging.

We are comprised of matter and carry electromagnetic magnetism as part of every single biological process in our bodies through which energy is liberated, moved and attached intercellularly and intracellularly. Our DNA stores, broadcasts and receives signalling communication throughout the body. This is the most important function of DNA. Sir Francis Crick first formulated back in 1953 the central dogma of molecular biology, about DNA's most important role in the body's genetics. He was also involved in the discovery of DNA's double helix structure.

Memory, learning, stress and healing are all continuous processes that run in modulated cycles. The environment, which activates our DNA and our genes, includes both the inner and outer milieu. The inner milieu consists of an emotional, biochemical, mental, energetic landscape. The outer milieu consists of the social network and several ecological systems expressed through water, air, food, poison and danger. Scientists tell us that close to 90% of all genes are engaged in a co-operation effort from the outer milieu. The other influence is within our control, via the informed choices we make; i.e., epigenetics.

Explanation: The piezoelectrical effect takes place through mechanical stress or electrical charge in materials like crystal, ceramic or biological tissue such as bone, protein or DNA.

Brothers Pierre and Jacques Curie first described this phenomenon. Candace Pert, PhD and well-known researcher in the field of neurophysiology expressed it clearly when she said, 'The molecules our emotions produce are intimately connected to our physiology. Consciously or subconsciously, we are our reactions and emotions. You are a result of your thoughts, feelings and being. The imprint may be of a positive or negative nature, whether the choice is food, water or air.'

Since water is 'the mother and matrix of all life', as expressed by Nobel Prize winner Albert Szent-Györgyi, it is natural to choose water of the highest quality of pureness and alkalinity with high ORP (oxygen reduction potential), antioxidant properties. The same goes for air: make sure that the air we breathe is fresh air loaded with negative ions, the health benefits of which have also been proven to be beneficial. What about food? Choose clean, nutritious food without additives or chemicals and prepare meals together with other family members, with tender love and care, ad modem Jamie Oliver. Family fun, education—learning by doing.

Epigenetics

Recent research in the field of epigenetics shows that we have a wonderful opportunity to make a decisive choice that will affect our health in one direction or another. The choices we make can either enhance the strength of the immune system and the body's innate self-healing systems, or reduce its dynamic capacity.

In the epigenetic toolbox, we can therefore choose thoughts, faith, feelings, energy, attitude, prayer, ionised vital water and air to lay the groundwork for waves of positive epigenetic expression that will modify our cells' DNA. Remember that 97% of your DNA's function is to receive, mediate and transmit signals. With this in mind, it is smart to make decisions that are in harmony with the physiological laws of nature. This will in turn set you free and contribute to better health and well-being.

Likewise, it is evident that you cannot expect optimal performance and health if you eat fast food, MSG, aspartame, 'lite' products and soy rapeseed oil—all junk!

Optimum health is your choice and responsibility and yours alone. Given the right keys and time-tested efficient solutions, you will be able to make responsible, positive choices that will change your health—and life—for the better.

Pure Energy Norway for You! Time to Celebrate

Is it not time to let all of your 600 trillion cells celebrate? If you follow the guidelines outlined in this book, you will make positive epigenetic modifications within your body and genes. Through positive thoughts, intentions, prayer, meditations and loving relationships, you have chosen to support the nurturing processes of your DNA. The resulting signals and frequencies that are transferred to the core of your being will reduce your stress levels and stimulate production of DHEA, serotonin, endorphins, oxytocin and thousands of other balancing and nurturing substances.

Equipped with this new knowledge, it is fairly easy to participate actively in redesigning your life. To quote our dearly beloved artist and songwriter Alfred Prøysen: 'A new, fresh sheet of paper with brightly coloured pencils...'

If you start with the single most important sources of all health and well-being—vital water and pure air—you will have laid the two most important cornerstones of your new body (temple) and life. Neglect this scientifically sound advice and you will deny your body the best self-defence system—i.e., prevention—and the best tool for reversing diseases.

One step at a time. We are all on a journey. I am reminded at this point of some wise words from St. Francis of Assisi, who said, 'Start doing what is necessary, then continue doing what is possible, and suddenly one day you begin to do the impossible.' (St. Francis of Assisi.)

The book *The Chemistry of Success: Six Secrets of Peak Performance* by Dr. Susan Clark MD and James H. Richards, MBA, looks at the advantages of alkaline water, stating that these go beyond increasing the pH value of our cells. Because water molecules have gained a considerable amount of free electrons through the process of electrolysis, these can be donated to active free oxygen radicals and become a super-antioxidant. In this way, the extra free negative electrons in alkaline water can block or neutralise oxidation processes—and therefore cellular destruction.

The ionisation and restructuring of water makes the rehydration process much quicker and more efficient. Because of the increased zeta potential, the altered water molecules pass faster through cell membranes. Zeta potential is the tiny electrical charge that exists in particles contained in a colloidal suspension. This is scientifically proven. The body is optimally balanced (Dr. Susan Clark MD and James H. Richards, MBA—*The Chemistry of Success*).

Ionised water is known by many names: Alkaline water, miracle water, Hunza water, electrolyzed water, et cetera. During the electrolysis process, water is passed through electrodes or titanium plates (the hardest known metal) covered in platinum, which is an excellent conductor. When the water passes through the negative electrodes (cathode) and the positive (anode) water is ionised. the water molecules are split and hydrogen (positive) and hydroxyl ions (negative) are created.

The separation of these two elements is the crucial point: the semi-permeable membrane, which separates the positive from negative ions and creates acidic and alkaline water, is one of the greatest inventions in water-and-health-advancement technology.

The health gain we are blessed with today is that the water is purified and has alkaline, rehydrating and detoxifying properties. This is a great blessing for both us and future generations.

The resulting increased and faster hydration and oxygen to the cells is also an antioxidant factor, which balances the body's pH. With this increase in alkalinity, the body is able to build a stronger immune system, prevent pain, inflammation and disease. In addition, this form of water offers the best detox and the most efficient rehydration. Wow! Here you really *can* have your cake and eat it too! (In Norwegian: *Få i pose og sekk!*)

A Powerful Antioxidant

Tap water is destroyed and dead, chemically treated and contains dangerous compounds, many of them carcinogenic:

- Dis-infection by-products (DBPs)
- Trihalomethanes, which can cause cancer
- Heavy metals including lead, arsenic, mercury, excitotoxins—neurological poison
- Other toxins
- Some parasites escape the chlorination process—

cryptosporidium and Lamblia Intestinalis are resistant to chlorine

Water-vitalising apparatus using purification and electrolysis techniques change water's structure and restore all the physical properties that have been lost. Water has a low atomic weight of 18,65. When it becomes ionised and the structure is altered, water can penetrate cellular membranes easily, faster and more effectively than other antioxidants, due to its greater zeta potential and lower surface tension. Other antioxidants have a higher atomic weight and larger molecules, which hinder absorption.

The normal ORP (oxygen reductions potential) for tap water is +300 to +400 mV. This kind of water cannot contribute anything to reducing the oxidation processes; on the contrary, it slowly drains your energy, devitalises the terrain, increasing cellular degeneration and accelerating the aging process.

When alkaline, antioxidant water with a high negative ORP comes in contact with other elements such as toxins, heavy metals viruses, bacteria and parasites, due to its opposite polarity, it has the ability to neutralise and remove these elements.

You Are Never Too Old to Become Younger—Mae West

Early aging—is it possible to reverse the aging process? Turn back the biological clock? Ray Kurzweil, author of the book *Fantastic Voyage*, claims that switching to drinking ionised water is one of the simplest and most powerful actions you can take to prevent and reverse a whole range of diseases.

Negative ORP reduces the oxidation processes, which is part of the aging process together with shortening of the telomeres. (A telomere is a region of repetitive nucleotide sequences at each end of a chromatid, protecting the ends of chromosomes from deterioration or fusion with neighbouring chromosomes.)

Alkaline ionised water with an ORP of between -50mV to -450mV (dependent on the source of the water and its mineral content) is highly efficient at reducing the oxidation process (aging) in the body. The structure surface fusion and zeta potential of new and improved water are brought close to perfection. The higher the ORP, the greater the ability to reverse the inner biological terrain. We are now talking about rejuvenation at the cellular level. The freeing of electromagnetic currents and increased zeta potential affects DNA in a positive way, restoring genetic structure to its optimum functioning capacity. (Zeta potential is the scientific term for electro kinetic potential in a colloidal solution.)

When ionised water is cooked, the free electrons are lost in the water and the ORP reduced. But it nevertheless remains alkaline, purified, restructured and easily absorbed by the cells. Still, we recommend that you drink vital water fresh in order to achieve an optimal antioxidant effect, counteracting free radical damage and cellular breakdown. Food, drink and air contain several harmful substances, which can cause oxidation, cellular damage and illness, and accelerate the aging process. In addition to drinking alkaline water, it is advisable to eat alkaline food, mostly raw food, preferably organic. Make sure that you rinse vegetable and fruit in vital water with a high alkalinity, pH 10. This will remove any impurities or pesticide residue.

Food that is grown and treated in this way will contain extra nutrients and electrons and is heartily welcomed by your body. You will find that you can each almost half the food intake and have more energy than before. See the book *Secrets of an Alkaline Body: The New Science of Colloidal Biology* by Annie Padden Jubb and David Jubb.

As mentioned earlier, we are bombarded by pollution, both in our external and internal environments, which accelerates the oxidation process, creates free radical connections and positively charged ions, thus accelerating the process of deterioration.

The Alkaline Body

By drinking ionised, alkaline water, breathing pure ionised air and eating more clean raw food, you increase the amount of great nutrients, enzymes, electrons and minerals in your body—building blocks that your body can utilise and transform without any added burden. Raw food is bio photonic food containing living enzyme systems and electrons created by the sunlight. It contributes to increasing bioelectricity and vitality for your body—more energy! The lack of bioelectric building blocks contributes to premature cellular damage and promotes the aging process.

By continuously supplying your body with alkaline, ionised water and vital raw food, you ensure your body is cleansed and recharged both electrically and energetically. This is the cellular life process, which makes the cellular metabolism run more smoothly and efficiently. Cellular communication is improved.

To quote Mae West, 'You're never too old to become younger.' By drinking alkaline, ionised water, breathing fresh ionised air with negative ions and eating more raw food you present your body with the optimum gift and opportunity: the ability to heal and build a better you! Take, for example, the liver: the liver is a very important organ with many functions, one of which is to detoxify your body. This job is performed much more efficiently when the cells of the liver receive extra ions from pure water and air, and photon-electrical particles from the food. Your liver will thank you! All cells live in a dynamic process and have a certain lifespan, depending on the type of tissue; bone cells take longer to replace than epithelium, for instance. Certain cells on the inner lining of the intestines are replaced continuously in a fraction of seconds. But cells' ability to change and regenerate is always best in an alkaline environment. 'Winning on vital water and air,' as we say at the Victory Clinic.

In nature, we find a degree of ionisation in brooks and rivers in the mountains, resulting in hydroxyl ions as the water moves over stones, gravel and mountains. Cascading waterfalls and ocean waves breaking onto the shore create the same kind of physical properties of ionisation. But negative ionisation is very temporary, cancelled out by positive hydrogen ions. In Daniel Reid's book *A Complete Guide to Chi Gung*, he claims that the best way to balance the inner terrain of the body, increase energy levels and transportation of vital oxygen to cells, is to drink ionised, alkaline and mineralised water. This will remove toxins, balance out acidity levels, and improve your health.

Vital water and air that has been purified and refreshed has regained all of the physical properties that had been lost and destroyed. Vital water and air is presently being integrated into many homes and is as natural as nutritious food, exercise and restitution. Two components prevent and reverse diseases, and slow down or reverse the aging process: Pure Energy Norway! Vital water and air!

Just to recall a few facts that we looked at earlier: a person who is properly hydrated with vital, living and restructured water is healthier, less toxic and more energetic; retains less water in the extremities (legs, feet, hands); is more alert mentally; and less prone to disease; and has better overall body, mind and soul function than the person who is not drinking such water and doesn't believe it matters what type of water is consumed.

The word *water* is mentioned 722 times in the Bible—many more times than *faith, hope, prayer* and *worship*, but nevertheless less than *God, Jesus, heaven* and *love*.

Genesis 1-3: 'In the beginning God created the heaven and earth. 2. And the earth was without form, and void, and darkness was upon the face of the deep. And the Spirit of God moved upon the face of the waters. 3. And God said: Let there be light, and there was light.

Vital Water and the Electromagnetic Field

In 1957, Nobel Prize winner Albert Szent-Györgyi (1893-1986), the father of modern biochemistry, postulated that 'the electromagnetic field, along with water, forms the matrix of life'.

Vital water in nature possesses a coherent structure as it moves in spiral formation, and because of the piezoelectric properties found in nature, energy is transferred to water. Circulating water in vortexes picks up information from light and sound. All this and more add up to what we can call *vital living water*.

Crystal-shaped, hexagonal clustered water molecules form the matrix of healthy DNA. These specific types of molecules are capable of receiving and transmitting electromagnetic signals: photo-phonon emission of intercellular communications.

Today, due to aging and the ever-increasing amount of intoxication due to stress and environmental pollution, these supportive water clusters are disturbed and malfunctioning. According to Dr. Lee Lorenzen, one of the world's leading experts in water technology, this is the primary underlying reason for aging and disease.

When vital, clustered water with hexagonal structures is consumed, a high-frequency wave of information is transmitted to proteins. This is a kind of 'wake-up call' for a wave formation to restore normal cell function (homeostasis). Almost imperceptible electromagnetic signals have the power to influence your whole body by supporting and activating the DNA system.

It is interesting that the 'tree of life', DNA's so-called *double helix*, has clustered water molecules supporting this structure— reminiscent of ancient and modern Sumerian art depicting the two intertwined serpents, the symbol of medicine and healing today, emulating the structure of the genetic code.

Despite the many thousands of happy testimonials from users of ionised water, there will always be those who try to debunk any great advances, come what may. The naysayers who frequently engage in negative banter, especially on the Internet, lack the knowledge of the facts about vital water. To close your eyes to the fact that all municipal water contains a cocktail of toxins, trihalomethanes, heavy metals such as lead, arsenic, cadmium, mercury, hundreds of chemical compounds, medicines, fluoride, and aluminium is a sign of ignorance. Fortunately, this can be remedied by an examination of scientific facts backed up by evidence, medicine and years of clinical practice. Yet some naysayers still say that vital water is too good to be true. Others state that it is impossible to verify the changes that take place when the minerals in the water are electrolyzed.

Research Using pH, ORP Meters, Infrared Spectroscopy, GDV Scanning (Electro-photonic Analysis ad modem Dr. Korotkov)

The scientific evidence in this field is measured using pH, ORP meters, infrared spectroscopy, GDV scanning (electro-photonic analysis ad modem Dr. Korotkov) and nuclear magnetic resonance—so there is plenty of scientific proof to back up this form of water treatment.

The scoffers of this new technology are dangerous carriers of incorrect knowledge—and if you don't recognise it for what it's worth, it will delude and poison you. George Bernard Shaw warned us all about this when he stated: 'Beware of false knowledge; it is more dangerous than ignorance.' And may I add: It is when people add and mix facts with fiction, and lies with truths that it creates a toxic cocktail that endangers your journey to health and wellness. When somebody with a scientific background claims that something is a hoax, people naively put their trust in these medical authorities, usually through fear-mongering from these quarters. Debunkers tend to be heavy on opinion and light on facts. It is not difficult to understand ionised water with minerals, but it seems difficult for some to accept that something so simple can have such a profound effect on our health.

There is 'nothing new under the sun', as the saying goes and in my forty years of practice in natural medicine I have witnessed these debunkers plying their trade in order to protect the status quo. This serves nothing other than to confuse the public about complex health issues and is especially disappointing and destroying when it comes to natural health.

When new ideas are introduced and presented honestly with all the available facts and scientific backup, it is usually met with resistance, ignorance and ridicule.

Examples: Classical and modern acupuncture; electro-medicine; magnetic field therapy; Dr. Voll's electro-dermal testing; Dr. John R. Lee (progesterone's role in reversing diseases); Professor Kahn's immunotherapy; alternative solutions to vaccines, oxygen therapies; Dr. Rife's technology and many others.

I believe that the technology of ionised water and the restructure of our water is yet another stepping stone towards better health and wellness that cannot be ignored. It is only a question of time before it is accepted into every home as a most valuable asset for maintaining total balance on a cellular level, this enhancing the efficiency of the immune system and preventing the lifestyle diseases that are so prevalent in society today.

At the time of writing, I have just received new and alarming reports on the scale of the huge environmental pollution from Fukushima. Every day, 300 tons of radioactive material enters the Pacific Ocean. This material is constantly building up in our food chain. Nobody knows for sure how many people will eventually develop cancer and other health problems as a result of the Fukushima nuclear disaster, but some experts are not afraid to say *billions*. It will take more than 40 years to clear up and there is nowhere in the northern hemisphere that you will be able to hide from it.

Iodine-131 can be ingested into the thyroid where it emits beta particles (electrons) that damage tissues. Reports show that 40% of all children living in the Fukushima area are already affected and the numbers are climbing. In youngsters, it can stunt both physical and mental growth. Among adults it can cause a wide range of ailments.

Cesium-137 from Fukushima has been found in fish caught near California. It spreads throughout the body, but tends to accumulate in the muscles.

Strontium-90's half-life is around 29 years, and it can cause cancer, especially in the bones. We are now looking at an environmental disaster of apocalyptical proportions—and with additional natural disasters such as earthquakes, subsidence and corrosion, this trend will increase dramatically.

Chemical pollution accumulates through bioaccumulation and bio-magnification. This is the number one reason you must regularly detoxify your body through the use of clay (bentonite), zeolite, minerals, herbs, chlorella and oxygen therapies.

Most importantly of all: drink ionised water daily. It has a strong detoxifying effect on your body. This is due to the small water molecules, which are restructured and negatively charged ions. Through the use nuclear magnetic resonance, it is possible to measure the altered molecular status and also observe that the water's surface tension is lowered, measured in dynes. A lower surface tension demonstrates the existence of smaller water molecule clusters (O. Teschke and E. F. de Souza) Chem. Phys. Lett. 403. (2005), C. J. Tsai and K. D. Jordan. Chem. Phys. Lett. 213 (1993).

Henry David Thoreau said, 'I believe that water is the only drink for a wise man.' Debunkers of vital water belong to a faux-intelligentsia that does not believe in field-testing before arriving at conclusions. Through testing and personal experience, you gain knowledge that formulas and theories could never have predicted.

Later in the book, I will describe how water has memory, can store and transmit messages. So, stay hydrated and level-headed— you may be in for a surprise or two!

I recall what Eve Taylor, a well-known aromatherapist from London, used to say: 'Don't forget your fluids!' She was of course referring to water, as the practice of aromatherapy massage has a tendency to drain your energy and water resources.

Had she been armed with knowledge on ionised, restructured *vital water*, she, her students and clients would have rehydrated much faster, and recovery-time levels would have been improved.

When a Man Is Tired of London, He Is Tired of Life (Samuel Johnson, 1709-1784)

You have probably discovered my affection for England, as evidenced in the many happy memorable moments sprinkled throughout this book.

One particular memorable story springs to mind. After

having completed many London Marathons in the eighties, I had an appointment with NRK (Norwegian Broadcasting) to be interviewed by Jostein Pedersen at Nitimen, Norway's most popular and longstanding radio programme, always broadcast at 9:00 a.m. from the marathon's finish line. As this programme is highly popular in Norway, I knew a lot of my patients and folks back home would tune in to hear what 'Gunnar the Runner' had to say. Naturally we'd decided to meet outside a pub, and there I enjoyed my first pint of beer of the year.

'Cheers! Well done and well deserved,' Jostein said smilingly.

Completing a marathon is quite an achievement in itself, and replenishing the body's fluid and electrolyte loss is imperative. 'For outside I felt invigorated and refreshed, as sweat ran down my back in rivulets.' William Wordsworth (one of the Lake Poets and Poet Laureate, 1983) came to me as I sat there, now in an exuberant mood. We chatted about general pleasantries on the beautiful spring weather. My Aunty Ellen, a colourful character known for her volatile temper and prone to distortion and exaggeration, heard the interview on Norwegian radio. She picked up that I was sitting in a pub drinking and not running a marathon at all, and spread her news to friends and relatives. To some it caused consternation and concern; others had a good, hearty laugh. It wasn't the first time Aunty Ellen had made a mountain out of a molehill. One pint of delicious beer before I hit the water wagon to replenish all the fluid loss. Vital water shortened the recovery period significantly. It always does. And it allows me to enjoy short and long runs well into my old age.

All of my patients were thrilled and happily shared the feat of yet another London Marathon under my belt.

'When a man is tired of London, he is tired of life,' said Samuel Johnson. I agree and will always come back for a visit or a marathon. A few years ago, strolling through a London park with my two oldest and now grown-up daughters, Camilla and Louisa, a beautiful rose tree caught my attention. Bending down, I was astonished to read, 'Poetry in Motion'. Serendipity? A fortunate opportunity for a prepared mind.

'What a dream it would be to run a marathon with one of you girls,' I said spontaneously—the rose tree having sown a seed on a beautiful sunny Sunday on a stroll through a London park. *Carpe Diem*. The dream started to unfold

In 2003, I shared the great joy of crossing the finishing line of the London Marathon hand in hand with Louisa, our oldest daughter. As she flung her arms around my neck, she exclaimed, 'This is the greatest thing we have done together, Dad—let's do it one more time!'

In the fall of 2003, we completed the Berlin Marathon, and by this time she had accumulated a wealth of knowledge about preparing for a marathon, including the importance of proper diet and hydration. Come pre-race day, she urged me to drink enough water—she even woke me up and ordered me to take another swig from the water bottle! I was a little anxious that we might suffer from water intoxication or delusional hyponatremia! The funny thing was, we were forced by the call of nature to dive behind some bushes just after the starting gun was fired—father and daughter in the Berlin trenches 'shaking hands with the old lady'! As we ran the marathon and passed under Brandenburg Tor, quite exhausted, my darling daughter Lulu, grabbed my hand, exclaiming, 'We can do it, Dad!'

Crossing the finishing line for a second marathon in 2003, this time 30 minutes faster, is one of the greatest shared moments of my life.

Who would have thought that our serendipitous encounter with a rosebush called 'Poetry in Motion' in a London park would be the beginning of a dream that went on to be shared and fulfilled?

Hydration

From my experience as a physiotherapist, trainer and naturopath, most people are dehydrated (90%), many not knowing. Living, restructured water rehydrates your cells faster and more efficient and has an added cleansing effect on your body. This is due to the fact that physical properties of this water are completely changed. By drinking this water, you are supporting and serving your whole body with the highest degree of purity, antioxidant capacity and detoxification factors possible.

A Sweet History of Victory, Against All Odds

As we have seen, stress, both from external and internal factors cause imbalance and disease. The following dramatic story serves to illustrate these points.

One of my patients, a young lady, came for physiotherapy treatment. She knew my background as a naturopath and a Christian, praying for the sick.

"You are a wonderful physiotherapist, Gunnar. But I don't want you to pray for me, - I just don't believe in that stuff. Just fix my muscles and joint pain! " She was very adamant about this issue and I obviously respected her opinion and I left the issue with the Lord.

Several months later I received a distressed lady's telephone call. It was her mother calling on behalf of my former patient. She was pregnant and serious complication had arisen, high blood pressure and pre-eclampsia. The life of mother and child was in danger. Remembering that I prayed for people, she had asked her mother to phone me requesting for my help. "Would you pray?" asked her mother. "But of course!" I answered. I cried out to the Lord Yeshua for healing and deliverance.

According to the doctor's report it took exactly 20 minutes from receiving the telephone to the mother being fully healed from life threatening high blood pressure and preeclampsia. The baby was saved, delivered by caesarean section, 3 months early, the smallest baby to be born at the University Hospital of Stavanger. Everybody was overjoyed by the happy outcome. A few weeks later I received another telephone from her mother of my former patient whom by now believed and asked if I would come to the hospital to pray for her baby who had been diagnosed with a heart failure and undiagnosed black spots on her lungs. Driving towards the hospital with our two young boys, Viktor and Daniel in the backseat, we prayed and rejoiced in God's many miracles. Daniel only mastered a little child's language, and together with his slightly bigger brother I heard them utter: "Please, dear Jesus, heal the baby and stop the blood running the wrong way through the heart!" What an endearing sight in the rear-view mirror, two mighty warriors in the hands of the Lord.

Holding the tiny and frail little baby, we all prayed in faith. The next working day ultrasound showed no heart failure and the black spots on the lungs had disappeared. A wonderful miracle of God!

Several months later I received a surprise visit at our clinic. A young girl, Sofie, her mother and granny. As I had not seen her since the day of healing at the hospital and knowing she was quite shy in front of strangers, we were much surprised as she without hesitation ran towards me and on her own initiative, flinging her arms around my neck and giving me a wonderful, heartfelt hug. We were all overcome by emotions as tears of love and gratitude rolled down our cheeks. Sofie is healthy and excelling at school.

Conclusion

Both external and internal stress reduces the immune system's capacity to fight disease. Any type of stress reduction is welcome: deep breathing, relaxation, dance and music, a positive attitude, exercise, just to mention a few possibilities.

Obviously, living water, restructured and brought back to nature's intended vibrant, hexagonal, restructured form, also has the power to reduce the stresses of everyday life.

CHAPTER FIVE

Acid-Ionised Water—The Other Side of this Miraculous Water

'Another glorious day, the air as delicious to the lungs as nectar to the tongue'.

John Muir

A water ioniser has many extraordinary uses and benefits. When you have ionised water on tap, it will save you a lot of money as it is an effective antimicrobial agent—killing bacteria. Instead of using sprays and detergents on your kitchen's work surfaces, you now have free access to a powerful natural detergent: acid-ionised water.

According to Dr. David Jubb, 'Acid-ionised water is generally best used externally as it acts as an antiseptic to the skin.'

Installing a water ioniser in your home can help to prevent and reverse ill health, as well as save you a lot of money. Families who have invested in a water ioniser find fairly quickly out that the children switch from drinking sodas and unhealthy diet and sports drinks to drinking only pure, vital water from the ioniser. Very often, the investment becomes the first stepping stone in an evolution and improvement of food and lifestyle changes overall in the family.

Acid-ionised water saves the family money on cleaning products for the kitchen, floor, oven, toilet and shower, as well as mouthwash and skincare products. Plus, when you take into account that super-strong alkaline water completely removes pesticides and chemicals from fruits and vegetables, you save money on other organic foods too, when necessary.

The bubbles on the acid side are hydrogen ions and, being an oxidant, should not be consumed—in addition to its high positive charge or ORP (+700 to 800 mV). We must avoid internal oxidation and free-radical damage. A water ioniser can achieve a pH of 4.0-6.5 depending on the mineral content of the source water. As with alkaline water, the temperature of the water and the flow rate through the water ioniser will determine its strength.

The effects of acid ionised water are easier to demonstrate than those of alkaline ionised water, because they tend to be more apparent and immediate.

Plant Growth—A Symbiotic Relationship

We live and breathe in a symbiotic relationship with various trees and plants. We breathe in the oxygen made available from plants, while they utilise the carbon dioxide that we exhale. A plant's growth and well-being is significantly enhanced through the regular use of acid ionised water, and the benefits are unmistakable. When you have seen it first-hand, you know it without any doubt in your mind. A wilted flower will return to its previous condition of rigidity, vibrancy and health within a couple of hours. Plants that look as if they should be on their way to the garbage bin can be resurrected in record time. The low pH properties are quite favourable to plants, which usually thrive in slightly acidic soil.

The adjusted pH in the water is quite helpful in this regard. The smaller restructured water molecules of acid ionised water are transported into the plant much more effectively than those of normal water, which helps increase the turgor of the plant. Watering the plant with acid ionised water, which contains an abundance of hydrogen ions, has a similar effect to fertilising it. This results in healthier plant growth, shinier leaves and richer colouring, as well as an increase in height. Acid ionised water can also be used effectively on lawns and golf courses as a combination of fertiliser and pesticide.

Impedes Bacterial Growth

Acid ionised water kills bacteria on contact. The efficacy depends on the pH (lower) and ORP (higher). For instance, an ORP of 1100mV and a pH of 2.5 are considered anti-microbial and anti-fungal, killing the offenders on contact. By comparison, chlorine, which is also an oxidant, has a one-second bacterial kill at 700mV. Mild ionised water in the range of 700-950mV is very effective at killing bacteria and slowing its growth. As with alkaline ionised water, the strength of acid ionised water depends on the flow rate and the temperature of the water through the water ioniser.

To demonstrate acid ionised water's antibacterial capacity, cut an orange in half and place the two halves side by side. Spray one half with acid ionised water 3-4 times a day, and leave the other untouched. The orange that is not sprayed with acid ionised water will decay much faster than the sprayed one, which will stay healthy and last several days longer. The bacteria on the sprayed orange is killed, thus the radical damage takes place much more slowly.

Skin, Hair and Scalp Conditioner

Acid ionised water has a wonderful conditioning effect on the skin and hair because they are both on the acidic side. Acidic skin is the body's first line of defence against bacteria. Human skin has a typical pH range of 5.4 in order to ward off bacteria and infection, and hair typically has a pH of 5.6, although this can vary slightly.

Applying acid ionised water to the skin works as an astringent to tighten and smooth wrinkles, leaving no chemical residue, as is the case with other astringents—just harmless water. Acid ionised water soothes the skin and helps remove acne and other blemishes. Because acne is caused by bacteria (propionic bacterium acnes), acid ionised water helps destroy the cause of the acne, since the smaller clustered water molecules can penetrate more easily into the skin pores, where they kill the bacteria.

Skin and hair, even animal fur, responds positively to the conditioning effect of acid, ionised water. The more you apply, the better the response, and there is no daily limit to the number of applications that can be made. Combined with drinking alkaline ionised water daily, which brings antioxidant properties to the body internally, skin conditions such as psoriasis, shingles and eczema are dramatically improved. However, the cause of the problem must still be addressed—which in these cases is often a food allergy/intolerance problem that requires a fundamental change to diet and lifestyle. Leaky gut syndrome, where undigested protein particles penetrate the intestinal walls and enter the bloodstream, causing several antibody reactions, can ultimately show up in the skin as psoriasis, and eczema. Toxins and Candida commonly follows in the wake of these disturbances. People with chronic skin conditions go through life using ointments and creams to alleviate the symptoms without ever treating their cause. Antibody symptoms can be tested accurately by eliminating foodstuffs that cause allergic or intolerance reactions (York Nutritional Laboratories, UK, and Immuno Laboratories, Florida). By switching to alkaline-forming foods, removing heavy metals and other toxins, and supplementing with probiotics and hempseed oil, for instance, a permanent and very positive result can be achieved.

Rashes, cuts, scrapes, even serious wounds, as well as athlete's foot and other fungal infections are dramatically improved with the application of acid ionised water. It soothes insect bites, alleviates the pain of stings from nettle, poison ivy, poison oak and jellyfish. It will even take down the swelling of a swollen lip.

It is highly effective as battery cell water, due to its strong conductivity thanks to its high positive mV (ORP).

Acid ionised water also acts as an astringent, which helps to tighten the skin and smooth out wrinkles, without leaving any chemical residue, which can clog the pores. Soaking the skin for 20-30 minutes is an excellent treatment for dry skin. Deep cuts near fingernails that people experience in extremely cold, dry weather will heal in a few days following a soak in acid ionised water for 20-30 minutes.

Scalp problems such as dandruff are improved with the consistent use of acid ionised water. Diabetic skin ulcers, open wounds and decubitus ulcers due to poor circulation and immobility respond favourably to acid ionised water, as do gangrene and amputation-related issues (remember my grandma I told you about earlier?). Soaking these types of ulcer in acid ionised water daily for 30 minutes has a tremendous healing effect on them—and so does ionised air by the way.

Doctors insist that diabetes ulcers must be kept absolutely dry, yet ionised acid water defies that rule completely with extraordinary results. Medical authorities are at a loss to explain the success of using water to treat diabetes ulcers. Also, drinking alkaline ionised water is highly beneficial for diabetics because it helps bring the body into pH balance and provides it with lots of oxygen, which increases circulation. This encourages the transportation of nutrients around the body into the tissues, creating homeostasis, a stable equilibrium which is key for fighting any disease. Changing the environment of the body with negatively charged hydroxyl ions (OH-) helps the body to restore balance, and healing can take place.

Applying Acid Ionised Water

Acid ionised water should be applied directly to the skin for it to work effectively. The stronger the acid ionised water, the better. It can be dabbed, splashed or sprayed on and allowed to dry, as often as possible. Use it directly out of the ioniser unit and apply to the skin, brushing your teeth or gargling to clean and remove bacteria from the mouth and gum area. This facilitates the removal of plaque from the teeth and promotes a good hygienic environment.

The smaller water molecules penetrate easily between the teeth and the gum line where bacterial growth can cause cavities. Many switch from using toothpaste to acid ionised water, which promotes good gum health.

Adding a gallon or more of acid ionised water to the bathwater, which is preferably cleansed using a charcoal filter to remove chlorine, trihalomethanes and other toxins, is a great way to soften and relax the skin and connective tissues. Fantastic after a workout! Swift recovery and renewed energy replenishment.

To Summarise—The Benefits of Acid Ionised Water

- Kills or impedes bacterial, viral and fungal growth
- Assists in healing cuts, blisters, scrapes, burns, wounds, sores
- Helps diabetes ulcers very effectively, especially when combined with drinking alkaline, restructured water

- Provides relief from mosquito bites and bee stings
- Provides relief from poison oak and poison ivy rashes
- Cleans and conditions the hair
- Relieves chapped hands and dry, itchy skin
- Kills microbes on toothbrushes
- Effectively removes plaque from teeth
- Kills bacteria on vegetables, fruits, meat and fish
- As a gargle, relieves sore throats and mouth sores
- Acts as an astringent to tighten skin and smooth wrinkles
- Leaves no chemical residue when used on skin
- Helps reduce acne, eczema and other skin and scalp conditions
- Excellent treatment for fungal infections such as athlete's foot
- Excellent cleaning agent
- Excellent for promoting plant growth
- Excellent to extend plant life for cut flowers
- Excellent to increase plant turgor
- Excellent for car, truck or boat batteries.

Super Acid Ionised Water

Super acid ionised water produces very strong acid, with a pH of 2.5. By adding sodium chloride to make hypochlorous acid, we get very strong acidic ionised water. Sodium is an alkaline mineral and chloride is an acid mineral. By using the sodium to raise the pH of ionised water on the alkaline side and chloride on the acid side, the result is very strong forms of both acid ionised water and alkaline ionised water. Super alkaline ionised water with a pH of 13.0-13.7 is an excellent degreaser. However, it is far too caustic for consumption, even though its pH may become as low as -1000mV.

Super acid ionised water, or HOP (high oxidation potential) water, is used primarily for medicinal purposes, such as advanced diabetic ulcers, gangrene and serious wounds or burns. At a pH of 2.5, it kills bacteria, parasites and viruses.

It is far too strong for plants; it should be used in hospital as a disinfectant to prevent MRSA (Methicillin-resistant staphylococcus aureus), the anti-biotic resistance bacterial infection.

HOP water can also be used in veterinary practices, for livestock, especially newborns, as it promotes cleaner working conditions and helps reduce mortality rates and veterinary costs.

Conclusion

By gradually removing harmful substances from your environment and reducing the overall toxic overload on your body, you have taken important steps in the right direction.

Explore the many aspects of the water ioniser and put this new knowledge into action. Your body will thank you for your choice to align yourself with the physiological laws that govern all life.

CHAPTER SIX

The Air

'What day is it?' 'It's today', squeaked Piglet. 'My favourite day', said Pooh.

"Your whole body system—step by step, brick by brick. You are building 'The New You'."
Gunnar V Espedal

'Love is in the air, everywhere I look around; in the whispers of the tree, in the thunder of the sea, in the rising of the sun…' The year is 1978, and these lines are being sung by John Paul Young, the Australian Scottish-born pop singer. These lyrics serve well as a reminder of how important love is.

But this chapter about air is probably best served by a reminder of what Dr. E. R. Holiday once said: 'Negative ions are the Vitamins of the air.'

As we all know, air pollution is a tremendous problem, not only for those with allergy and lung problems, but for all of us, as it is a constant onslaught on our body's defence system. 40 % of all asthma cases and 30 % of all respiratory diseases are linked to air pollution. Measurements show that the quality of our air indoors is four times worse than that outdoors, sometimes 100 times worse. What can we do about this sad state of affairs? Air ionisation: solid science; thousands of happy and truthful testimonials.

A quick reminder of some strategic points for staying in vital good shape:

- Make sure you have 'the oxygen magnets in place'. Ref.: Dr. Warburg, Dr. Peskin.
- Don't fall prey to the water, food and pharmaceutical industries' deceptive marketing strategies. They will kill you softly.

On average, we breathe approximately ca.: 10,000 litres of air on a daily basis. The quality of the air we inhale is therefore very important for the correct functioning of our bodily systems. Polluted air with an excess of positive ions affects the respiratory system and the blood circulation.

An air ioniser provides clean air with negative ions and will clean indoor pollution. As we spend 80% or more of our time indoors, the quality of the air you are breathing in is of paramount importance. Negative ions will help your body to carry more oxygen to the working cells. After just 10-15 minutes of breathing fresh, purified and ionised air, the red blood corpuscles, which transport oxygen, will have regained their normal and congruent form. Prior to this, they were clumped together with a bulky, irregular appearance. But with ionised air, these red blood cells, if viewed under a microscope, will have regained their normal shape and form will be moving freely in the bloodstream. The overall surface for oxygen transportation is increased tremendously, giving the body a great advantage, which it did not have when breathing 'normal' air with its pollutants.

Fresh, Ionised Air

'Negative ions are the vitamins of the air,' said Dr E. R. Holiday. There are numerous accounts of people who regained good health by moving to the mountains or to the sea. Sanatoriums were traditionally built for the treatment of tuberculosis in the Alps, and doctors worldwide prescribed 'a change of air' for their patients. In Sandnes, close to Viktorklinikken, a sanatorium was built for TB patients. It is now run by the Seventh-Day Adventist Church, who preach, among other subjects, the health message from the Bible on vital air, food and water, sunshine and exercise.

Dr Herman Brelimen, a German medical doctor, was diagnosed with TB. Through the use of vital nutritional food and fresh ionised air, he was declared cured and wrote, 'Tuberculosis is a curable disease.' He later founded the first German sanatorium for the systematic air treatment of TB.

In 1873, Dr. Edward Livingston Trudeau from New York arrived at the Adirondack Mountains very weak and with no hope of a cure—prepared to die peacefully in beautiful surroundings. To everybody's astonishment, however, he regained his health and became completely cured from TB. The recipe: fresh mountain air, some sun and beautiful surroundings.

So what is the secret of this kind of air? Why should the air in the mountains and by the sea be any different than that in cities or indoors? The answer is to be found in the small, electrically charged particles called *negative ions*. Certain areas have an abundance of these ions: near to waterfalls, rivers, and the sea and pine forests. The freshness of the air here resembles the freshness of the air following thunder and lightning.

Several thousand scientific documentations exist showing a clear connection between negative ions and healthy cells, tissues and body. Medical research has concluded that negative ions have a definitive positive health effect.

Environmental pollution, both indoors and outdoors, has increased over the last years—one of the major reasons we see an almost epidemic proportion of increased incidence in coronary heart disease, cancer, diabetes, asthma, COPD, autism, obesity, et cetera.

The beneficial effects of negative ions:

- They improve asthma, allergies, lung diseases and infections
- They promote a longer and better quality life
- They act as antioxidants and reduce the ravaging effects of free radicals
- They alleviate depression, lack of energy, lethargy
- They improve mood and mental stability
- They improve sleep quality

- They prevent migraine and headaches
- They promote faster recovery and healing of burns and sores
- They improve ADHD and autism
- They improve learning, focus and memory
- They increase wellness.

Lack of free negative ions can lead to:

- A disharmonious state and accelerated aging process
- Increased stress levels
- Worsening of symptoms related to asthma, allergies, lung diseases, ear, nose and throat problems
- Mental problems and instability
- Learning and concentration problems
- Fatigue, lack of initiative

Murderous Winds

Professor Albert Krueger, a member of the medical faculty of the University of California, found that positive ions increased the production of the hormone serotonin in the blood. This is a nerve transmitter hormone and affects well-being, mood and mental outlook. Negative ions have been shown to reduce and normalise the production of serotonin. The results are less irritability, and a relaxed and less stressed state.

Dr Felix Sulman at the Hebrew University in Jerusalem has confirmed these findings and has discovered interesting facts regarding the seasoned desert winds (Sharav winds). During these conditions of strong winds, the air is filled with positive ions, which increase serotonin in the blood, often resulting in migraines, heart cramps, breathing problems, allergies, sleep disturbance, hot flushes, stomach cramps, irritability, anxiety and lack of energy. For the duration of these desert winds, traffic accidents increase by 100% and shoe sales increase by 300% due to people's feet swelling so much that they have to buy new shoes.

There is an old saying: 'The weather's changing; I feel it in my bones/joints'—the explanation being that an increase of positive ions will lead to an increase in serotonin production, which affects the weakest point in the body. In this way, a person with asthmatics feels increased pain in the joints and the connective tissues for as long as the positive ions prevail.

In the Arabic countries, the desert wind is known as Hansien or Khamsin, which refers to the 50 days it lasts, from spring to autumn. In the Bible, it is described as the East wind. In the Alps, it is called the Foehn wind. All of these winds bring with them the same physical and psychological disturbances. The good thing is that they only blow during a portion of the year. Far worse is the scenario of increasing pollution of which we are all a part, both indoors and outdoors. In addition to positive ions, we have a tremendous pollution problem due to chemicals, viruses, parasites, bacteria, dust, et cetera.

Many of the so-called stress-related diseases have their roots in the 'sick building syndrome'. Is it possible to create a healthier indoors environment in the place we spend more than 90% of our time? Is it possible to reverse the many disease-causing agents? Create a balance between negative and positive ions?

According to the US Environmental Protection Agency, indoor air contains five times more pollution than outdoors air. Modern homes, institutions, hospitals and kindergartens all face the problem of infection being easily transmitted in these indoor environments. The increase of antibiotic-resistant bacteria in today's modern hospitals is a major issue, and patients die as a result of this pollution problem. We know that air conditioning increases the amount of positive ions. Particles in the air, microbes, viruses and dust have a positive ionic charge. The sources of pollution are numerous and it is natural and smart to look for effective ways to reduce pollution and increase negative ions.

Fresh Indoor Air using an Ionisation Unit

One of the smartest and most effective ways to enhance indoor air quality is to install an ionisation unit that produces negative ions.

Several very interesting facts have come to light in this field. At St. James's University Hospital in the UK, several ionising units were placed in the intensive care unit. Measurements showed a 100% elimination of resistant Acinetobacter microbes from the air. These bacteria can cause serious infection and even death.

Microbiologists at the University of Southampton confirmed these findings. In addition, they found that E-coli bacteria was eliminated using ionisation units. E-coli can cause serious food poisoning.

As we know, infection is a huge problem for hospitals; it is estimated that 110,000 people die every year in the US due to infections picked up in hospitals.

We are all like a big alkaline battery. Don Tolman, known as the 'Whole Food Medicine Cowboy', has said that if we attached ourselves to an ECG, electricity could be measured, as with any battery. Healthy cells with an abundance of negative ions and a steady supply of negative ions from vital, fresh air and water will increase nerve conductivity and cellular communication. Energy will increase and the immune system is strengthened.

Negative ions from an ionisation unit will cleanse the air from pollution and positive ions. Viruses and bacteria with the opposite electrical charge will bond to the negative ions, clump together and fall out of the atmosphere. Negative ions have a positive effect on the cilia in the respiratory tract, too; the respiration is improved and oxygen capacity is increased.

We receive daily reports from happy and grateful clients, customers and patients who have regained their health, often after enduring years of misery.

After just 15 minutes of breathing ionised air, it is evident from examination of the red blood corpuscles, which transport oxygen throughout the body, that these cells have regained their round form. They no longer clump together and they have a much greater surface area for transporting oxygen. Many sportspeople have discovered the health advantages of breathing ionised air, including a decreased risk of infection and breaks in training, increased oxygen-carrying capacity, and speedier recovery times.

Children at kindergartens are vulnerable to airway infections. An air ioniser can solve this problem.

The 'Fresh Air' units from Vollara come with NASA certification and cover an area of 280 m2, with many technological advantages, too.

Geographic Stress

I would like to share with you the story of Fred who worked for an American multinational company in New York before he moved to Geneva where he lived for eight years. Whilst there, he gradually lost his energy, libido and had frequent digestive problems and colds. A doctor specialist suggested removing his gallbladder. But before having the operation, he went on a vacation to New York and noticed that his symptoms disappeared. Upon returning to Geneva, he got worse again. Another specialist said he had an underactive thyroid gland. He was put on medication for this plus tranquilisers for his nervousness and sleeping pills for his insomnia. Most of the time he suffered colds, throat infections and had very low energy levels.

But every time he had to go abroad and leave Geneva, he noticed a clear improvement in his condition. On a return visit to his medical doctor, he was diagnosed as psychosomatic. He attended psychiatric counselling, but got gradually worse as he became more and more depressed. In his diary, after eight years in Geneva, he wrote:

- 'Very sick, very depressed. More dead than alive.'
- 'Lacking in energy.'
- 'Sleeping very badly.'
- 'No sex life.'

In the end, he came to Dr. Wissmer who had many patients with a similar history. Foreigners coming to Dr. Wissmer's clinic also had noticeably high divorce rates, high alcohol consumption, reduced libido, eating and sleeping disorders, and were generally more prone to upper chest, ear, throat and nose affections, depression and weight problems. Dr. Wissmer also noticed that these patients came at the same time of the year, as if they were 'under the weather', as the saying goes.

In Shakespeare's *Othello* there is a line which goes like this: 'It is the moon's biggest mistake. She comes closer to the earth than she should. And makes mankind mad.'

These dry 'Witches Winds', as they are called, often start before a full moon and storms, and have been known since prehistoric times. They are even mentioned in the writings of Hippocrates, the father of medicine, and Talmud: 'You shall not judge when the Sharav winds blow.' This wind exists worldwide:

- In Switzerland, Germany and Tyrol it is called the Foehn wind.
- In the Toulouse region, France: Vent d'Autan
- In Provence and the Riviera: Mistral
- In California, US it is called Santa Ana
- In Italy: Sirocco
- In Argentina: Zonda
- In Canada: Chinook
- In Egypt: Sharkije
- In Spain: Levante
- In India: Thor
- In Australia: Northern Wind
- In the Middle East: Sharav or Khamsin

During these winds, increased numbers of suicides, criminal acts, car accidents, divorce rates and several symptoms of stress and disease occur.

Benjamin Franklin, one of the founding fathers of the United States, discovered many aspects of electricity in the 1750s, and several research studies have subsequently discovered how this affected the plant and animal kingdom. In 1775, Father Giovanni Battista Beccaria at the University of Turin wrote, 'Nature makes use of electricity to stimulate vegetation.'

In 1899, Elster and Geitel discovered the existence of ions. But it wasn't before 1930 that an American researcher called

Hansell discovered how an electrostatic generator could affect mood fluctuation. When the polarity was positive and emitting positive ions into the atmosphere, he became moody, depressed and aggressive. When switching to a negative polarity, his mind and mood altered to become more positive and alert.

In the 1970s, around 5000 scientific research studies were conducted in this field and they showed that negative ions had a positive impact on health and wellness, whilst the positive ions had an opposite, distressing effect.

As we all know, atoms consist of a positively charged nucleus surrounded by negative charged electrons. A balance between positive and negative polarity means a neutral atom. When electrons are released from the nucleus, the atom becomes positive—a positive ion. But if the neutral atom catches an electron, it becomes negative—a negative ion. If the positive or negative ion is part of a molecule, it becomes an ion, positive or negative, and can be part of a larger group of molecules in smoke, water or droplets of water. In the following text, all small particles carrying an electric charge will be called ions.

In nature, the most common ratio of ions is 12 positive to 10 negative ions. But these proportions vary a great deal depending on area, air pressure, wind conditions, radioactivity in surrounding areas, and of course air pollution. Areas with high concentrations of negative ions are the seaside, waterfalls, rivers, mountains, trees, and woods. Before an electric storm when the atmosphere is charged with positive ions, the air feels heavy and the organism becomes stressed. After the storm, the air feels fresher and one feels more invigorated. Taking a deep breath of negatively charged ions will increase the feeling of health and wellness.

During rush hour in cities, the air is almost completely lacking negative ions, even inside the cars. The so-called 'Faradays cage effect' makes the air stuffy, and the lack of negative ions means less oxygen being transported via the red blood corpuscles, which clump together and have considerably less surface area for transporting oxygen. A little negative ionising device for use in the car or when travelling on trains or by plane will remedy the situation wonderfully. With this method, you can breathe fresh, ionised air wherever you go and thus prevent being infected by fellow travelling passengers. Airplane cabin air is unhealthy because of the lack of negative ions, which leads to an unbalanced/unhealthy body and decreased well-being.

By carrying a negative ioniser, a friendly Buddy around your neck, or a slightly larger ioniser device for your car, you will have taken an absolutely positive action towards better health and well-being by eliminating air pollution around you.

Fred, the executive director I mentioned previously, told me a story about a newlywed couple from Montreal who went to the South of France for their honeymoon. Soon after they had arrived, he became very tense and started to argue with his wife. He felt moody, lacking in energy, thirsty, had no interest in sex, and was very short-tempered.

It was the height of the mistral wind season in that region.

Shortly after, the couple decided to move away from the region, with the immediate result that his health and wellness returned. It is a well-known fact that Winston Churchill was very particular about when and where he travelled to the South of France, to avoid the mistral season.

On the west coast of Canada and the US, the Chinook wind from the mountains during the spring causes the same health problems. This is common knowledge as medical doctors report a higher incidence of upper respiratory tract infections and mental disturbances of various degrees.

The Santa Ana winds in California blow from Hollywood and Los Angeles down to San Diego. The knowledge that this wind, with its positively charged ions, tends to cause an increase in criminal activities, suicides and murder, has inspired film editors to produce a TV series in which the wind features prominently as a factor in crimes and distress.

The Foehn, Sharav and Khamsin winds have been studied extensively, in particular through research conducted by Dr. Felix Sulman at the University of Jerusalem. As mentioned above, people's feet swelled due to oedema, with shoe sales increasing 300% during the Sharav wind season. Psychiatrists noticed a change of moods towards more depressive states; insurance brokers reported a 100% increase in accidents; whilst the police noticed in increase in domestic violence during this period. Military personnel reports showed an increase in depression, lethargy and restlessness. In certain translations of the book of Isaiah in the Bible, there are warnings concerning the destructive effect of this wind.

Dr Felix Sulman's research in gynaecology showed that serotonin affects the body and emotional disposition. In a four-year study, he examined serotonin production in healthy persons who were not sensitive to the Sharav winds. He monitored serotonin levels through daily urine tests. The conclusion was that serotonin production increased only in response to high levels of stress, especially emotional stress.

After this study on normal, healthy subjects, Dr. Felix Sulman conducted research to determine how sensitive persons would react. Urine samples were tested twice a day for one year. The study showed that these people produced 1000% more serotonin when the Sharav wind blew! Even though their bodies doubled the capacity to break down serotonin to the harmless substance called 5HA, there was a huge increase of serotonin in their bodies.

But how could this wind cause this physiological increase of serotonin? During the 1950s and 1960s, the American researcher Krueger made an association between positive ions and the body's production of serotonin. Based on Krueger's theory, Dr. Felix Sulman recruited physicists and meteorologists to measure electrical conditions during the Sharav winds. The conclusion was that the only variable factor, the Sharav wind, was responsible for the increase of positive ion concentration.

The 'Witek winds' are all loaded with positive ions, with practically no negative ions. These winds start in the upper atmosphere, and disturb negative ions as they approach the earth. Some of the winds, such as the Sharav winds, travel over landscapes where they whirl up a lot of dust. Negative ions, which are by and large oxygen, attach to dust particles, with the result that very soon, only positive ions are left in the wind. The negative ions now leave an unbalanced, ion-depleted air. The negative ions are attached to dust and moisture, and the air feels heavy. Because the earth is negatively charged, it will attract the positive ions. Thunder and lightning clear the atmosphere, and with the rain that ensues, an overproduction of negative ions makes the air feel refreshed.

This is the same phenomenon that occurs by rivers, waterfalls and the sea. Small drops of water are charged with negative ions in these places. Similar effects are observed during thunder and full moon. Dr Shealy, neurosurgeon, and in charge of the pain clinic in La Crosse, Wisconsin found that cases of serious bleeding (haemorrhaging) were worst during a full moon. He also found that blood transfusions were much higher during a full moon.

Dr Edson Andrew at the Tallahassee Hospital in Florida observed that in 1000 patients he operated on, 82% of serious cases of bleedings during operations happened during a full moon.

Dr F. Sulman also discovered that spontaneous miscarriages were affected by the ionic changes in the air during the full moon cycles. About 30% of the population is sensitive to these weather changes according to Dr. F. Sulman.

By ionising the air at home and when travelling, the negative ionic balance can be controlled. The teaching of correct breathing and relaxation in addition to this will stop the dramatic and unwanted increase in the production of serotonin.

Today there are reliable instruments for measuring the quality of negative and positive ions. Due to electrical apparatus, PCs, TVs, mobiles, Internet and other sources of indoor electrical and environmental, particle, dust or microbial factors, and well-insulated, 'sealed' houses, we have a 'sick building syndrome', an ionic imbalance that disturbs our health and well-being.

The Good Life

Maybe we have an inbuilt knowledge, an inner wisdom, because when we go on holiday, we choose to go places where negative ion concentration is at its highest; for example, near to the sea, mountains, running water, forests. Another very important source of negative ions is during the process of photosynthesis of chlorophyll, the green pigment in the grass and leaves in nature. When this is exposed to sunlight, oxygen is produced, which is negatively charged. This is the chief reason country and forest air feels fresher. This fact underlines the importance of parks in cities.

Running water, cascading waterfalls and waves lapping the seashore make us happy and exuberant. We appreciate green parks and water fountains, and feel refreshed and relaxed after a shower (preferably without toxic chlorine).

All of these places have an abundance of negative ions because of the so-called *Lénard effect*, which builds up through the friction of water drops splitting up in the air.

Around 1700, Saussure observed that people who lived within close proximity to waterfalls lived a healthier life. The wellness properties of warm springs are mostly attributed to the quality of the water and its mineral contents—but another reason could possibly be the movement of the water molecules and friction, causing increased production of negative ions by fountains and pools.

Love is in the ionised air

As we have seen, systematic research into the air's electricity began around the 1930s. After the war, we see a lot of research coming from Russia, as they were particularly interested in finding out how negative ions affected the development and progress of athletes and respiratory diseases. No ions—no life! In Russia, Dr. Tehijewsky tried to raise small animals in oxygen-rich air which did not contain ions. After a few days the animals died. Tehijewsky concluded that we needed oxygen with ions to survive.

Dr Krueger likewise proved that a high concentration of negative ions is necessary for energy and endurance, health and well-being.

Negative Ions for Athletes

After World War II, the Russian researcher A. A. Minkh performed a whole series of trials on high-level athletes. In one experiment the athletes had to lift 3-5 kg weights at the rate of one lift per second until exhaustion. Then the test persons were given:

- Supplements with negative ions
- Supplements with negative and positive ions
- Ordinary air

The group who received negative ions recovered fastest followed by the group who got a mix of both negative and positive ions. Those who breathed ordinary air needed the longest recovery time. The conclusion was clear: athletes recovered fastest when breathing negative ions.

In another experiment, the athletes had to run on the spot at a pace of 180 steps per minute until exhaustion, to test the body's oxygen capacity uptake. One group performed in air with enriched negative ions, and the other group were tested in ordinary air. To begin with, they both exhibited the same results. But after a month, the group who performed in the air with enriched negative ions improved their endurance by 240%! This high level was maintained 10 days after the experiment ended and, without any negative ions, added and stabilised at a 38% improvement.

The endurance (oxygen uptake capacity) for the reference

group increased from 7% to 24%. The reduction of endurance level decreased significantly faster compared to those who received air enriched with negative ions.

The reaction time for visual signals was also measured. This variation, although small, can mean the difference between a gold medal and no medal at all for Olympic athletes. A 10% improvement was measured in the athlete's reaction time when negative ions were added.

Several other researchers achieved similar results measuring visual and audible signals. Also strength, using a dynamometer, showed significant improvement in strength when the test persons performed in air that was enriched with negative ions.

Killing Bacteria, Viruses and Parasites—Improved Plant Cultivation

A priest named Nollet conducted the first studies on electricity on plants in 1748. He and many others showed that plant growth was enhanced using a high concentration of negative and positive ions.

Studies conducted by Elkieg on cereal grown in an atmosphere of 400,000 negative ions per cubic centimetre showed a 15% increase in growth and an 18% increase in dry weight. In greenhouses, a significant increase in growth was noted, and also fungus and insects disappeared. The farmers were able to stop spraying their crops with pesticides and insecticides. Negative ions act as an antibacterial and anti-fungal agent, as well as an insect repellent.

The first discoveries made by Dr. Krueger, a famous American researcher in the field of ions, were that negative ions, even in small quantities, disturb bacteria and other microorganisms. In this way, they prevent infections of the ear, nose, throat and respiratory organs.

Professor Krauss at the Hygen Institute, University of Hannover, Germany, noticed an 87% reduction of bacteria in a room that had had negative ionisation during one hour, and a 97% reduction within 100 minutes.

Dr Kellogg studied the frequency of survival of staphylococcus bacteria, which is prevalent in skin infections. Bacteria with a concentration of one million particles per ml. were placed in a bottle. After five hours in non-ionised air, the concentration had increased to one million fifty-two particles per ml. In the negative-ionised air, all the bacteria had disappeared.

Studies conducted on the spread of virus infection among chickens who were given 0.3 ml of a mixture containing 100 million Newcastle virus per ml revealed that when these chickens were later placed among non-infected chickens, all the injected chickens died. In normal air conditions, 75% of all the chickens died who were placed among those that were infected with the virus. In ionised air, the virus was not transferred to other chickens, which all survived.

One of the conclusions from these studies is that both ions have an effect: the positive ions have a solely electrical effect, while the negative ions have a more chemical-biological effect, which kills the bacteria. This effect may be due to the fact that the majority of the negative ions are oxygen ions and that oxygen disturbs these microorganisms.

A Happy Testimonial

Camille, a colleague of mine, gave an ionisation unit to her sister who had leukaemia and was on regular chemotherapy. After each chemotherapy treatment, she was sick with fever and got infections, which lasted several weeks. A weakened immune system is one of the side effects of chemotherapy.

But with the instalment of an ionisation unit in her room, she no longer got any fever or infections. Her medical doctors were amazed. The nurses who treated her said they had never witnessed anything like it during their work with cancer patients. In 1998, she had a bone marrow transplant. She was the only patient at the hospital who recovered without fever and complications. The wonderful gift given by her sister proved beyond any doubt to be a very precious one for which she was so happy and grateful.

All Creatures Great and Small

The above is the title of a British television serious based on the books of the British veterinary surgeon Alf Wright, who wrote under the pseudonym James Herriot and filmed in my favourite English countryside of North Yorkshire, 'God's own County', as it is fondly called. One of his first books had the title *If Only They Could Talk.* Yes, indeed—if animals could talk, they would have a word or two to say about the quality of air they were made to breathe. If given the choice between negatively charged ionised air and ordinary air,

James Herriot—and, indeed, all animal lovers—would opt for the former, because negative ions in the air make a whole lot of difference to the health and well-being of our beloved animals.

Research has shown that if you have three cages, one with positive ions, one with ordinary air and one with negative ions, the mice will never choose the one with positive ions, but will go for the cage enriched with negative ions.

Had James Herriot, and for that matter all veterinary doctors, known about the power of ionised air, it would naturally have been part of his veterinary surgery and his practice.

For farmers and others, it might be of particular interest to know that research has shown the following: After five weeks in ionised air, the weight of the turkeys increased by 5% even though food consumption decreased by 4%. Seven weeks later, the relative increased weight was 5% but food consumption decreased by a further 8%. After 26 days of treatment with negative ions, the weight of rabbits had increased by 20%. Pigs showed an increase of 23% after 14 days.

Apart from the definitive improvement in health and well-being for both animals and humans due to less microbiological burden, there is the added bonus of better oxygenation, improvement in blood quality, an increased feeling of relaxation and decreased stress levels for the organism. This again leads to a better-functioning immune system, creating a win-win situation on many frontiers.

Research has shown that animals become more stressed and aggressive when they are exposed to positive ions. In another experiment, old and young mice were placed in a labyrinth. In normal air, the young mice managed to get out of the labyrinth much faster than the old ones. When the air was changed and charged with negative ions, the old mice got out of the labyrinth just as quickly as the young ones! In experiments using T-labyrinths, the researchers noticed that old mice made three times more mistakes in normal air compared to the young mice. In negatively ionised air, the difference was equalised. The old mice had been revitalised and solved problems on par with their younger relatives.

On behalf of all animals and animal lovers: 'Give us air enriched with negative ions and we will give you tenfold back.'
'If only they could talk', James? They just did!

All things bright and beautiful,
All creatures great and small,
All things wise and wonderful,
The Lord God made them all.
He gave us eyes to see them,
And lips that we might tell,
How great is God Almighty,
Who has made all things well.

From the poem *Maker of Heaven and Earth (All Things Bright and Beautiful)* by Cecil Frances Alexander)

It Shouldn't Happen to a Vet is the title of another famous book by James Herriot. *A touch of serendipity, dear James*—the rest is up to you, dear friends. You see, I can lead a horse to water, but I cannot make it drink. *Right, James? Right on, Mr Espedal*—though I guess Chuck Norris could force the horse to drink!

Negative Ions and Healing of Burns—A Treatment Revolution

The earliest systematic study on burns injuries was conducted in 1958 by Dr. Igho Kornblueh at the General Northeastern Hospital in Philadelphia. The study involved 187 patients suffering from various degrees of burn injuries. A group of 49 patients received ordinary medical treatment; the remaining 138 patients were treated with negative ions. 79 patients experienced pain relief (57.3%) when treated with negative ions, while 22.5% experienced relief with ordinary treatment. The researcher was astonished by the results. Dr Minehart, who participated in the study, exclaimed, 'First I thought it was voodoo. Now I am convinced that it is really a revolutionary treatment. The results were so encouraging that the hospital has installed ionisation units in all post-operative wards.'

Despite this enormous progress with burns victims, and the positive results in terms of pain management, danger of infection and reduced recovery times, the new discoveries had not been taken up by other hospitals, even by 1971—much to the disappointment of Dr. Igho Kornblueh who initiated the first studies in this area.

The Philadelphia study also demonstrated that burns victims experienced less bronchitis, asthma and other respiratory distress when using negative ionisation. Encouraged by these results, Dr. Kornblueh started a series of investigations at the University Hospital in Pennsylvania. This time, he focused on patients suffering respiratory conditions. 63% of his patients made a complete or partial recovery using negative ions. Because of this, Dr. Kornblueh described negative ions as the *vitamins of the air.*

Breathing Problems, Asthma and Allergies

All over the world, respiratory diseases are increasing at an alarming rate. This is due to increased pollution, internal stress, lack of vital minerals and vitamins from food and, last but not least, chemicals in water and food, lack of oxygen and enzymes, and heavy metals. In the US, approximately 40 million Americans suffer from a respiratory disorder or allergies that affect the respiratory organs such as smoking, pollen and pollutants. Over the last 10 years, there has been an increase of 80% among women, 50% in children and 30% in men. Because indoor air quality is about four times worse than outdoor air, and we spend most of our time indoors where diverse chemicals contribute to the overall picture, these figures should not come as a complete surprise.

We have received numerous happy testimonials from customers who are using the ioniser on a daily basis, particularly with regard to allergies, respiratory problems, obstructive pulmonary disease,

asthma and sinusitis.

How do negative ions have a health positive effect for these people? Respiratory canals are covered by cilia, tiny hair-like projections in the mucous membrane of the nose, which usually move approximately 800 beats per minute. Positive ions reduce this movement to 200 beats per minute, and reduce the production of mucous. The net result is that dust enters the airways and, because of the inefficient cilia movements, typical allergic reactions can occur. An environment with a lot of circulating pollution and positive ions is an added stressful burden for the body, which tries to get rid of the accumulating toxins. But in an environment with a surplus of negative ions, with added oxygen supplied to the blood, the cilia are reactivated, moving faster and more efficiently and thereby reversing symptoms of pulmonary distress.

Pollen has always been in the environment. Why has pollen allergy increased so dramatically over the last years? The dominance of positive ions can explain a great deal, as they are detrimental to the movement of the cilia, to the mucous membrane and its blood supply. These figures should not come as a surprise. Particles of less than 10 microns stay floating in the air—such as detergents, which have particles of between 0.05 and 5 microns in size. Heavy metals in food, air and water are another important health-degrading factor.

A professor who lived in Tunbridge Wells south of London

became allergic to dust following the birth of their first child. She became so dysfunctional that she was unable to tend to the chores at home. Even preparing meals would cause distress and symptoms of strong headache, running nose and breathing difficulties, triggered by allergens in food (flour, et cetera.). Her husband, who worked in electronics, bought an air-ionising unit. She sat close by and the effect was immediate, like a miracle. The negative ions enabled her to work indoors without any problems. She remained well.

Monica developed sinusitis and had a constant running nose. None of the medicine she tried helped. Her boss was about to install an air-cleaning system, but Monica had heard about negative air ionisation devices, which she suggested. Her boss promptly bought and installed this in the office, and after half a working day, Monica's symptoms all cleared up.

Thus the first line of defence had already weakened. But another aspect to consider in this respect is the link between pollen allergy and food intolerance. Due to the pioneering work of Immuno Laboratories in, Florida, and York Nutritional Laboratory in the UK, we now have a high-performing, accurate tool for determining whether food intolerance is the main culprit in preventing optimum health and wellness. Lastly, let's not forget the importance of *vital* ionised water here, purified and free of chemicals. This factor should always be seen as one of the major building blocks for good health and great well-being.

By eliminating the negative factors, which undermine the strength and balance of the immune system, and by gradually rebuilding the body through proper nutrition, minerals, vitamins, enzymes and probiotics, the body will be able to regain balance.

Negative Ions and Your Sex Life

Many people report on a lack of sex drive during the 'Witches Wind season'. Many a happy wife has reported back on the renewed zest in their men's libido when they come home from work, having spent the whole day breathing in enriched negative ions at the office. Based on this happy experience, the decision is made to invest in an ioniser for home use. Many a marriage has been improved—and, indeed, saved—thanks to negative ions!

Animal studies have shown that negative ions increase the production of testosterone and sperm, and regulate the menstrual cycle. In several countries, negative ionisers are the norm in birth clinics, and negative ions are used to improve lactation and encourage breastfeeding.

Rheumatism

Acute rheumatic inflammation has been treated with negative ions since 1940. Tehijevshi reports that 20% of his patients were completely cured after 10 treatments. After 25 treatments, 40% showed a great improvement. 28% had an average improvement. 10% had no improvement. 2 % got worse.

Tehijevshi observed that treatments with negative ions

resulted in pain relief in 80% of cases presenting acute joint inflammation.

Learning Difficulties

The effects of negative ions on teaching and learning ability have also been studied. All research shows conclusively that negative ions increase energy levels, alertness, concentration and reaction. Negative ions work very well for restless children (ADHD) and in stressful circumstances. The effects observed in this area are very pronounced and encouraging.

In summary, scientific studies show that we can assuredly say that negative ions improve:

- Endurance
- Physical strength and stamina
- Mood
- Reaction time
- Vitamin and mineral uptake
- Pain
- Attention—students, drivers, pilots
- Allergies
- Burns
- Healing time

- Sleep
- Sex drive
- Tiredness
- Vitality
- Rehabilitation
- Recovery time after exertion, operation, chemotherapy
- Asthma
- Allergies
- Inflammation
- Stress
- Pulmonary disorders
- Stroke
- Heart attack
- Depression
- Low metabolism
- Reproductive function
- Gastritis
- Cholesterol
- Immune system
- Urine dysfunction
- Skin
- Headache
- Anxiety

Our World—A Generator of Positive Ions

The natural phenomena that produce positive ions are transparent and transitory. A full moon, for example, does not occur every day; the 'Witches' Winds' don't blow constantly; and storms are not always lurking on the horizon.

But in our modern-day society, we have created an atmosphere that is saturated with positive ions and depleted of negative ions. Roughly 6000 particles are present in the country air—as opposed to indoor air, which consists of *millions* of particles per millimetre. Maybe this imbalance is one of the major reasons we see such a dramatic increase in violence, crime, suicide, depression, ADHD, allergies, lung diseases and cancer. Coupled with an unnaturally high level of continuous stress, this leads to a further imbalance. Very often we see that alcohol is used to counteract this stressful state of affairs. Alcohol consumption rises and the use of antidepressants and tranquilisers increases.

Antidepressants are often prescribed to patients who are sensitive to changes in the weather and ionic changes in the atmosphere, with the side effect of reinforcing the symptoms. Instead, one should aim to look for the cause and seek out natural solutions—which always produce better and more consistent results.

Many factors contribute to the detrimental effects of increasing amounts of negative ions inside of our homes, including heavy metal toxicity from food, air and water.

Conclusion

If you reduce the chemicals, detergents, aerosols and sprays, you minimise the toxic burden, which is always a good thing to do. Using vital water and air ionisers with proven and patented technology can easily do this. The body, lungs and cardiovascular system suffer from an added burden of toxicity when exposed to polluted air. Arterial constriction can be measured after a person is exposed to smog for just two hours. Think about the small arteries around the heart; they are also under assault not only through the food we eat, but the water we drink and the air we breathe.

The World Health Organization, in conjunction with the European Society Congress in Stockholm, 2007 stated that one billion inhabitants suffer from chronic lung disease, and that by 2020, this will the world's greatest cause of death. Chemical air-spraying is part of this picture. We can do something about this! Take responsibility!

You can take control over how air pollution affects your health—today.

CHAPTER SEVEN

House Insulation—Sick Building Syndrome

'The righteous will flourish like a palm tree; they will grow like a cedar in Lebanon.' Psalm 92.

Geopathic stress including microorganisms, viruses, bacteria, parasites (mould), air pollution, electrical apparatus, from microwave ovens to PCs, TVs and wireless represent a significant worsening of the quality of our life indoors. Depression and added stress are often the result of a dramatic shift in the electrical environment from negative ions to an excess of positive ions, which reduces and impairs all bodily functions.

In order to be energy-efficient and save money, our modern-day houses are tightly insulated, which again predisposes them to produce more positive ions. Modern buildings, banks, schools, et cetera, are fitted with insulating materials and ventilation systems that contribute towards positive ions and hence allergies, pulmonary disorders, concentration and learning problems.

When the school authorities in two of Toronto's schools decided to install ionisers in the classrooms (1997-98), the students scored overall much better in their examinations, had less days of sick leave (both teachers and students) and reported back with more clarity and energy—all thanks to negative ions.

The same experience occurs when ionisers are installed in

nurseries, which often tend to be breeding grounds for infections of the ear, nose and throat, as well as chest complaints. Very noticeable positive results have been achieved when ionisers with negative ions enhance the indoor environment: less sickness and pain, less distress and tiredness—both for children and their caretakers.

Chemicals and Aerosols

Louis Pasteur taught us that microorganisms are living entities that reproduce and increase in number. Every day we use cleaning detergents; particles from these can float in the air and circulating, and in our quest for a cleaner indoor environment, we use more cleaning detergents, which again makes the whole air quality worse. Today, our indoor air is at least four times more polluted than outdoor air.

This is likely the reason why lung diseases among women have increased by 80% over the last 10 years. The natural solution: Install a negative ioniser and exercise outdoors—regularly. And have fun doing your workout!

Electrical Apparatus

Microwave ovens, PCs, TVs, stereos and wireless appliances all produce positive ions. A TV or a PC screen produces about one million positive ions per minute. The concentration is of course greatest closest to the apparatus, and PC screens emit more positive ions than does a TV.

South Africa's Standard Bank had its data register department in the cellar. Ninety-two people worked in a high-stress environment registering huge amounts of money daily. Depression and stress levels were very high. More out of desperation than conviction, the management had negative ionisation units installed. Shortly afterwards, the management reported an overall greatly improved state of health amongst the data personnel, and the operators' margin of error fell from 2.5% to 0.5%. Another bank in Johannesburg reported the same results—all thanks to negative ions.

In Norway, the electrical environment around PCs was measured. In normal room air, people receive a positive electrical charge of three volts. When seated in front of a PC, 45 cm away from the screen the positive charge is 150 volts—50 times higher. Unfortunately, the positive charged ions attract negative ions to the screen, whilst at the same time positive ions are driven towards the user of the PC with a speed of 1 million per square centimetre per minute.

To improve the working environment—and subsequently productivity—it is smart to install negative ionisation units in offices in which PCs are used. In our office and clinic, we have installed an ionising unit with NASA-certified technology to purify and let the patients experience first-hand the freshness of the air and the benefits of negative ions. Our patients comment on the freshness and energy they get just by being there. Plants thrive and flowers bloom.

Synthetic Materials

When walking on mats and carpets, the friction of the soles of our shoes produces static electricity. Furniture polish also tends to do the same, as do clothes containing untreated synthetic materials and chemicals. Mr Bach, chief of the Danish Ionisation Institute, worked in different hospitals treating patients with respiratory problems. He told me of a woman who had asthma problems while at home, but not when she visited her friends' home. He was puzzled as to why the ionisation did not make a clear difference to her problem, until one day Mr. Bach found the source of the woman's problem. She used furniture polish that contained silicon-producing positive ions. When she changed to ordinary wax, which does not generate electrical charges, and treated the furniture with an anti-static medium, as well as continuing with the negative ionisation, the woman's problem with asthma disappeared.

Everybody has experienced an electrical shock of some form—be it electrostatic through synthetic clothes or electrical wire, or worse (I still remember to this day peeing on an electrical fence, as I was encouraged to do when I was a little boy, unaware of the imminent danger—the ensuing shock causing my hair to stand on end, *à la Einstein*). Mineral ions lead the electrical current. The lesson here: don't pee on an electrical fence, even if your older friends promise you superman status if you do!

To get permanent, great results for asthmatics, it is sometimes necessary to change clothes, bed linen, et cetera, as well as other environmental and food trigger elements. A radical approach will be beneficial. Negative ionisation and *vital water* with antioxidant properties (instead of regular water) is a must in overcoming asthma and other pulmonary problems. Detoxification, herbs, minerals and electro-medicine therapy are all effective, together with retraining your breathing (Buteyko method) and relaxation.

Chemical Pollution and Dentists

Of all of the medical occupations, dentistry is the one that causes the greatest pollution. A research study by H. Robert showed that dentists often work in small, poorly ventilated rooms. They are in an environment with at least 1500 particles per square centimetre, which consists of viruses, bacteria, pollen, dust, mould, and dental materials including heavy metals, medicines and other materials. Static electricity can accumulate because of synthetic clothes and other sources.

A high degree of concentration using ultrasound instruments is stressful, often resulting in tiredness, headaches, irritation, digestive and concentration and memory problems. These problems can be reduced or eliminated through the use of negative ionised air and restructured electrolysed water.

Chemical Pollution and City Life

We all know about pollution from industry, which has become a vast and increasing problem over the last 200 years. Many of these aspects have been described in this book, including the tools, which will reduce and eliminate the problem. There is no need to become a victim.

Rush hour is a particularly intensive period when air pollution reaches a culmination point. Whether you work in Paris, London, Berlin, Rome, Madrid, Tokyo, New York, Los Angeles, Bangkok, Manila, Cape Town, Sidney, Rio de Janeiro, San Paulo, Mexico City or Beijing (the latter two being some the most polluted cities in the world), the problem is the same: Rush hour is a nightmare. The pollution from cars and buses is of a huge magnitude.

According to one of Norway´s largest newspaper the researches tell us that the mortality rate is significantly increased in days where the air pollution is measured containing NO_2 and air-borne dust pollution above the legal limits. (VG 08.12.2014, Folkehelseinstituttet). ESA (European Space Agency) has reported that the limits of NO_2 have been exceeded since 2008. Approximately 7 million are killed every year because of air pollution according to figures from WHO.

An improvement of the air quality will increase life expectancy larger than previously thought, according to new research from 51 American cities, (Published in New England

Journal of Medicine). Particle pollution was measured. These are air-born dust pollution, which can cause asthma and cancer, respiratory and heart problems. By improving the air quality and reducing the amount of pollution in the air, a decrease in the above health was registered and a nations overall health was improved. Outdoor air pollution is bad, but indoor air pollution, which wreaks havoc invisibly with your health, is much worse. Luckily you can take effective steps to improve your indoor environment. According to EPA, our indoor environment is 2 to 5 times more toxins than outdoor environment. In some cases, the air measurements indoors have been found to be up to 100 times more polluted than outdoor. The International Agency for Research on Cancer and WHO have concluded that 80% pf all cancers are due to environmental factors, including exposure to many carcinogenic chemicals found in household cleaning products. As we spend 80% of our lives indoor, it is imperative that the toxic burden is decreased significantly in people's homes.

Researchers have found that childhood diagnoses of allergies, autism, Asperger's and Tourette´s syndrome are linked to indoor pollutants like dust, phthalates, PVC flooring, formaldehyde, detergents and second-hand smoke. Multiple chemical sensitivity (MCS) is increasing, also known as environmental illness or multiple allergy syndrome. This heightened immune reaction can be debilitating.

The symptoms of MCS include:

- Burning eyes
- Breathlessness
- Cough
- Chromic running nose
- Digestive problems
- Dizziness
- Fatigue
- Headache
- Memory problems and poor concentration
- Muscle and joint pain
- Rash
- Sensitivity to light and noise.
- Sinus problems and sore throat

Solutions and recommendations:

Eliminate the source. Ventilate. Install air ionizer. Use natural cleanses, baking soda, citrus and essential oils. Wash all your clothes with Laundry Pure Technology, without using washing powder and only cold water. You save money and the environment. Get indoor household plants for air cleaning, such as:

- Areca palm
- Reed palm
- English Ivy

- Rubber plant
- Weeping fig
- Dwarf date palm
- Boston fern
- Australian sword fern
- Dracaena

Chemical Pollution Inside the Car

When I was a kid, I remember my dad had a rubber lead that hung down from the car and touched the ground. With this contact, the car could get rid of the excess positive ions that build up inside the car, often called the 'Faraday Cage Effect'. The friction of air against the car causes a build-up of positive electrons. This is then added to air conditioning, static electricity and surface polish used inside cars, which all accumulates to produce an inordinate amount of positive ions. As we have seen with the 'Witches' Winds', some people are more sensitive than others, but the build-up of positive ions with its accompanying pollution has a very health-damaging effect for everybody.

Could this be part of the reason some drivers become so aggressive when driving? The latest research, which is now available, shows that sensitivity towards positive ions and a disturbance in the production of serotonin is the most plausible explanation for this health problem. It is also a safety problem, which the traffic authorities have to deal with.

Have you ever thought of new car's smell? The smell is a mixture of solvents, volatile organic compounds (VOCs), phthalates and plastic softeners (plasticisers)—all of which are bad for you!

A French study, conducted by the Research Institute for Transport and Safety together with Prost Transport Co, showed that negative ionisation units improved drivers' alertness and safety during long-distance driving, air quality was improved and pollution eliminated. Talk about a win-win situation! And may I add: Make sure you always carry a bottle of vital, restructured, ionised water with you. *Bon voyage*!

Love is in the Pure Ionised Air! More Happy Testimonials

Tore was diagnosed with asthma and allergies 28 years ago and used strong cortisone medicines on a daily basis. After having installed a Fresh Air Ioniser, he noticed an immediate effect and stopped using the nasal spray straight away.

'I was very dependent on using my spray daily, but now I don't miss it at all. My asthma problems have improved considerably and everybody comments on the freshness of the air in our house. I can warmly recommend this air ioniser,' says Tore.

Jorun writes in a letter to us: 'My husband and I are very grateful that you advised us on the indoor climate problem. After we started using our Fresh Air Ioniser, we felt a new lease of life had been given to us. Both of us had asthma and used a lot of medicine. But thanks to your advice, we now function wonderfully well without medicine and our sleep has improved as well. Our friends comment about the freshness and the lack of dust. We are so happy, and think this unit should be in every home.'

Frida contacted us and told us her story: 'Lately I moved to a basement flat where I have been very tired, no energy, experiencing disturbed sleep and respiratory allergies, according to my doctor's findings. I had the flat tested for fungus, and it did contain a lot of fungus. After I had a Fresh Air Ioniser installed, the air changed immediately, and on retesting for fungus, it had gone completely— amazing! This unit has really given me a new life. My sleep is back to normal and once again my energy levels are up! Thank you!'

The Norwegian Church sent us a short letter thanking us for the great improvement in the air after a Fresh Air Ioniser was installed in the crematorium. 'We are very happy and satisfied with the unit as we no longer have any smell —the air feels fresh and healthy. Thank you!'

From **Ullevål University Hospital, Oslo**, we received this letter: 'Thank you for sending your excellent Fresh Air Ioniser, which works very well indeed. As I explained to you, we have had very bad indoor air due to odour, probably fungus, from the basement, which spread upwards to all the floors. All the floors now have fresh air, thanks to the ozone capacity and the new NASA-certified technology, bringing the ions through the walls. We are very happy with our investment.'

From a secondary school in **Stavanger, Godalen Videregående Skole**: 'Thank you for recommending your ioniser to us.' The smell from blood and meat is totally absent now and this had caused a great deal of concern because many of the pupils felt sick because of the smell. The same experience for the bakery and hairdressing classes: A clean and fresh environment, which we have never had before. Both the pupils and the teachers are very, very satisfied.'

We could have filled a whole book with happy testimonials like these, from homes, hairdressing salons (a lot of chemicals there), printers, paint and other industries, nurseries, schools, bakeries and homes where you spend most of your indoor time using chemicals. These are, just to remind you, neurotoxins which build and accumulate in your body.

Fresh Air, which we use and recommend, has five elements that work in synergy:

Negative ions: Negative ions from the unit attract dust particles which, as they become heavier, tend to fall to the floor. You will quickly notice a reduction of dust in the air, which you can quite easily see when the sun is shining through the window. The dust particles will move away from the breathing zone and some particles will be oxidised with other cleansing functions from the unit. You will notice less dust in general.

'Radio-wave particle reduction': This is a unique function. Energy will charge air particles and bind them together, like the needle ionising device does. The device works for about 20 meters in all directions from the unit, independently of air circulation.

Ultraviolet light: The bulb used is of a high-quality, durable design. It is called a UVX bulb because the frequency emitted is at the high end of the spectrum, just below x-ray. The light produced from this bulb has the same effect as the oxidation, sterilisation and ionising effect of sunlight. This light works in synergy with the other elements in the unit.

RCI, Certified Aerospace Technology: RCI, Radiant Catalytic Ionisation is a technology developed by NASA to cleanse the air in the space shuttles. This system is only used in Fresh Air Ionisers and is a new technology for home use. A 'certified in space logo' means it is issued by NASA's Space Foundation. The RCI technology duplicates the cleansing effect from the sun using the powerful UVX bulb, which transmits light signals to a catalyser cell constructed like a beehive, which is coated with a special alloy consisting of four precious metals. The RCI beehive acts like a 'cleansing plasma', much like the sun, transmitting out into the air, where air and surfaces are purified. Independent analysis shows a reduction of

99.9% of all microorganisms, E-coli and other bacteria and viruses.

Active Oxygen (Ozone): is used when the air needs to be refreshed and purified quickly from microorganisms including moulds. Ozone will be emitted from the unit when pushing the button labelled 'Purifier'. The great advantage is that cigarette smoke, food smells and animal smells will quickly disappear. The unit also has an 'Away mode' enabling you to use it even when you are out of the house or building.

The synergy effect of all these functions and exclusive design means that the unit can purify 280 square metres of indoor space.

For active people interested in health and fitness, as well as professional athletes, the indoor ioniser and air purifier will be a natural aide in:

- Preventing airborne microbes that cause respiratory infection and thus interruption of training and competition
- Improving performance—scientifically proven
- Shortening and improving recovery times
- Ensuring optimum health: A must for athletes in continuous training and competition. Cyclists on the tours (Tour de France, et cetera), skiers, et cetera.

Look Around You and Rejoice!

Stavanger Aftenblad, one of the larger papers in Norway, ran a series of stories accompanied by beautiful charcoal drawings by a local artist Henry Imsland (1900-1981) called: 'Look Around You and Rejoice'. These gems were inspired by the nature of Rogaland, my home county, and brought a lot of happiness to the regular readers.

Wherever you are, these pearls of nature's artistry are everywhere. Once you start training yourself to observe, wonderful and unexpected things may happen. I wish you good luck (enlightenment) in your earnest endeavour to uncover the treasures in your life.

The Viktorklinikken is situated in a tranquil location by a park, near a river that flows from the lake to the fjord. This is the spot where I tend to do my workouts. In the lower part with its magnificent trees lies a set of various apparatus where you can do some calisthenics and strengthening exercises. On many of my runs through the park, a beautiful property by the river caught my attention. I would often stop in that spot to do some stretching, just to admire the tiny island in the middle of the river, with its two miniature bridges from either side of the river towards the island. Gorgeous rhododendrons on one side of the property. Immaculately mowed lawn. After many years running past this house and wondering who lived there, I got a telephone call from a man who introduced himself. He'd heard my health programme on the radio and wanted advice about betting a water and air ioniser.

'I live by the park on the most beautiful property in town,' he said. So then I knew exactly where he lived. A gem of a tiny island in the middle of the river, with two sweet, connected bridges. He told me briefly about the history of the park and the activities that used to take place on the river in days gone by.

Along the river, there used to be15 mills where the local farmers came to grind their grain. As many as 34 bridges cross the river from the lake to the fjord. The river is home to fish—trout mostly—and ducks, which you can see everywhere. Elegant white swans with their bobbing, grey cygnets in tow adorn the area where the river meets the steely-blue fjord.

Serendipity favours the prepared mind. Both this and the following story serve to illustrate this point—and they both happened in the same park.

On a very wet and rainy day, I was out on my regular morning run when all of a sudden I spotted a bunch of small children a few hundred meters in front of me. They were dressed properly for the rainy weather, for an outdoor activity. Obviously from a nursery school, a group of 10 or so kids and three adults. As they headed towards me, I saw them jumping up and down to land in the water puddles with a big splash. Oh, what delight and joy! As I approached them, they all of a sudden stopped jumping, obviously tentative and a little apprehensive of this oncoming jogger. Then, in a split second, I leapt in front of them, jumped up and landed in the water puddle, with a huge splash. The startled expressions of mild shock, utter disbelief, and sheer delight when I, in the blink of an eyelid, did a run, jump and then ended with each foot firmly planted on dry land, was a delightful moment of pure joy as I saw their smiling, laughing faces. The kids and adults were obviously very relieved and surprised at this unexpected and sudden chance encounter.

A delightful moment of serendipity and joy—a memory to treasure for the rest of my life. A priceless picture remains embedded in my heart: if the ducks swimming happily up and downstream in the river next to us could talk, I am sure they'd tune in to this famous tune:

Joy to the world! The Lord is come,
Let the earth receive her King.
Let every heart prepare him room,
And heaven and nature sing,
And heaven and nature sing,
And heaven, and heaven, and nature sing.
Joy to the world the Saviour reigns;
Let men their songs employ.
White fields and floods, rocks, hills and plains
Repeat the sending joy
Repeat the sending joy
Repeat, repeat, the sending joy
No more let sins and sorrows grow
Nor thorns infest the ground.
He comes to make his blessing flow
Far as the curse is found,

Far as the curse is found,

Far as, far as, the curse is found.

He rules the world with truth and grace,

And makes the nations prove

The glories of His righteousness,

And wonders of his love

And wonders of his love

And wonders, wonders, of His love.

Isaac Watts (1674-1748), 1719.

With the ripples of laughter from exuberant children still echoing in my ears, beautifully resonating with the slapping waves of the river water, trees waving jubilantly, songs of joy energised my final home-stretch run like never before! Homo Ludens, the playful human did a few Kangaroo jumps like Skippy from the famous TV series, much to everybody's delight as I overflowed with ebullient excitement.

I love kids, especially when they play and use their imagination—don't you? I think that's why God blessed me with seven wonderful children! Exuberant and playful children are a wonderful sight to behold. 'Imagination and playfulness is more vital for your well-being than knowledge' (Albert Einstein). You are both a thinking human being (Homo sapiens) and a playful one (Homo Ludens), and without imagination and somebody revealing these mysteries, you can easily get lost in the wilderness. See Proverbs: 29:18 King James: 'Without vision (imagination) the people will perish.' The kingdom of Yeshua has revealed itself through children—and seven wonderful arrows he bestowed upon me in my youth! Oh, what a blessing—*and how I luv 'em!*

Leaving the park that day, bursts of endorphins still rushing through my body, I was reminded about the unusual background for *Joy to the World*, written by Isaac Watts with music originally by, it is believed, George Fredric Händel (though Händel did not compose the whole tune). As a child, Isaac was mostly home-schooled. He showed a great aptitude for theology and language at a very young age. At age five, Isaac learnt Latin, and at age nine Greek. At age 11, he learnt French and proceeded to Hebrew at the age of 13. In Isaac's opinion, church music was boring. When he complained to his father, he challenged his son to write something better. The result was a revolution in church music. In 1719, Isaac published *Psalms of David,* imitated and inspired by the language of the New Testament. *Joy to the World*, Isaac Watts paraphrased the second half of Psalm 98. He was born in Southampton in 1674 was recognised as 'The Father of English Hymnody', and is credited with some 650 hymns. Despite his genius, he was unable to go to either Oxford or Cambridge on account of his non-conformity.

Resonating joyful music, laughter and kids' play and banter spread like ripples in the water. Come to think of it, what are music, language and joyful noise made by kids?

In scientific language: Electromagnetism, a fundamental physical force that is responsible for interactions between charged particles which occur because of their charge and for the emission and absorption of bio photons; light energy (Webster's Dictionary). Creating sound waves, music, as with the kids making laughter, noise generates visible crystalline, cellular water structures. Peter Petterson, an expert in 'cymatics', the study of sound on matter, pointed out that Ernst Chladni was the first to observe that various shapes and forms were produced as a result of sound vibration.

In 1787, Chladni published 'Discoveries concerning the Theory of Music' and laid the foundation, which is called acoustics, the science of sound. The Chladni figures were produced as a result of striking a violin bow perpendicularly across the edge of flat plates covered with sand. Different shapes or geometric patterns were formed according to the frequency, or oscillations per second. Nathaniel Bowditch, an American mathematician, expanded this discovery further in 1815: 'Bowditch curves' or 'Lissajous figures' after French mathematician Jules-Antoine Lissajous.

If you apply the knowledge to electro-medicine and how it affects healing at the cellular level, optimising the restructuring of water molecules and resonating perfectly with DNA's main function—to receive and transmit frequency signals 528 Hertz, or the love frequency—you will discover vibrating and radiating healing energy waves, as we experienced on that serendipity encounter with the kids and their teachers. And long after they got back to nursery school, they continued talking and laughing about that crazy old jogger, and his joyful little banter. By now I was sure that even the kangaroos 'down under' had received the quantum banter of ebullient energy vibrations.

This is the phenomenon called quantum entrainment, where two or more interacting, oscillating systems begin vibrating in harmony (synchrony). This scientific principle appeared in chemistry, neurology, biology medicine, astronomy and more. *Example*: In 1656, Dutch scientist Christian Huygens found that if he placed two unsynchronised clocks side by side on a wall, they would slowly synchronise to each other. In fact, the synchronisation was so precise not even mechanical intervention could calibrate them more accurately.

Entrainment

Harmonious sound waves created by the river in the park on that rainy day had the power to set up and produce a striking difference in humans. Bio-sonic vibrations, which are at the core of the Universe, or standing life-wave, a standing gravitational wave (time-space wave). And the core, the very essence of this, is your heart centre in love and overflowing of love, like an endless stream of living water, John 7.38: and Yeshua said: 'He who believes in Me, as the Scripture says, from his innermost being, will flow rivers of living water.' Every time without exception.

Every day, I pay a visit to my favourite park with the calm and beautiful river and six waterfalls—jogging, walking or just sitting still to meditate and ponder with an open and grateful heart. Did I say *calm*? Well, the other day the river muscled its way under a bridge, breaking it up, close to the Victory Clinic, eroding so much so that a whole area had to be sealed off. But thanks to a swift-acting local bridge builder, my entrepreneur friend Kjell, whose office is situated next to our clinic, a new bridge has now been built, much to the relief and delight of strollers, joggers, and runners alike… 'He comes to make His blessing flow, far as the curse is found.' (From *Joy to the World*!).

Conclusion

Reclaim and restore your health by installing units with RCI, radiant catalytic ionisation, a technology developed by NASA to clean the space shuttles, 99.9 % of all microorganisms, E-coli, bacteria and viruses disappear. Superb for athletes, and for preventing ear, nose, throat and respiratory infections when travelling. We have testimonials from numerous clients including banks, hotels, offices, industry and dentists who suffered from bad indoors pollution prior to installing their units.

CHAPTER EIGHT

More Testimonials and Stories

'What's water but the generated soul?' William Butler Yeats

'No food or drug will ever do for you what a fresh supply of air will do for you'. Tony Robbins.

Testimony: Healed Psoriasis

You have probably heard one of the many sayings along the lines, *'The greatest joy you can have, is to make other people happy.'* At the Viktorklinikken, the Clinic by the Park, we have ample opportunities to put these words into practice—always bearing in mind, of course, *Nil nocere* ('First do no harm')— and that the role of a doctor, naturopath or healer role is that of a teacher/counsellor of positive steps towards better health and happiness.

Many great healing stories have come our way at the clinic, and just recently Jurgen, who had been suffering from a bad affliction of psoriasis for 40 years, told me his story. 'Forty years ago I was diagnosed with psoriasis. I tried numerous different medicines and natural remedies, but they only gave temporary relief of my symptoms. Then I was advised to drink ionised alkaline water. At the start, 90% of my body was covered with psoriasis, and my therapist taught me the importance of detoxification and alkalinisation. Now, nine months after, 70% of my body surface is healed. I have no itching or bleeding sores at all, which is wonderful, and the acidic water I used externally really sped up the recovery process. And yet the last words my doctor had said to me were that I was going to have to live with this for the rest of my life and use hydrocortisone and moisturising lotions. I am living proof that the doctor's prediction was wrong. I am medicine-free and almost all of my psoriasis has gone.

My therapist tells me he's confident that the rest will disappear with a little practical naturopathic treatment and oxygen therapy. He tells me to continue the daily vital water therapy, internally and externally, and never to stop. You can bet I will heed his advice!'

Fit as a Fiddle

I must confess that I quite like idioms and metaphors. And 'fit as a fiddle' is a good one when you are asked, 'How are you?' The term *fiddle* typically refers to a musical string instrument, such as a violin. As with most musical instruments, violins require frequent cleaning and maintenance to remain in good working condition, not to mention prime, mint or peak condition.

It is the same with your body. We need to clean, detoxify, de-acidify, oxygenate and practise our workouts. Training. Power.

Speed. Endurance. We were built so that physical training would benefit us—all of our faculties: body, mind and soul.

You Don't Get Owt for Nowt

'Use it or lose it' is another expression of which I am fond—telling us that lack of exercise is a shortcut to slowly destroying your body, wasting away, so to speak. The same thought has been expressed wonderfully by many others, such as Disraeli, the British Prime Minister (1845), who said, 'To do nothing and get something, formed a boy's ideal of a manly career.' (B.T. Barnum, *Struggles and Triumphs*.)

'When people expect something for nothing, they are sure to be cheated. You don't get something for nothing. If you want the lovely things, you can't have them unless you are prepared to pay for them,' said Stravinsky and Auden.

And then one of my favourite Yorkshire expressions, as I mentioned before: 'You don't get owt for nowt.'

Richard Branson on Working Out

You've got to invest some time and effort in keeping active—and remember that 'A journey of a thousand miles begins with a single step.' Even if you just spend a small amount of time exercising daily, you will reap the benefits down the line, and your body will be profoundly grateful.

When Richard Branson, the famous billionaire, founder of the Virgin Empire with more than 300 companies, more than 50,000 employees, and 45,025 billion per year in revenue, was asked, 'How do you become more productive?' his answer was, 'Work out!' He then elaborated on this, explaining to his audience that working out gave him at least four additional hours of productive time every day!

Back to the Violin

Violin strings must be replaced if broken; tiny pegs need to be kept tightened, and the bridge needs to be positioned properly to ensure for optimal sound. Additionally, to prevent dust build-up, the violin needs to be diligently cleaned every so often. All of these factors contribute to the violin's health, keeping it in a playable condition. One might even describe the violin as being 'healthy' or 'fit'.

I believe that this could be at the origin of the expression, 'Fit as a fiddle', in that musical instruments are kept in a 'state of good health'—it would appear that a person's health was directly compared to that of their instruments. A person in a state of good health and fitness was as fit as their fiddle.

I have made a vow to stay fit and healthy for as long as I live, because it gives me great joy to exercise. I am for mental clarity, fitness and well-being that is on a par with or beyond that of my boys—who are in their twenties and, I may add, are in very good shape!

But it didn't used to be like that. As a child, I was very sick with infections and was given a lot of antibiotics. At school, I was generally last in gymnastics, track and field—much to my embarrassment. One day, I looked at myself, made a swift assessment and decided to change. I started to train, and in my mind's eye, I set my goals to excel in sport and decided to train. On my own, aged about 12, I persevered to reach my goals of achievement: I lost weight and got healthy, winning top prizes for the school's best all-round track and field athlete. A complete transformation. From being a chubby, lazy loser in sport, my body responded gratefully—it was *fit as a fiddle,* performing at the highest level in both sports and academics.

Later, I went into compulsory army training as a physiotherapist and while there, conducted a research study on the physical fitness status of my fellow army friends. These guys were in their early twenties and in poor physical shape as far as strength, speed and endurance were concerned. Almost nobody trained! I decided to do something about it and opened a physiotherapy centre with a training facility, and welcomed everybody. Gradually I formed a runners' group and a badminton club, and began competing in races.

From being sick, chubby, lazy, and absolutely un-sporty to being *fit as a fiddle*.

Keeping Fit

Hopefully, this book will inspire you to get out of your chair and move a little. Tuning the fiddle to play a harmonious tune is like tuning your life, through exercise, detox, de-acidity, and energising, so that it works in a harmonious balance, as your creator intended.

Today, as of writing these lines, I am always ready and on the go for the next move. Take, for example, the telephone call I got from Louisa, one of my seven kids, 12 years ago:

'I want to do a marathon with you, Dad!'

'Really? Are you serious?'

'You know me Dad—once I've made up my mind…'

Yes, I know my eldest daughter. Once she has set a goal, there is no looking back. I was exuberant and did a little Indian dance on the spot! 'I'm ready and fit as a fiddle!'

And my long-term goal: To run a marathon or two in London with my grandchildren at eighty-plus. Oh, what fun! And knowing that even a Stradivarius won't sound good unless the strings are at the proper level of tautness, now, in my prime, I am playfully renewing my life daily through my workouts, prayer and meditation, knowing full well that 'Old age ain't no place for sissies' (Bette Davis).

A Double-Decker Bus and a Medical Doctor

Both short-term and long-term goals act as stimulating milestones along the way, motivating and inspiring you. The great thing is that you can do all your workouts practically everywhere: in your own home, outdoors or in a studio; standing in a queue, doing heel raises, walking upstairs or skipping the elevator.

This reminds me of the ground-breaking scientific study done by Dr. Jeremy Morris, who proved that exercise is healthy for the heart and blood circulation. Through his study, J. Morris, a British epidemiologist who died aged 99½ of pneumonia and kidneys failure ('He always insisted on the ½,' said his daughter Julie Zalewska), laid the groundwork for the modern aerobic exercise. He compared the heart attack rate amongst double-decker bus drivers and conductors in London in the late 1940s/early 1950s.

You can go way back to the ancient physicians and philosophers like Hippocrates, the father of medicine, and Siddhartha, the founder of Buddhism, who all said that exercise is good for you, but lacked the data to back it up. Stephen N. Blair, a professor of exercise science and epidemiology at the University of South Carolina, said about Dr. Jerry Morris's work that his impact was huge and that he was the inventor of the whole field of physical activity epidemiology. Other authorities in the field, such as Terence Kavanagh, an internist and professor at the University of Toronto, have confirmed this statement.

Dr Morris surmised that the proof could be found in the stairs of the double-decker buses. The conductors climbed 600 stairs a day, whilst the bus drivers were seated during 90% of each shift. In 1953, he published the data, which showed that the conductors had fewer than half the heart attacks of their sedentary colleagues.

In a follow-up study, he found that the lower incidence of heart attack among people doing physical work was not related to body type. The protection against heart attack was the additional amount of exercise—independent of body size or whether a person was, slim, average or portly.

To corroborate his findings, Dr. Morris conducted another study, this time of postal workers.

Comparing those who delivered the mail on foot or by bicycle with the clerks who sat behind desks, he found that the deliverers also had a lower incidence of heart attack.

Then, in the 1960s, he conducted an eight-year study of the overall physical activity of 18,000 men in sedentary civil service jobs. The data showed that those who engaged in physical activity like aerobic exercise—fast walking, cycling, swimming or other sports—reduced their risk of heart attack by half. In 1972 in Atlanta, Dr. Morris, together with Dr. Ralph S. Paffenbarger, Jr. were awarded the first International Olympic Committee Medal in sports science.

Jeremy Noah Morris was born in Liverpool on 6 May 1910, into a family of Jewish immigrants who had fled eastern Poland. His father, Nathan, was a Hebrew scholar. After arriving in England, the family took the last name of the captain of the ship that had brought them to Liverpool. Jeremy was born within weeks of their arrival. The family then moved to Glasgow.

Jeremy began to exercise early in his childhood. His father

would take him on four-mile walks, and then reward him with ice cream. I think many parents recognise themselves in such a situation—rewarding, tricking, bribing and encouraging—we have all done it, I guess.

After attending the University of Glasgow and completing his medical degree at University College London Hospital in 1934, he served in India and Burma in World War II, rising to the rank of lieutenant colonel. In 1984, he was appointed director of the social medicine division of the government-financed Medical Research Council where he began his research studies of exercise and heart attack.

The studies Dr. Morris started more than 60 years ago not only showed that those who exercised had a reduced risk of heart attack, but promoted the concept that those who had a heart attack should exercise as well.

In 1973, seven heart attack and bypass patients who had been rehabilitated by Dr. Kavanagh, the exercise professor at the University of Toronto, ran the Boston Marathon. Twelve years later, 20 other patients, one of whom had had a heart transplant, ran the marathon. 'Back in the sixties and seventies, once you had a heart attack you were side-lined; people thought your life expectancy was limited,' Kavanagh said.

The work of Drs. Morris and Paffenbarger changed everything, however, when they went on to conduct follow-up studies of longshoremen in Los Angeles. 'Without their work and data, we wouldn't have had the groundwork to show that the heart patients who exercise are less likely to have another heart attack, and those patients are no longer considered invalids,' said to Dr. Kavanagh.

Great Inspiration

Almost every day, well into his nineties, Dr. Morris swam, pedalled on his exercise bike or walked for at least half an hour. That carrot-and-stick ice cream reward his father Nathan had promised him when he went for those four-mile walks must have worked very well indeed!

A physical impairment need not stop anybody from exercise—as demonstrated by many people, through their role-model achievements. Kjetil Moe, from Norway, was born with cystic fibrosis, which thickens the mucous in the lungs. He had physiotherapy throughout most of his 32 years, to help him breathe. In 1983, against his doctor's advice, he ran his first marathon. He went on to run the New York Marathon a staggering 14 times! In 1995, he completed the New York Marathon with Johan Olav Koss, who had won four Olympic gold medals at the 1994 Olympics at Lillehammer, Norway, running alongside him carrying his oxygen bottle.

'I'll never forget how he joked with me during that race and encouraged me to keep going,' said Johan Olav Koss, who was *Sports Illustrated*'s 1994 Sportsman of the Year. Kjetil Moe kept running after his lung transplant in 1997, and did much to help change the way cystic fibrosis patients are treated: doctors had long told them to avoid strenuous exercise but began to change their approach after seeing how Kjetil's running enriched his life. At the 1994 Lillehammer Olympics just before Johan Olav's 1500-metre race, Kjetil told his friend, 'Johan, you can do it. We believe in you. Do it for the less fortunate in the world. I wanted to show him anything was possible, just as he had shown me'.

The two last times he finished New York Marathon, he had had two lung transplants—a world first. The dramatic life of this hero and role model from Lillesand became internationally known through books, TV documentaries, Chinese TV series and an opera musical, *Some Sunny Night*. 'I wonder how medicine can explain a heart such as Kjetil's,' said his friend Johan Olav Koss.

Conclusion

One of the oldest proverbs in the English language springs to my mind: 'You can lead a horse to water, but you can't make it drink' (recorded as early as 1175 in *Old English Homilies*). It encapsulates many mindsets better than most other sayings.

All lifestyle changes start with a joyful and enthusiastic thought of 'Yes, I can and I will'. Taking on a new mindset, believing in the power of a change, is 'very much a matter of the heart' (Kjetil Moe, a real hero and a great source of inspiration).

CHAPTER NINE

Training Trends

'I don't measure a man's success by how high he climbs, but how high he bounces when he hits bottom'. George S. Patton.

- Train but don't strain, (G.V.E)
- You don't get owt for nowt (Yorkshire saying)
- God helps those who help themselves (Benjamin Franklin)

It is funny to think that I used to be a coach potato. But that was many, many years ago. Out of shape, short of breath, and with an increasing dislike for my bulging 'love handles', I decided to change. I started walking, 'wogging' (a run-walk), and jogging—a little at time: I could not jog more than the distance between two lampposts at first. Realising that you 'don't get owt for nowt', and discovering the joy of being able to move freely out in nature opened up a treasure chest of health benefits for me. Plus, it didn't cost me a cent—just a little effort, putting one foot in front of the other.

Some people seem to hate exercise. But a timely reminder from Edward Henry Stanley (1826-1893) could put this important issue into a sharp perspective: 'Those who think they have not time for bodily exercise will sooner or later have to find time for illness.'

Colin, a local barman, simply hated exercise. 'I would not

touch that with a ten-foot bargepole. That's the reaction I got from Colin when I struck up the following conversation:

'Hi Colin, what's up? I see you're limping.'

'Yeah, Gunnar. I've strained and twisted my ankle. It's *** painful and swollen.'

'I can fix that. Come to my clinic tomorrow. And why do you need that asthma spray you're using?'

I knew that Colin had asthma, was significantly overweight—and now also had a painful ankle injury. 'Tell you what, Colin: let's make a deal! In six months' time you and I will run a half-marathon. I will fix your ankle, your breathing problems, get you fit, reduce your weight and train with you. But I will only do this for free if you commit yourself to my programme and at the end of it. We will enjoy a half-marathon together!' Now, Colin looked exhausted just at the thought of this. A little perplexed, he asked, 'Do you think I can do it?'

'Yes! Just put your mind and heart into it! Remember, Colin: It's your attitude, not your aptitude, that determines your altitude!'

Many years later, I met Colin again, and he proudly beamed a broad smile as he remembered his 'unthinkable achievement', finishing a half-marathon. In the process of his preparation, his ankle injury got fixed, he lost weight and his asthma was almost cured.

Training trends

High-intensity interval training: According to the American

College of Sports Medicine, a study done by 3,800 professional trainers worldwide working in sports organisations showed for the first time that high-intensity interval training of maximum 30 minutes' duration is the most efficient form of exercise—and today is number one on the top ten 'trendy training list', probably with a view to attracting those who want to get maximum output with minimum effort. For this type of training, it is important to use the guidance of competent training personnel.

Weight training using one's own bodyweight: This is also on the list of 'trendy training methods', although physiotherapists and trainers have practised this for many years. Today's commercialisation of this old concept is welcomed as this form of training is cheap, easy to perform and can be done alone, practically anywhere you wish.

Strength training, weight reduction, personal training coaches, lifestyle changes, functional training, group training, yoga, dancing, et cetera—the list is long and indeed trendy, though many are old concepts dressed up in new, smart outfits, *à la* emperor's new clothes! And yet, one thing is missing from the above list—and that is:

Rebound Exercise/Workout on Your Mini-Trampoline

Rebounding on a mini-trampoline activates all of your body's cells in a way that no other training form does. Figures from NASA show that rebounding exercise is 68% more effective than jogging or running! Why does NASA care about trampolines? NASA laboratory researchers were looking for efficient ways to restore muscle bone balance and strength for the astronauts after the prolonged periods of weightlessness during their space travel.

When you hit the bottom of the trampoline's canvas, all of your body cells compress, and the piezoelectrical forces spread throughout your body—which is what happens during the rebuilding process of the muscular-skeletal system and the inner organs. At the top of the jump curve, for a fraction of a second you get expansion, which augments cellular and lymphatic flow. This contrast facilitates healing on many levels. Rebounding is suitable for everybody, from old grandmas to trained athletes.

A group of champion cyclists from my hometown didn't see much use in the rebounding exerciser, believing it was more suited to housewives. Indeed, their expressions of disbelief when I instructed the whole group to follow my programme specifically designed for top athletes were a sheer delight to behold! A pulse-meter enabled us to monitor everyone's pulse rates, and driving this up to their maximum rate was no problem at all. They soon changed their minds about the trampoline and conceded that it had multiple uses as a tool to train:

- Endurance
- Strength
- Interval

- Flexibility
- Co-ordination and much more!

First and foremost, it is fun, effective, cheap, and you can do it indoors or out. It stimulates all of your body—you can even strengthen the pelvic floor muscles, the bladder and the sphincter control function.

Several years ago, I composed a whole training programme for the trampoline, using music and improvising several moves as I listened to the music. As I love to train outdoors, I had my mini-trampoline on the veranda. My regular workouts in the morning attracted the attention of neighbours walking past on their way to work. Many years later, I had a patient from my neighbourhood who came to the clinic. She told me about 'this crazy man who jumped on his trampoline every morning in his pants or shorts' whom she saw as she passed by his house on her way to work. 'Crazy?' I burst out laughing: 'That's me! I used to live on that street!' The poor lady blushed, but I assured her I didn't mind her reaction, thanked her and gave her an improvised trampoline instruction on the spot, explaining how it would benefit her health and well-being. She was convinced. Relaxed and laughing, she decided to take up rebounding exercise herself!

As part of my research into the physiological effect of rebound training, I started a group training on mini-trampoline three times a week for six weeks. The aim was to see whether rebound exercise could influence the eyesight. Everybody came to the first session with a recent report from their ophthalmologists (eye specialists). My group ranged in age from 6 to 65, and had a variety of different eyesight problems, including farsightedness and near-sightedness, for which they all wore glasses or contact lenses.

After four weeks, everybody had greatly improved eyesight. Some were able to stop using their glasses; others needed adjustments because of the improvement in their eyesight. The exercise involved rebound exercise combined with specific acupressure holding points whilst bouncing on the trampoline.

Later, I repeated this method with the same amazing results. Rebound exercise is a little more than just jumping up and down. So how do you do it? There are four basic categories:

- The health bounce
- The aerobic bounce
- The strength bounce
- The sitting bounce

There are also specific programs to improve lymphatic drainage and improve eyesight, as well as for the elderly. The above are more or less self-explanatory. You can incorporate them all into a fun-filled rebound workout. However, as a word of caution, please do not overexert yourself when first using a trampoline. It can be tempting, because it seems like an easy exercise, but moderation is the key, especially in the beginning. Rebounding has a profound effect on your body, so take it slow. After all, when was the last time you exercised your liver, kidneys and spleen? Don't shock your system.

If you feel pain anywhere, stop bouncing and try again later, or bounce lightly by just flexing and extending your knees whilst maintaining an erect posture. If you feel any tingling sensation in your arms, legs, buttocks—or anywhere really—this should not concern you. It is actually a good sign that circulation is returning to these areas.

The first couple of times you start exercising on your rebounder, you might find a call to the toilet interrupts your routine. This is normal and is caused by the bouncing, which helps to get things moving along in the digestive track. Once your body gets accustomed to the exercise, your bowels will behave themselves.

The Health Bounce

As the name implies, this is a bounce for your health and well-being. Stand on the mat, barefoot or with shoes, your feet shoulder width apart. Lightly bounce up and down, making sure that your feet do not even come close to leaving the mat. This is a small, relaxing bounce. If you are unsure of your balance, place a couple of dining chairs either side of the trampoline, to give you support if needed.

Do this for a few minutes a few times a day. This will flush your lymphatic system and energise your immune system. This bounce should also be used as a warm-up and cool-down for your other rebounder exercise.

Do not wear socks as they are too slippery while bouncing!

Socks could turn your health bounce into a hurt bounce…

The Aerobic Bounce

The aerobic bounce is way better than a regular aerobics routine or step class. Why? The rebounder mat absorbs 87% of the shock of the bounce! It is **very** low impact. Rebounder exercise actually stimulates healing processes for the knees, ankles, hips and back, and the inner organs and eyesight as well. Other activities such as jogging or running can exert wear and tear on these areas, especially with the wrong types of shoes.

The aerobic bounce is whatever you want it to be. Follow the music. Make a few dance moves. Improvise. Have fun! Want to jump like a bunny rabbit? Do it!

Why not exercise in front of your favourite show on TV? Use the commercial breaks to do some serious bouncing and stimulate those dormant cells. Let every nook and cranny of your body feel that you care. Feel the tingling; feel the energy and clarity of mind rush through your body.

As you get used to your newfound, efficient exercise rebounder, you can increase the speed and height of your jumps, incorporate twists and turns, do some sideways jumps, et cetera. The bottom line here is that the possibilities are endless. Make sure you build up slowly and progress as you improve balance, posture and co-ordination, therefore gaining more confidence.

The Strength Bounce

This is an easy rebounder exercise in theory, but in practice it's quite hard. The purpose of the strength bounce is—yes, you've guessed it! —to build strength. Make sure that you have good balance. Increase the effort and height of each jump to as high as you can comfortably go. Your body tissues, bones, ligaments, muscles, cartilage and the connective tissue or fascia become stronger as you bounce higher, because you are subjecting them to increased gravitational pull. Remember, the more you resist gravity, the stronger you will become. This bounce is both challenging and rewarding. Practise deep breathing as you bounce, and also when you lie down to relax.

The Sitting Bounce

This bounce serves two purposes. The first is mainly for those who are in a weakened condition and cannot stand on the trampoline. The person remains seated whilst another person bounces gently up and down behind them. Or, if the person is up to it, he can bounce lightly himself. This small bounce will flush the lymphatic system and boost immune system health. Next, progress to standing with the support. The second purpose of the sitting bounce is to strengthen the inner core muscles, your stabilising muscles in your abdomen, back and legs. Sit on the mat, lean a little backwards and take your feet off the ground. Hold your arms straight out and bounce. Deep breathing. As you get stronger, hold your legs straight out and up so that your torso and legs form a V-shape. Only your butt will touch the mat. It's not a good idea for beginners to do this bounce—it's better to start slow, then progress as you gain confidence. More advanced performers often use this last exercise near the end of their rebounder workout. Finish this off with a minute or two of health bouncing and congratulate yourself on mastering these rebounder exercises.

Bouncing for Athletes

As we have seen, elite athletes can use the rebounder to train sprint, interval, strength, endurance and high-intensity cardio workout as well as speeding up the recovery process. The rebounder is an excellent tool for flushing out metabolites such as lactic acid and its derivatives. If you combine the rebounder with lymphatic drainage exercises whilst gently bouncing and performing deep, diaphragmatic breathing, you will speed up the progress dramatically.

Every serious athlete competing in a progressive event such as skiing, cycling, running, decathlon, et cetera, should use it. Combine it with vital alkaline, restructured water and purified, ionised air, and you are on to a: Pure Energy Norway Winner! (Vital Water and Air).

Conclusion

A chance meeting in a bar. An Englishman in Norway in a health crisis—which turned into an opportunity for renewed health. Six months later, Colin and I completed the Stavanger Half-Marathon together. The holistic health programme had worked once again. The joy and pride was written all over his face. Wishing him well, I encouraged him to keep up the good work he had just started. My last words before parting: 'Sláinte Mhath' (Gaelic, pronounced Slaanche Vaa, meaning 'good health'). It seemed to be a fitting farewell to Colin, originally from Scotland, after a serendipitous meeting in an ordinary bar in the southwest of Norway. Time to celebrate.

As I pondered on this story, I was looking out at the North Sea—the same sea that my ancestors, the Vikings, had crossed on their raids to 'burn, pillage and plunder'. The same sea on which the heroic and lifesaving 'Shetland Bus', a nickname for special operations and part of the Royal Norwegian Navy (from 1943), had operated as a link between the Shetlands, Scotland, and German-occupied Norway. The same sea I crossed many times 'to be drawn from ignorance'—i.e., to get a good education in lovely Yorkshire.

According to the World Health Organization, a sedentary lifestyle is one of the ten leading causes of death and disability in the world. Combined with effective lifestyle changes in food intake, living, vital, restructured water and ionised air, the health benefits are enormous.

Just a quick review of the many health benefits of exercise:

- Reduces premature death
- Helps control body weight, blood sugar levels, blood pressure, blood cholesterol
- Builds healthy and strong bones, thus preventing osteoporosis
- Reduces stress, anxiety, depression, colon cancer
- Improves circulation. Helps heart, lungs and other internal organs to work more efficiently
- Improves sleep quality, thus giving you more energy

CHAPTER TEN

Remarkable Discoveries

'A sense of humour is a divine quality of man'. Arthur Schopenhauer.

Most people respect the laws of society, including traffic rules. They are made to protect us. The outcome of breaking traffic rules—for example, driving through a red light—can be immediate and catastrophic. When driving your car, you check on the petrol, oil and water status, right? And what about maintenance service? You do that, too?

What about the maintenance service on your body? Time for a holistic check-up?

As the saying goes, 'Idle hands are the devil's tools' (from the Bible Ref. Proverb 18:9). It is your responsibility to respond to your body's calling for a change, that will give you joy, blessing and good health, a call to follow the physiological rules of health. Much the same as you'd respect the traffic rules. Break these and face the consequences. As you sow, so you shall reap. It is that simple. The rewards are almost seen and felt immediately. Especially if you combine and follow the joyful discoveries outlined in this book. Pure Energy Norway! *A votre santé! Sláinte Mhath!*

More and more people realise that refined sugar in its many

forms and artificial sweeteners like aspartame, Splenda and sucralose are dangerous chemicals; toxins causing havoc with your heart, circulation and brain function.

Diet sodas are losing popularity as more people switch to water. During the last five years, we have seen a decline in the consumption of diet sodas, with 7% drop in sales as at the end of 2013. People are finally waking up. To prevent further decline in sales, the $61-billion-dollar industry is considering replacing artificial sweeteners like aspartame with Stevia, as consumers are becoming more health-conscious. The fundamental shift in consumers' preferences, habits and behaviours when it comes to diet soda has happened so quickly that the industry leaders are worried. Not only are people now aware that artificial sweeteners are detrimental to our health, but they are waking up to discover many of the other health myths that have been instigated and kept alive by fraudulent science. *Example*: The great cholesterol myth, and why lowering your cholesterol won't prevent heart disease. The dangerous energy here—and elsewhere—is sugar. Artificial sweeteners are defined as neurotoxins (ref. Russell Blaylock's *Excitotoxins: The Taste That Kills.*

Switching from diet soda to ordinary water is a good step in the right direction. But the full health benefit is first felt when you start drinking ionised, vital, alkaline water with the ability to detoxify and supply your body with antioxidant, energy-rich water.

Dangerous Chemicals in Sodas and Sports Drinks

During the last couple of years, people have become aware that citrus-flavoured soda drinks contain a flame retardant known as brominated vegetable oil (BVO). Beverage companies use BVO to weigh down the citrus flavouring, preventing it from floating to the drink's surface. In addition to aspartame, you will find many diet sodas contain:

- Phosphoric acid
- Artificial caffeine
- Acesulfame potassium
- Potassium benzoate

This is just to name a few. Putting a dash of Stevia together with all the artificial, chemical toxins is not going to change our opinion. Diet sodas should be banned. But before that: Take responsibility for your own health, choose healthy, vital water—and feel the difference. Choose wholegrain sprouted bread, and naturally fermented relishes and condiments instead of sugary substitutes.

Many misconceptions exist around so-called 'primitive people', their culture, nutrition and state of health. We could learn a great deal if we laid aside the myths and images around our ancestors as being primitive, savage, undernourished, plagued by illness and ignorance. In truth, many of our ancestors experienced robust health until death.

A high percentage of people in primitive societies died during infancy or while still young, due to lack of hygiene and sanitation. Again, the Jewish people were the significant exception because of their adherence to God's sanitary and hygiene guidelines.

Many researchers have written extensively about the absence of modern lifestyle diseases in primitive cultures. As long as these people stayed away from modern diets, they avoided cancer, rheumatoid arthritis, heart disease, obesity, diabetes, osteoporosis, Alzheimer's, et cetera. But when modern lifestyle habits were adopted by these people, they contracted the same diseases that are now of epidemic proportions in Western society. This transition from their own native way of eating and living to a 'modern style of diet' has deadly consequences.

Nobel Prize Winner Dr Albert Schweitzer

In 1913, Albert Schweitzer, the Nobel Prize winner physician and missionary, visited Gabon in Africa and was astonished that he did not encounter any cases of cancer.

'I saw none among the natives. The absence of cancer must have been due to the difference in nutrition of the natives compared to the Europeans.'

While on his expeditions exploring the Arctic, the anthropologist Vilhjalmur Stefansson searched in vain for cancer among the Inuit people. In his book on cancer, *Diseases of Civilisation*, he describes how a whaling ship doctor, George Leavitt, found only one cancer case in 49 years among the Inuits of Alaska and Canada. After 1970 when these people started to adopt a modern diet with toxic chemicals from our food, breast cancer malignancy started to spread in the Inuit population.

Another example, this time from the other side of the planet, 'down under': Diabetes used to be very rare among the native Aborigines. With the change of diet to a refined, toxic, nutrient-deficient diet, diabetes level has increased tenfold. The Australian Aborigines used to eat a great deal of fermented sweet potatoes, a natural source of probiotics and soluble fibre, which is a great foundation for the friendly bacteria of the gastro-intestinal tract. When eating these sweet potatoes in fermented form, they reduce significantly the blood sugar imbalance. Sadly, sweet potatoes in any form reach our plates as our favourite food.

The Amazing Discoveries of Dr Weston Price

Dr Weston A. Price was a Harvard-trained dentist, often referred to as 'the Albert Einstein of nutrition'. His wakeup call came when the numbers of young patients with numerous cavities, crooked teeth and deformed dental arches started to alarm him.

Price believed that dental health was a good indicator of physical health. The abnormalities in the mouth cavity could be caused by nutritional deficiencies, also causing heart attacks and cancer.

Together with his wife Florence, he embarked on a six-year expedition on five continents to explore primitive cultures, just as many of these societies began adopting modern diets as a result of being exposed to 'outsiders'. Price and his wife collected a huge amount of data on the dental status, diets and lifestyles of thousands of people in primitive cultures. In this way, Dr. Price could compare people who had grown up with the primitive diet against those who ate modern diets. He studied isolated villages in Switzerland, Gaelic communities in the Outer Hebrides, the Inuits and Eskimo people of Canada and Alaska, the native American Indians of North America, Melanesian and Polynesian South Sea Islanders, African tribes, Australian Aborigines, New Zealand Maori and the Indians of South America.

The surprising discovery Dr. Price found was the traditional diet produced beautiful, straight teeth, with no trace of decay. These people had normal arches, strong and resilient bodies, and a remarkable resistance to disease. Dr Price documented his amazing findings in the book *Nutrition and Physical Degeneration:* that the choice of food and nutrition was the deciding factor.

Modern diets produce physical and psychological degeneration. Dietary deficiency was responsible for the physical degeneration he observed and also poor brain development followed a poor, modern diet, indicating that social disorders such as juvenile delinquency and high crime rates could be attributed to the deficient nutritional status. When the primitive diet was analysed, Dr. Price found out that it provided at least four times the water-soluble vitamins, calcium and other minerals, and at least ten times the fat-soluble vitamins such as A, E and D compared to 'modern' diets!

The primitive diets derived their nutrients from animal foods such as butter, fatty fish, wild game and organ meats.

Most people with common sense understand the importance of good nutrition during pregnancy. Dr Price's research showed that members of primitive cultures practised 'a pre-conception nutritional programme' for both prospective parents. Many tribes also required a period of premarital nutrition for youth who were planning to wed. Special foods were given to maturing boys and girls and lactating women. These foods were abundantly rich, fat-soluble vitamins A and D—nutrients found only in animal fats. The couple plan forward and space their children to allow the mother to regain full health and vigour to ensure physical excellence and safety for subsequent offspring.

Freedom from degenerative ills, healthy physical bodies, emotional stability, and homogeneous reproduction was part of their culture. This is in sharp contrast to modern individuals existing on impoverished foods such as sugar, white flour, pasteurised milk, and convenience foods packed with chemical preservatives and additives. An ironic twist of fate.

Dr Price discovered, virtually without exception, that the primitive diets provided exceptionally high levels of phosphorus, calcium, iron, magnesium, fat-soluble vitamins, (A, D, E, K) and water-soluble B vitamins (foliate, pantothenic acid, thiamine, riboflavin, niacin, B6, B-12) and vitamin C.

Nutrition and Physical Degeneration was first published in 1939 and Dr. Price provided solid empirical evidence that primitive people did not suffer from degenerative diseases such as diabetes, obesity, heart disease, digestive disorders or cancer, as did those on 'modern diets'. The level of vibrant vitality of these communities has virtually been lost to modern-day civilisation.

Why is it that most people are still unaware of this giant and his remarkable findings? Dr Price became very unpopular because his observations and recommendations flew in the face of the 'politically correct' view on nutrition—both then and now. For many decades, Dr. Price's work was buried and forgotten. However, due to the diligent work of the Price-Pottenger Nutrition Foundation and the publication of Price's book for the public, this is, fortunately, starting to change.

Today, several prominent nutritional doctors and naturopaths have traced their heritage back to Weston Price and his work. Abraham Hoffer, founder and developer of orthomolecular psychiatry, Dr. Jonathan Wright, noted author, Alan Gaby, medical columnist and Professor Melvyn Werbach, nutritional author of *Nutritional Influences on Illness* and other doctors all commend the brilliant work of this ingenious dentist. Nutritional anthropologist H. Leon Abrams, Associate Professor Emeritus at the University System of Georgia and author of over 200 papers and eight books, points at Dr. Price as a giant, **ahead of his time with a message relevant to us all.**

Price's conclusions and recommendations were shocking at his time. He advocated a return to breastfeeding when such a practice was discouraged by Western medicine, and considered fresh butter to be a supreme health food. He warned against the use of pesticides, herbicides, preservatives, artificial colourings, refined sugar, and hydrolysed vegetable oils—in short, all the things modern agriculture and nutrition have embraced and promoted the last few decades. W. Price believed that margarine was a demonic creation.

With recommendations like this, he really became unpopular. But the results of his research speak for themselves. Knowing that his data flatly contradicted everything that is 'politically correct' in terms of nutrition, it is common to find his work belittled. If Price's studies are correct (which they are), then the low-fat school with its constant brainwashing advertisement on 'the dangerous saturated animal' and their glorification of vegetable oils, must go the way of all flesh: Into the graveyard where it belongs! To rot forever!

The message is clear: If you want to prevent and reverse degenerative diseases, avoid the politically correct nutritional advice and follow Dr. Price's recommendations: All of the foods that we eat should be whole, fresh and unprocessed.

Westerners live in countries where food is readily available, unlike in other parts of the world where people routinely starve or are malnourished. We live with a choice between two ways of eating: the way of whole foods and the way of processed junk food.

With such a privilege, we owe it to ourselves and our children to choose the way of vital life and food with optimum nutritional value. By making such a choice, we can stem the tide of chronic disease and embrace the ways of our ancestors who had the wisdom of traditional diets and lifestyles.

Good Health, Good Luck, God Bless You

The above phrase is from a well-known song, and is the tune played every time we broadcast our weekly radio programme on health. Good luck is attainable by everybody, and I have written about it earlier in this book.

Concept number one for achieving good and vibrant health, and a happy and long life is to avoid 'stepping on the landmines', or 'driving through a red light', to use a couple of metaphors from our daily life. Say that you avoid unnecessary death from road accidents, predators and the obvious: avoid smoke, don't do drugs, avoid chemicals and industrial wastes in food, air and water. Avoid going to the doctor, educate yourself and prevent diseases. Modern medicine kills. Death by doctoring is number 3 or 4 on the health list.

Have you ever thought about this: Why is it that Mormons and Seventh-Day Adventists live on average to 82 years of age, about seven years longer than others? What's their secret?

Most important is what they *don't* do: they avoid caffeine, a drug in itself, soft drinks, ice tea, tea, alcohol, smoking and fried foods; pork, catfish, shrimp, sugar. And now that you have avoided the most important landmines, and drink vital, alkaline, restructured water, your next step is to supply your body with the 90 or so essential nutrients, each and every day.

This is the raw material your body requires. Vital, fresh food, supplementation and daily exercise like rebounding, walking, jogging, cycling or swimming—preferably outdoor activities.

Remember, plants can't manufacture minerals like they do vitamins. And nothing works in the body without mineral co-factors—nothing! Vitamins, DNA, RNA, chromosomes, enzymes, hormones, energy, not even oxygen works without mineral co-factors. Minerals and vital water and air are the limiting factors for health and longevity. This is in fact 'the fountain of youth'.

Unfortunately, most Westerners have been taught that our health system is of superior quality, as long as you stick to the government advice on diet and eat from the four food groups. But in fact this could be compared to putting dirty oil or petrol in your car, and a little more dirt in your cars' engine. How about that? Even a village idiot would not do that to a 20-year-old Volkswagen.

Yet every Westerner has been 'trained' directly by their respective governmental institution to throw away half of their health and longevity potential just by eating and following the politically correct dietary advice. 'You can get everything you need from our good Norwegian/American/English/Swedish or… four food groups—and by the way, supplements are only expensive urine!' How many times have we heard this brain-washing, indoctrinating gibberish on TV's health debate?

This blind faith in the medical system's way of advising its people has killed more Americans than have all the country's foreign enemies during its 220 years as a nation.

The so-called 'Western' diet pattern—high in red and processed meats, refined grains, potatoes, and sugary drinks, and low in fruits, vegetables, whole grains and healthy fats—is associated with higher risk of heart disease and other degenerative diseases.

The traditional Mediterranean Diet pattern appears to lower the risk of heart disease, stroke and metabolic syndrome. This diet is high in fat, but most of the fat comes from olive oil or plant sources, such as nuts and seeds. Saturated fats are low. The diet is also characterised by a plentiful intake of vegetables, fruits and beans, nuts and whole grains, as well as some cheese and yogurt. If you are concerned about heart health, it is smart to pay attention to your overall diet, not only the type of fat.

You Are What You Eat, Drink, Think, Digest and Breathe

Most medical doctors, 'nutritional experts' and the food industry tell us that we don't risk anything if we eat 'normal, balanced food', a favourite expression used in this field for many years now. It is a phrase devoid of a precise meaning, a cover-up designed to hide the fact that the refined foods produced today are nutrient-deficient and lacking in vital vitamins, minerals and enzymes.

Lifestyle diseases like diabetes, coronary heart disease, metabolic syndrome, allergy, obesity et cetera, can be traced back to the hazardous effects of the utilisation of modern food technologies, refined sugar and flour, environmental toxins, stress, genetics, mental and emotional factors—processed food to increase shelf life. Artificial additives, pesticides and herbicides, irradiated food, GM 'Frankenstein Food'—the list of health-damaging food factors seems never-ending—and all in the name of profit.

The Divine Art of Health

In an unpublished book entitled *The Art of Health*, Dr Peter Rothschild, M.D., Ph.D. points out some interesting facts:

'It suddenly dawned on us that God, the greatest master nutritionist of all time, has given us an all-purpose diet more than 3000 years ago. There is abundant historical evidence that the Israelites, up to the end of the last century (19th) lived much longer than the average Gentile; i.e., the Israelites up to the end of the last century, when an overwhelming majority of Jews obeyed God's law on the whole.

'However, beginning with World War I, both diet and hygiene began to slacken among the children of Israel all over the planet, until only a small fraction remains true to biblical tradition. Worldwide statistics confirm the changing eating habits. The trend of longevity is gradually vanishing among the non-observant. It appears that God indeed knew what nourishment to recommend.'

In Genesis 1:29, God says: 'I give you every seed-bearing plant on the face of the whole earth and every tree that has fruit with seed in it. They will be yours for food.'

In this provision for food there is an abundant richness of vitamins, minerals, enzymes, protein, healthy fats and 'phytochemicals'.

Many religious people in the Western world have, by an odd twist of logic, dismissed the Jewish dietary laws as outdated legalism at the same time they embraced the Ten Commandments as fundamental, universal and timeless. The moral and dietary guidelines were given to the Jews at the same time. These moral laws were used by America's founders and were built into the Norwegian Grunnlov (Constitution) from 1814, based on the proven principles of the Ten Commandments. The dietary was advice given by a loving God to save his people from physical devastation long before the scientific principles of hygiene, viral and bacterial transmission, infection or molecular cell physiology was discovered.

However, after the exodus from the Garden of Eden, God approved eating clean animal protein (Leviticus 2, Deuteronomy 14). Why did God create unclean animals? They were created as scavengers. As a rule, they are meat-eating animals that clean up anything that is left dead in the fields. The flesh of swine is mentioned by many health experts as being one of the prime causes of much of our declining health, resulting in blood diseases, liver troubles, allergies, tumours, et cetera.

The scavengers of the sea—scaleless fish and shellfish—can harbour toxins and germs due to their inefficient excretion systems. The meat of unclean animals is about ten times more perishable and more difficult to preserve than that of other animals.

The second reason is the scary fact that the by-products resulting from the ingestion of scavenger meat are highly poisonous, especially dead enzymes such as cadaverine and putrescence. These death enzymes are extraordinarily effective and useful in nature. Without them no flesh would revert to dust as they are extremely useful at breaking down a corpse, but terribly inconvenient in a living human body.

Essentially, clean animals have 'three stomachs' to digest or chew the cud, to process and refine their clean vegetation—basic food that usually takes more than 24 hours to digest.

Pigs, on the other hand, will eat anything they can find, including rats, faeces and their own young, sick and dead piglets from the same pen. Their digestive system is simple and four hours after the pig has eaten his polluted swill and other putrid offensive matter, man may eat the same second-hand off the ribs of the pig.

Pigs are sometimes used in sewage plants to remove faeces and toxins from the plant before the sewage is further cleansed to become drinking water for the cities. This way, sewage plants save millions of dollars annually, since the pigs will eat anything. Certain parasites survive in pig's meat even once it is fried. The Bible, science and experience tell us that nothing has happened biologically to swine since the time of creation.

A former flight surgeon named Michael Jacobsen, from the US Army, noted that during the bubonic plague in the mid fourteenth century, one-fourth of Europe's population was wiped out in just one year. This repeated over the next 250 years, killing nearly a fourth of London's population in 1603. England lost nearly half of its population to this plague.

It is very interesting to see how the Jews fared in face of this epidemic. As the scourge continued, it became evident that the Jewish people somehow escaped its death grip, which led many to persecute them, accusing the Jews of being behind the plague since they were the only ones who were not dying.

But the truth was that hundreds of years prior to the discovery of the deadly Yersinia pestis microbe (the cause of the bubonic play), the Jews had been protecting themselves through good hygiene and cleanliness, which the Creator had laid down more than 3000 years before man discovered bacteria. The detailed instructions were to be found in the Torah, and if followed, would prevent the spread of such deadly communicable diseases. All but the Jews had forgotten the rules of hygiene and the sanitary conditions necessary to prevent diseases. Sanitary conditions, especially in the large cities of Europe, were quite appalling at that time.

God's dietary guidelines do not contain any refined, processed or artificial food or beverages. Take sugar, for example: this insidious refined product sneaks into almost all kinds of food, baby food, cereals, bread, cakes, biscuits, et cetera, and because it acts as a preservative, it can be found in ketchup, mustard, herring, anchovies, et cetera.

During World War II, a noticeable improvement of people's health occurred in England, which came as a surprise to the majority working in the health service system. The same happened during World War I. The reason was that sugar consumption fell drastically because of the sugar blockade by the colonies. Sugar is addictive, and until recently has been mostly confined to industrialised nations. But the trend is that food containing sugar is slowly destroying poorer nations' health now, too.

An excellent analysis of the toxic effects of white sugar is to be found in the books *Sweet and Dangerous* and *Pure, White and Deadly* by the scientific researcher Professor Emeritus John Yudkin of Queen Elizabeth College in London. He recommends that sugar should be forbidden. But even if the government were to implement a reduction to the same levels as England experienced during the two wars, there would be significant improvement in people's health. I strongly urge you to read Dr J. Mercola's well-researched book *Sweet Deception*, which reveals the secrets that the big sugar industries don't want us to know.

The unfortunate fact is that most pre-packaged and fast-food products overload our bodies with adulterated fats and refined sugars such as that found in baked products and refined grains. Even the terms 'Enriched with vitamins' and '100% natural/organic' are more a gimmick than the truth—nothing more than marketing tricks.

Even *organic* doesn't necessarily mean *toxin-free* or *clean;* i.e., not containing heavy metals.

Over the following pages, I will introduce some guidelines for a healthy lifestyle plan involving eating natural game rather than artificially fattened and estragon-enhanced feedlot-raised beef. Naturally fermented raw products. Wild fish with fins and scales.

Runners, Fitness and Health: Many believe that they get all the nutrients from their food and that supplementation is only contributing to 'expensive urine'. To explain this in greater detail, we will look at international athletes as well as ordinary people, keep-fit runners, and couch potatoes.

Jim Fixx, who started the whole running movement with his bestselling books, died at the age of 52 following multiple cardiomyopathy attacks due to a simple selenium deficiency. Fixx had this strange idea that if he took supplements, the water would be muddied and people would not know if it was the exercise or the supplements that got him to the age of 100.

Both he and George Sheehan, a medical editor for *Runner's World Magazine,* thought that running was the elixir of health and the foundation of longevity. Dr Sheehan is quoted as saying, 'As long as nutrition and supplements did not interfere with running, it was all right.'

Dr Sheehan died of widely spread prostate cancer at the age of 76. All that sweat and running and pain without supplementation bought him six months longer than the average classic American 'coach potato', who averages 75.5 years. According to the medical school at the University of Arizona, JAMA 1996, selenium supplementation of 250 mcg/day will reduce the risk of developing prostate cancer by 69%.

The legend Jesse Owens, 1913-1980, who won four gold medals in track and field at the 1936 Berlin Olympics, died at the age of 66 of lung cancer, after smoking for 35 years. Selenium-deficient Joe Lewis, the 'Brown Bomber', died at the age of 66 of cardiac arrest. He had previously been operated on for aortic aneurism, due to a copper deficiency.

None of the 'Flying Finns'—Paavo Nurmi, Hannes Kolehmainen (smiling Hannes), Ville Ritola, V. Iso-Holla—the track team from Finland who dominated long-distance running in three Olympics during the '20's and '30's, reached the age of 70.

Athletes sweat out more minerals in five years than couch potatoes sweat in 50 years. If you sweat out all of your copper and become depleted in this vital mineral and don't replace it by supplementation, you are at risk of dying of a ruptured aneurysm. If you sweat out all your selenium and don't replace it by supplementation, you're at a high risk of developing cardiomyopathy, heart attack or cancer. If you sweat out all your chromium and vanadium and don't replace it by supplementation you're at a high risk of developing adult onset of type 2 diabetes. If you sweat out all your calcium, magnesium and sulphur and don't replace it by supplementation, you are at a high risk of developing arthritis, osteoporosis and kidney stones. Still think supplementation is only expensive urine?

Essential nutrients are called *essential* because our bodies cannot manufacture them. We must consume essential nutrients through our food and supplements on a daily basis. If you lack any of the 90 essential nutrients for any length of time, your body will break down gradually and you will end up with one or several illnesses. Remember that depleted soil (as documented in the 1930s) cannot supply vegetation with enough nutrients—and that is precisely one of the reasons we should take supplementation.

An analogy of our genetic potential for health and longevity is the sturdy energy of, let's say, a Porsche, a great in German automotive engineering. The engine is designed to run 300,000 miles before it needs a major overhaul. But if you, the owner or driver, don't maintain the car's engine by changing the oil, fuel and air filters, coolants, lubricants and motor oil, the wondrous engine will break down very quickly indeed, and not reach the 'genetic potential of health and longevity' it had the capacity to do. Through neglect or ignorance, you may well drive your body—and therefore your life—to a grinding half. You were not built and intended to end your days in this way.

There is much well-documented data that shows an association between maximum longevity and intake of optimum and essential nutrients. The correlation between essential nutrient intake and state of health is well proven in the laboratory for many species, in so-called primitive cultures and naturopathic clinics such as the Viktorklinikken and thousands of others worldwide. Illness of longstanding duration is reversed using the principles of:

- Detoxification - alkalinisation - oxygenation
- Electro medicine – exercise - essential nutrients supplementation

It is interesting to note, as mentioned previously, that the longest-living cultures lived close to permanent good sources of water and often drank 'glacier water'. Glaciers move up and down mountains and rocks due to their sheer weight. These rocks are ground to 'rock flour' each year, which often contains as many as 60-72 minerals which are suspended in the water as small particles. The water is thus restructured and the resulting liquid is known as *glacial milk* because of its whitish appearance. These long-living cultures build canals and aqueducts to carry the glacial milk to their valleys. These healthy folks don't only drink the mineral-laden glacial milk, but have their fields flooded by it, which replenishes the soil with mineral-rich silt every spring. Their grains, vegetables, fruits, seeds and nuts convert the inorganic minerals in the fields to plant-derived colloidal minerals.

'Mens Sana in Corpore Sano!' Benjamin Franklin, one of the founding fathers of the United States of America, 'the land of plenty', showed a keen interest in health habits and longevity. Most people have an image of Benjamin Franklin being an obese man due to a famous portrait painted of him in his mid-seventies when he was living in Paris, France, eating rich food and fraternising with old ladies. This remarkable man was a publisher, statesman, diplomat, scientist, inventor, postmaster, musician, writer and fitness guru! He was also an all-round original thinker, a true 'Renaissance Man'. In his forties, he was a tall, lean, muscular figure.

His motto was, 'Mens sana in corpore sano' (A healthy mind in a healthy body). This was his core value regarding his person. He firmly believed in and practised regular exercise, leaping being one of his favourites. He would have enjoyed my trampoline aerobic classes! He was rigorously abstemious about food and alcohol. Franklin's long and healthy life was a consequence of the way he chose to live. Besides his genes and natural brilliance, Benjamin Franklin was able to excel in so many fields because of his lifestyle. Unlike many of his fellow citizens at the time, he didn't walk around in a stupor from excessive heavy meats and sugar, not to mention intemperate alcohol consumption. His eating and exercise habits were light years ahead of his time, and he passed away at 84—almost twice the age of his contemporaries.

Conclusion

'A stitch in time saves nine.' Procrastination, putting off doing something until later, creates more work in the long run—and along the way you may stumble upon more roadblocks than you can handle. We are talking of course about prevention being both smarter and better, as the saying goes: 'An ounce of prevention is worth a pound of cure.' Actions speak louder than words.

CHAPTER ELEVEN

Fun, Fitness and the Fountain of Youth

'You've got to dance like there is nobody's watching, Love like you'll never been hurt, sing like there's nobody's listening, and live like it's heaven on earth'. William W. Purkey.

As you have discovered, you can be fit and still be unhealthy. The sad story of Jim Fixx, who is credited with helping to start the fitness revolution through his bestselling book *The Complete Book of Running*, is just one example.

To neglect the scientific evidence of vitamin and mineral supplementation, proper nutrition, vital water and air, is like the blind leading the blind. Both fall into the ditch. Over four decades, I have first-hand witnessed erroneous advice being dished out by incompetent doctors and trainers: 'Don't worry; you get all the vitamins and minerals you need from your food.' Wrong. You don't get sufficient vital nutrients in your food. Mineral soil depletion has been well documented since the US Senate conducted their study in 1936.

'Lacking vitamins, the system can make use of minerals; but lacking minerals, vitamins are useless' (Senate document 246.74[th] Congress, 1936).

Another cause of mineral deficiency is diet and blockages in the intestines. One of the prime functions of the colon is to reabsorb water, in order to prevent dehydration. Both water and minerals are lost because this function is partially blocked. And a further cause of mineral deficiency is mineral competition. An excess of one mineral can cause a deficiency of another, because minerals compete for the same binding sites, like a molecular Musical Chairs. Drugs and lack of bio-availability are further causes.

Benjamin Franklin—Fun, Frolic and Fitness

Franklin's fascination with fitness began at the young age of seventeen. Working as a typesetter in London, he garnered physical stamina by running up and down stairs with heavy trays of lead. Sometimes he would carry two trays of lead, which must have impressed colleagues. He eschewed alcohol, preferring water, his favourite drink. Just think about it: He touted proper and healthy diet, lifestyle and exercise two hundred years before the USDA (United States Department of Agriculture) constructed their 'Food Pyramid'.

In an age where few people know how to swim, Franklin taught himself and remained a competent swimmer all his life, even having plans to become a swimming instructor himself. Franklin is the only founding father in the Swimming Hall of Fame.

Later, Franklin returned to the colonies, and in 1733 began to publish the famous *Poor Richard's Almanac* in Philadelphia. In this publication, he often offered advice on health matters.

- 'Early to bed and early to rise, makes a man healthy, wealthy and wise.'
- 'Eat to live, live not to eat.'
- 'A full belly makes a bad brain.'
- 'To lengthen thy life, lessen thy meals.'

This approach was honest, simple, scientific and biblical. When old age restricted his activities, he would focus on lifting and swinging weights. 'No gain without pain,' he quipped, probably hobbling from muscle soreness the following day.

He certainly would have laughed at modern man's unwillingness to move and exercise. As the comedian Joey Adams put it, 'If it weren't for the fact that the TV set and the refrigerator are so far apart, some of us wouldn't get any exercise at all.'

In a letter to Joseph Priestly, a chemist and scientist (1733-1804) who discovered oxygen, Benjamin Franklin stated, 'Agriculture may diminish its labour and double its produce. All diseases may by some means be prevented or cured, not excepting that of old age, and our lives lengthened at pleasure even beyond the antediluvian standard.'

Dr Alexis Carrel (1873-1944) received the Nobel Prize in Physiology or Medicine in 1912 in recognition for his work on 'vascular suture and the transplantation of blood vessels and organs'. He managed to grow fibroblasts, connective tissue cells, from chicken hearts in flasks fed with extracts of blended chicken embryo; the cells kept multiplying and growing for 34 years, two years beyond Carrel's death. This resulted in the theory that cells are inherently immortal if fed a perfect diet and kept in a perfect environment. His colleagues got bored with the experiment and threw the fibroblasts out.

Then Dr. Leonard Hayflick came along and used artificial growth media with major mineral deficiency. In this experiment, bound to fail from the beginning, human fibroblasts could only replicate 50 times before dying because of lipid peroxidation and a selenium deficiency. Poor and limiting nutrition resulted in the fifty replication limit of fibroblasts known as the 'Hayflick limit'.

The Quest for the Fountain of Youth

James Hilton made 'Shangri-La' famous through winning the 1934 Pulitzer Prize for his novel, *Lost Horizon*, in which people lived healthy, loving, productive and long lives. The novel was made into a classic movie of the same name in 1937, starring Ronald Colman and Jane Wyatt, directed by Frank Capra. In the original novel and movie, the people of Shangri-La attributed their youthfulness, health and longevity to a Spartan diet, peaceful attitude, a work ethic devoted to gardening and farming, and a rich Christian faith and lifestyle.

Fontana di Trevi, Dancing Water Molecules, and Structured Water

A remake of the film *Lost Horizon* was produced in 1973, directed by Charles Jarrett and starring Peter Finch, Liv Ullmann from Norway and Sally Kellerman. The film portrayed an Eastern form of meditation being the basis for their health and longevity, which contributed to a passion for Eastern meditation by the 'hippie movement', a deviation of sorts. The quest for a long and happy life continues. Everlasting dreams lead people to ancient wells and sacred places of healing fountains, Lourdes being the most famous. One of the most frequently visited fountains is Fontana di Trevi in Rome, at the junction of three roads (*trevi*). At 85 feet high and 65 feet wide, it is enormous, situated at the end of one of Rome's *ancient* aqueducts,—the Acqua Vergine. The original fountain was destroyed but was rebuilt under Pope Clement VII by Nicola Salvi, based on a design by the famous sculptor Bernini called Oceanus, who's seen riding on giant oceans and lakes. The figure of Triton, Poseidon's son, who is most often depicted blowing a conch shell, is easy to recognise to the right side of Oceanus. The horses represent the ever-changing nature of the sea. One is calm, and the other is restless.

To the left of Oceanus sits the statue of Abundance, and to the right sits the statue of Salubrity (health). Abundance holds the horn of plenty, full of fruit, and water spills from the urn at her feet. Salubrity wears a wreath of laurels on her head and holds a cup from which a snake drinks. Above each statue is a bas-relief, and above Abundance we see the general Agrippa who commanded his soldiers to build the aqueduct. The bas-relief above Salubrity depicts the origin, pointing to the water source of the spring.

Every day, some eighty million litres of water flow through the fountain to supply several other fountains in Rome, including the Fountain of the Four Rivers, the Tortoise Fountain and the Fountain of the Old Boat in front of the Spanish Steps. Legend has it that if you throw a coin into the Trevi, with your back to the fountain, using your right hand to throw over your left shoulder, it guarantees you a return trip to Rome. A second coin leads to romance, and a third leads to marriage. Thanks perhaps to the film *Three Coins in the Fountain*, the staggering amount of around 3000 euros daily is collected from the Trevi Fountain (1.26 million annually) and distributed via charities to the needy. The fountain offers a beautiful setting, to just sit down by this stunning masterpiece, rest your legs and contemplate on the symbolism of the fountain's intricate features, all of which are found in the Scriptures.

And now for a sweet little bonus legend for you, just to enchant and pull at your heartstrings: There is a miniature fountain to the left of the Trevi Fountain. Legend has it that if a couple each drink from this small 'Fountain of Lovers', they will be forever faithful to their partner.

You may recall the famous scene from the film *La Dolce Vita* (1960), directed by Federico Fellini and starring Marcello Mastroianni and a buxom lady, the former Miss Sweden, Anita

Ekberg, who jumps into the Trevi Fountain, and Marcello (the main character) wades after her, idealising her into the ultimate woman who remains forever just out of reach. This multi-layered film can be viewed as a portrayal of the seven deadly sins taking place on the Seven Hills of Rome, involving seven nights and seven days. Or perhaps a cautionary tale of an unbalanced man missing the mark, as an archer misses his mark. Or maybe an even deeper meaning; a definition of sin—but that's another story, as the saying goes.

As a touching side note, when Marcello Mastroianni died of pancreatic cancer in 1996 at the age 72, the city turned off the water in the Trevi Fountain for one day and draped the whole ornamental sculpture and fountain in black as a tribute to the actor.

Dr Benveniste and Dr Emoto—'Water's Memory'

Whilst you may think of the tossing of coins and well-wishing as pure superstition, this nevertheless gives us an interesting starting point for further exploration. As I mentioned briefly earlier, water has memory (Benveniste, Emoto). You may well feel that this is a rather odd and doubtful notion, despite the fact it is scientifically validated. Let us look at this idea from a slightly different angle.

Recently, scientists found out more about one of the most intriguing mysterious of water: how it can contain and store information about its inhabitants. Organic molecules trapped in the water can be stored for a long time. This is strange because, in theory, the imprinted information should immediately disintegrate—but for some reason it does not.

Typically, a water medium transmits odours less efficiently than air does, especially over longer distances, as the signalling molecules in water tend to disintegrate quickly, even in distilled water. In addition, because of the constant motion of currents (which are even present in standing water), the concentration of odour decreases dramatically and quickly as molecules quickly spread in all directions.

Biologists and chemists know that the olfactory organs in aquatic animals are much better developed than their other receptors. It has been long known that a shark can smell its victim at a distance of several hundred metres—and this is in seawater, where the ocean currents are more rapid and strong than in freshwater, due to the high concentration of salts.

Professor Boris Koch at the Alfred Wegener Institute of Polar Research recently resolved this paradox. By using spectrometry analysis, he was able to show that single molecules of organic matter remain in water a long time after the breakdown of the organic matter. 'Water has a 'chemical memory' that retains the information about organisms that were once in that water,' says Professor Boris Koch. Spectrometric analysis can accurately determine the atomic structure and the proportion of carbon, hydrogen, nitrogen, et cetera. 'Based on this, we can reconstruct the original molecule itself, and even determine what part of the organism it used to be.

According to Koch's study, water often retains

carbohydrates and organic acids. These substances are found in most secretions emitted by the body's surface, such as mucus in fish and many invertebrates. The composition of mucus and other excreta is specific to each species. This could be the reason sharks are able to effortlessly locate their victims from a far distance; they simply follow the trail of organic molecules that remains in the water for a long time, sometimes several days. The specific odour will immediately inform the predator as to whose trail it is—harmless tuna or not-so-harmless dolphins.

Some molecules of decaying bodies can be found in places where the animal suffered death a very long time ago. Many marine scavengers such as hagfish and crabs, which have poor vision, will pick up these signalling molecules and thus can easily detect dead creatures.

Professor B. Koch's discovery seems to contradict some of the laws of chemistry that state that any organic molecule, upon exposure to seawater, should quickly decompose into simple components such as carbon dioxide and water. But in this case, it does not happen. Why? Maybe the excretory substances are leaving behind an electromagnetic imprint capable of forming complex links with water molecules resistant to any 'destroyers'.

How long can these stable compounds live? The paper suggests a few days, but this may be possibly because of the limited time of the experiment. Perhaps molecular information can be stored for mortals for years. This technology can be used to track migration routes of various marine animals. 'Can these animals navigate using smell?' is the next question researchers are asking. Finally, researchers can find out the ocean's capacity for storing CO2, as well as what portion of C02 is produced within the ocean and how much comes from the outside. This will assist in helping to understand the notorious greenhouse effect.

Beauty Is in the Eye of the Beholder (From 3rd Century BC Greek)

Still contemplating on the remarkable fusion of architecture, sculpture and water, The Trevi Fountain, its symbolism and metaphor, the Acqua Vergine was the only aqueduct that supplied the city of Rome, and its water was sold and carried everywhere. Water has, throughout history, and especially in Rome, been used to express the generosity and power of rulers, both secular and spiritual. The pure water of Acqua Virgo of Antiquity (later renamed Acqua Vergine) arrived triumphantly at its terminus in the city, where the masterpiece of the Trevi Fountain is situated.

Did you know that water falls from the sky and takes sometimes hundreds of years to seep into the groundwater? Former professor Joan S. Davis of Zurich Technical University has conducted research for over thirty years into flowing water, and refers to it as 'juvenile and wise water', as the water picks up information from stones, rocks, silt and people's attitudes and feelings towards it, expressed explicitly or by intention. So when the water enters the Fontana di Trevi and gushes over the sculpted carvings, it spins and spouts over the fascinating details of rock formation and plant life. There is even a snail carved on a marsh marigold. The spiral formation of the snail's house and the spiralling of the water molecules: a universal phenomenon that results in structured and revitalised water. With all the love, joy and grateful well-wishing from people tossing coins, making a wish, or saying a prayer, these positive intentions are picked up by the water, as water is the most excellent carrier of information in the universe.

No wonder Anita Ekberg and Marcello Mastroianni were mesmerised by the flow of cascading water in perfect spiralling harmony—restructured and hexagonal. Wading into the fountain, Mr Mastroianni, beguiled by the exuberant, voluptuous and tantalising Anita Ekberg, was simply hypnotised! *Oh, la Dolce Vita!* 'Beauty, like supreme dominion, is but supported by opinion', according to Benjamin Franklin in *Poor Richard's Almanac 1741*.

A rare moment producing 'a resonance transcending the culture and age that conceived them.' (*The Trevi Fountain*, by John A. Pinto).

But then again: Beauty is in the eye of the beholder ('The Duchess', Margaret Wolfe Hungerford, an Irish novelist).

An Exceptional Dancer, Poetry in Motion: BCN—Best Cure Now

It was a sunny afternoon in Rome. The cascading water molecules danced a poetry in motion dance as they fell into the Fontana di

Trevi, creating a resonance in the air and a surplus of negative ions, the vitamins of the air. Raymonde, a brilliant dancer from Beirut, and I headed down the Via Delle Muratte.

The warm Sirocco wind from the southeast ruffled her summer dress, which fluttered as she swirled elegantly down the pavement, onto the road and back onto the pavement again. An exuberant joy to behold as she smiled, moving rhythmically, circling and spiralling effortlessly, tiptoeing as if she were floating along a river. In the eternal city of Rome, an Oriental belly dancer expressing her gratitude and joy of life. Pure artistry. Demi-pointe, pointe technique—I had been taught some of the finesse of the dance moves.

Mesmerised by all these magical and gracious moves, I observed something fascinating: those same movements Raymonde performed in her impromptu dance along Via Delle Muratte I had observed many times as free-flowing water in rivers and brooks. Circles and spirals which have the power to restructure the water and are so essential for the water's vitality, and hence life-giving properties. Joy and gratitude are always the best recipe for the right attitude to reach new altitudes!

It is the very same phenomenon that Victor Schauberger, the Austrian forest caretaker, philosopher and inventor, and Henry Thoreau, the writer and naturalist, had observed and described. But, to my knowledge, nobody had made the connection between a belly dancer's kinetic movements creating vibrating energy and being transferred to every cellular structure. Like ripples on a lake spreading outwards.

There was no music in Via Delle Muratte, just the tune that came from within her heart as she was almost carried and lifted by the gentle breeze of the warm Sirocco wind. Past wartime memories from Beirut, when she herself was shot and almost killed by a sniper in the roads of Abdel Wahab El Inglizi, were buried in the sand that afternoon by this dancer of divine origin who has performed for members of the Norwegian Royal family, the military and government ministers.

Is she dancing with the Sirocco wind from Africa, as it sweeps up into her dearly beloved Lebanon before swirling between the Seven Hills of Rome? Is it the water molecules of pure poetry in motion? Although not a professional dancer myself, I flew with the wind on this memorable afternoon; I flew, running, singing and gesticulating along Via Della Muratte. *Bella! Bella!* And I was reminded of some wise words from Albert Einstein: 'If you can't explain it simply, you don't understand it well enough.'

Michael 'Misha' I imagined myself dancing like Michael `Mish`Baryshnikov, playfully being in a ballet scene. *Bella! Bella!* 'Imagination is more important than knowledge' (Albert Einstein).

The famous song *Nella Fantasia* ('In My Fantasy'), based on the theme 'Gabriel's Oboe' from the film *The Mission*, 1986, composed by Ennio Morricone, with lyrics by Chiara Ferraù, expressed our sentiments perfectly as we celebrated Raymonde's fiftieth birthday in Rome. *Cin cin!*

In my fantasy I see a bright world,
Where each night there is less darkness.
I dream of souls that are always free
Like the cloud that floats,
In my fantasy exists a warm wind,
That breathes into the city, like a friend.
I dream of souls that are always free,
Like the cloud that floats.

As a physiotherapist and coach for many years, I have never seen anything that brings so much exhilarating joy as dancing—from ballet to hip-hop, from classical to contemporary. If you are feeling a bit down in the dumps, just tune into *SYTYCD* (*So You Think You Can Dance*) on the Net and feel yourself becoming energised as you attempt some of the moves yourself. Immerse yourself in the choreography by the legendary Mia Michaels, the reigning queen of contemporary dance. There are routines that will make you laugh, cry and scream out in utter disbelief about how they can possibly move their bodies like that. Still unsure? Rest your eyes on the beautiful Cat Deeley and laugh along with the witty comments from Nigel Lythgoe and Mary Murphy (*'If you're not riding on the Hot Tamale Train tonight, you're certainly on the platform'*—Nigel Lythgoe). She can enchant anybody with her charming metaphors and her exuberant way of being!

These performances, I hope, will inspire you to take your 'work-out' seriously, with a smile and a laugh, no matter what kind of exercise appeals to you.

Remember we were created to move. Every day. But don't forget the fluids—and living water, restructured and with high redox potential, is the only fluid that can reach the innermost parts of your cells, rejuvenating, rebuilding and strengthening your immune system.

Remember what Henry Thoreau said? 'Water is the only drink for a wise man.' And so spoke The Pure Energy Norway Man.!

A Young Dancer and Her Dream

Some time ago, a young girl of sixteen, Jasmine, came to our clinic desperate for help. She had contracted a serious liver infection and I was shocked to see her yellow, jaundiced colour. Despite being on heavy medication, her liver had been gradually getting worse and both the girl and her parents were obviously very anxious, not knowing the progression or the outcome. During our conversation, she told me about her favourite hobby and passion: ballet dancing.

Immediately one of my many heartstrings was pulled into life and I intuitively knew how to proceed. The Holy Spirit has guided me many times before, but not like this. This is what happened: First, I asked her if she was disappointed and maybe angry because she was unable to practise her favourite ballet routine. 'Oh, yeah! You bet I am!' she answered. She was so angry at her condition and her liver dysfunction that she could scream. Before proceeding any further, I explained about how her anger and hatred put her body in a cul-de-sac of a non-healing modus. And according to old Chinese medical therapy, and as proved by modern-day research, emotional states persisting for long periods of time will weaken the immune system and lead to physical symptoms of breakdown. Typically, we see a connection between anger/hatred/un-forgiveness and liver/gallbladder dysfunction. I explained about forgiving herself and her liver, which had become the target for her anger and hate. Continuing, I talked and prayed for forgiveness and finished by saying, 'Let me talk to your liver'. Whereupon her eyes nearly popped out of her head as if saying *'What is this, poco-loco?!'* Steadfastly I proceeded and we both heard a remarkable noise of a sound resembling the crunching of dry paper!

'Hey, that's your liver saying he's accepting your apology and is forgiving you!' Jasmine thought this was most odd.

'But I don't want you thinking that was just a coincidence—let me repeat it one more time,' which I did and the same thing happened again: a sound of crackling paper.

'Praise the Lord!'

The day after, new tests at her doctor's office showed a tremendous fall in the liver readings. We repeated the process again, she was off medication straight away, her liver tests normal, her skin colour returning to normal, and the sclera (the white of the eye), which had been very yellow, glowing bright white again. She was full of energy super-fast—and best of all, she was back dancing ballet again.

Was I talking and praying to God? The water? Her liver?

Jasmine? In faith, Let His Kingdom come and His be the glory! A miracle that spread like ripples on a water's pond.

Lebanon, The White One

'A garden fountain, a well of living water, and flowing streams from Lebanon.' (Song of Solomon 4:15)

For many years, I had a dream to visit Lebanon, the land of the Canaanite and the Phoenicians. My knowledge of the country consisted mainly of impressions of a nation that had been war-torn since the seventies, suffering both civil war and occupation by foreign countries. But my curiosity grew when I read the many (71 altogether) beautiful biblical descriptions about Lebanon, especially in the Psalms and the Song of Salomon.

'The righteous shall flourish like the palm tree; he shall grow like a cedar in Lebanon.' (Psalm 92:12).

The Lord must have seen my heart because this is what happened: During one of the bleakest periods of my life, a beautiful woman from Lebanon came to our clinic with a longstanding and serious health problem. It became my privilege to restore health and balance into her life, for which she and her family expressed their gratitude by inviting me to Lebanon, to the Cedars of Lebanon, the Cedars of the Lord. I was warmly greeted by her family and enjoyed the famous hospitability for which the Lebanese are well known. During my whole stay they insisted on calling me 'Dr. Viktor' (my middle name)—probably because my first name, Gunnar, sounded too much like a gunman, a bad association for the peace-loving Lebanese, but also as a sign of respect and gratitude for having helped Raymonde to a better health in Norway.

Teta Montaha, the Incomparable Grandmother in Abdel Wahab El Inglizi

My first meeting with Teta Montaha, when she was 96 years of age (now 103), is best described as a warm, electric and illuminating event. The petite old lady radiated kindness and vibrating energy as is rarely seen at her age: beautiful, strong blue eyes and a wonderful smile. She thanked me profoundly for having helped her granddaughter Raymonde, the apple of her eye, to a new lease of life. During the festive dinner and celebrations, she insisted that 'Dr. Viktor' had to sit next to her. I was honoured. And I was able to ask her my most pertinent question: 'What is your secret, Teta?' (*Grandmother* in Lebanese.) 'How have you managed to stay so healthy and happy all these years?'

She had survived five wars in her beloved Lebanon and experienced the massacre in Damour, her hometown, on 20 January 1976, during the 1975-1990 Lebanese Civil War, when PLO units attacked the citizens of Damour. Those who were not killed on land were forced into the sea, where they drowned. An estimated 582 civilians died, many of them close family members of Teta Montaha.

An eyewitness, Father Mansour Labaky, a Christian Maronite priest who survived the massacre, said, 'Thousands upon thousands were shouting 'Allahu Akbar!' (*God is great*). 'Let us attack them for the Arabs. Let us offer a holocaust for Mohammad!'

One can only begin to imagine the trauma of five wars and massacres, including witnessing her grandchild Raymonde being shot and almost killed by a sniper just outside Teta Montaha's ground-floor flat. Two innocent people were killed on that same spot the same day Raymonde was shot.

Here I was sitting next to a very remarkable woman, enjoying sumptuous Lebanese cuisine. The Spanish have their tapas, the Romanian their mezeluri, the Italian their antipasto, but the Lebanese mezze beats them all! An array of small dishes placed in front of you full of different colours, flavours, textures and aromas; fresh fish and meat, usually lamb, with garlic, olive oil, herbs and spices, according to the season. A typical mezze will consist of an elaborate variety of thirty or so hot and cold dishes, and will always include tabbouleh, the queen of the table, and hummus, baba ghanoush, kebbeh and sambusac, baked pastry with a savoury filling such as potatoes, ground lamb and beef or chicken with onions, peas and lentils; pickled vegetables, baba ghanoush and bread; fresh fruit or baklava, a rich, sweet pastry filled with chopped nuts and sweetened by honey or syrup. Ever heard of Ashta? This original Lebanese recipe, fit for a king—and yes they did make me feel like a king, the first Protestant Maronite Cedar King! *Ashta* is a slang word for 'Kashte' in classical Arabic, which refers to clotted cream prepared with rose water and orange-blossom water. Ashta is used in desserts like knafeh, znoud, atayef, and many others.

As the conversation flowed and laughter filled the room, Teta Montaha reminisced about the days back home in Damour when she used to pluck oranges and rosebuds to make rose-and-orange water. Nobody could replicate the delicate aroma and taste that flowed from Teta's loving, caring hands. Until this day—and she is now 103 years old and still going strong with a clarity of thinking and memory that much younger people have a hard time keeping up with—her orange-and-rose-blossom water recipe is still a secret.

The Cedars of Lebanon

As a little child, I was always fascinated by nature and the biological diversity so purposefully created, beautiful to behold—from the tiny little sprouting bud to giant trees. But the Cedars of Lebanon overwhelmed me completely with their majestic splendour. Great natural monuments, described many times in the Bible, especially in the Psalms and Song of Solomon: 'Well watered are the trees of the Lord, the Cedars of Lebanon, which He planted' (Psalms 104:16).

The breath-taking natural beauty of Lebanon with its cedars has inspired poetry and religious writers for centuries, and the people in the Orient entertain a traditional veneration for these trees.

Vegetative powers are attributed to them, together with an 'intelligence' which causes them to manifest wisdom and foresight, enabling them a profound understanding of seasonal changes. They stir their vast branches by lifting them towards heaven or down towards earth as the snow is falling or melting. It is said that the snow has no sooner begun to fall then the Cedars turn their branches to rise, pointing upwards, forming, as it were, a pyramid or a parasol. Assuming this new shape, they can withstand the immense weight of the snow settling upon them.

The Cedars of Lebanon have been used by many civilisations throughout the ages. The Egyptians used its resin to mummify their dead and called it the 'life of death'; cedar sawdust was found in the tombs of the Pharaohs. In pagan rituals, cedars were used with their offerings. Jewish priests were ordered by Moses to use the peel of the Lebanese Cedar in circumcision and treatment of leprosy. According to Talmud, Jews used to burn Lebanese cedar wood on Mount Olive, announcing the beginning of a new year.

The Phoenicians used it to build their ships and military fleets, as well as their temples, houses and doorsills, because of its superb quality for resistance to insects, humidity and temperature. The most famous buildings constructed with Cedars of Lebanon are the Temple of Jerusalem and King David and Solomon's Palace. King Solomon sent 30,000 workers to Lebanon to obtain the cedar for the temple. (1. Kings 7:2-5). Forty years prior to the Temple's destruction (70 AD), first-century Rabbi Yochanan ben Zakkai, the last survivor of the Grand Sanhedrin, saw the Temple doors open by themselves. He related this incident, in which he saw Lebanon as a symbol of the Temple, to Zechariah, a prophet, (11:1-2). Zechariah prophesised that one of the places to which God would bring back the scattered children of Israel would be to Lebanon (10:6-10). Maybe Lebanon one day will be part of Israel?

In the opulent Palace of Alhambra, Spain, 8000 pieces of cedar wood from Lebanon crown the dome of the Salon de Embajadores (Hall of the Ambassadors), evoking the seven levels of heavens noted in the Scriptures, the seven heavens of the Muslim cosmos (*heavens* is always plural in Hebrew). As we once stood there, craning our necks to absorb the breath-taking artistic and natural beauty of the dome's cedar work, and thinking about the blood, sweat and tears that had gone into creating this, tears filled our eyes, and a line by K. Gibran, Lebanon's famous writer, came to my mind: 'A tear to unite me with those of broken heart; A smile to be a sign of my joy in existence.'

The Many Wonders of Snow and Water

Admiring the magnificent cedar trees of Lebanon and staring at the snow-capped high mountains, my thoughts drifted off to winter's secret beauty: snow and snowflakes—so wonderfully captured in the works of Wilson Alwyn 'Snowflake' Bentley in 1885.

I think Henry David Thoreau put it admirably well when he said, 'How full of creative genius is the air in which these are generated! I should hardly admire them more if real stars fell and lodged on my coat.' The famous writer and naturalist was of course talking about snowflakes.

Once again, water, now in the form of snow, talked to me. A snowflake, or rather snow *crystal*, is a temporary work of art. Nature produces a great many variations, each exhibiting elaborate and intricate patterns. A snow crystal refers to a single crystal of ice— so how do they form and develop into such intricate six-branched structures? Snowflakes form when water vapour in the air condenses directly into solid ice. As more vapour condenses onto the snow crystals, it grows and an elaborate pattern emerges. Snowflakes are the product of a rich synthesis of physics, mathematics and chemistry. What fun to catch on your tongue! These and many other pictures flashed across my mind as I admired the snow-capped mountains of Lebanon and how fun it was to be in a country where you can ski on pristine snow one moment, and a short hour later swim in the warm Mediterranean Sea. These intricate patterns formed by the snow crystals—i.e., water—have mystified scientists for years, and still cause a lot of headaches for those preparing the ski slopes for the Olympics in Sochi 2014, but not for the world-famous violinist Vanessa Mae competing in the Giant Slalom for Thailand. What a joyful sight to behold!

'Was Life's history ever written in more dainty hieroglyphics!' (WA. Bentley and G.H. Perkins), *A study of Snow Crystal*, 1898. Lucky is the man who can catch a snowflake on his tongue and feel the exhilarating joy as you touch one of life's great mysterious!

I felt in good company when I learnt that in 1637, even René Descartes, the French philosopher and mathematician, was absorbed in the study of snowflakes and the science behind it. Most people remember his name for his metaphysical dictum '*Cogito ergo sum*' (I think, therefore I am). We are all thinking (*Homo sapiens*) and hopefully playful (*Homo ludens*). Both of these faculties should be exercised in various ways, as they will give you a great deal of joy and strengthen your immune system by increasing your life's vitality.

So, next time you see snow falling on the ground as glittering crystals, try to catch one or two, then do the following exercise: Alone or with your kids and friends, make snow angels. Absorb the moment and enjoy it fully, and your thankful heart will send good, healing vibrations into each power station mitochondria and DNA of every one of your 600 trillion or so cells. And thank you with a smile. This is mindfulness: as you lie on your back, arms and legs flapping, gazing towards the sky and maybe catching one or two snowflakes. Who knows, maybe Jim Reeves' *Snowflake* will come dancing with you:

Hey, hey, hey snowflake, my pretty little snowflake,
Hoo, hoo, hoo the change in weather has made it better for me.
Hey, hey, hey, snow flake, my pretty little snowflake,
You've got me warm as fire with a burning desire for you.

Jim Reeves recorded this on 15 October 1959 and, thanks to Mary Reeves, his wife, who loved it and kept the tape to release it posthumously in 1966, it became a great hit.

I did exactly like this some years ago, just before going onstage to hold a lecture in Denmark. Greatly inspired by the snow and the angels I made on the snow-covered ground, the lecture flowed elegantly and effortlessly—one of the best lectures I've ever delivered. The audience was astonished and greatly inspired.

'*God moves in a mysterious way His wonders to perform.*' These are the first two lines of the hymn by William Cowper (1731-1800). Ref Psalm 77:14-19:

You are the God that does wonders; you have made known Your strength among the peoples.

By Your arm you have redeemed Your People, the sons of Jacob and Joseph. Selah.

*The **waters** saw You O Elohim, the **waters** saw You, they were afraid, the depths also trembled.*

*The clouds poured out **water**, also, Your arrow flashes back and forth.*

The voice of Your thunder rolled along; the lightning lit up the world.

The earth trembled and shook.

*Your way was in the sea, and Your path in the great **waters**. And your footsteps were not known.*

Teta Montaha in Abdel Wahab El Inglizi

Back to my story of this lovely lady. After dinner and a few improvised dancing steps with my companion, the wise and graceful Teta Montaha revealed her secret of a long and happy life. What follows is a short summary (more to follow)

- 'Have faith in your Lord Yeshua, Dr. Viktor. He has carried me through all sorrow and travail and never let me down.' She emphasised her faith several times; she belonged to the Maronite Church on Beirut, which she attended on a regular basis.
- Water. Clean and vital water to drink. Immaculate hygiene throughout the house.
- Nutritious food prepared with tender love and care, from fresh vegetables and fruit; a little meat and fish, but never pork; whole grains, seeds, herbs and spices; highest-quality olive oil; natural butter, never margarine, light products or hydrolysed vegetable oils; animal fats, whole milk products, yogurt. Total absence of additives, preservatives or chemicals in air, food and water. Daily consumption of natural salt when cooking vegetables, meat and fish. Olive oil and vinegar used every day on salads.
- Keep active in and around the house. Walk daily.
- Eat regularly but relatively small portions each mealtime.

- Peace of mind. Despite the shock of massacre, yearlong wars, bombs and grenades, and having lost her nearest and dearest, she was surrounded by a loving, calm peacefulness. 'Have faith, Dr. Viktor,' she emphasised.

- Rest. 'Forty winks' in the afternoon. De-stress; do not worry.

- Lots of laughter. Here I might add that the Lebanese people have a great sense of humour and their language is colourful and rich on puns as they play with words. They are masters of self-irony.

- The importance of good, supporting and loving family relations. Every day, Raymonde's mother Georgette would visit her in the quaint ground flat, which she shared with Aunty Laudy, Georgette's sister. When their brother Eli became seriously ill and needed kidneys transplantation, Aunty Laudy volunteered to give her brother a kidney, as tests showed good compatibility. Out of necessity, Eli had to keep a keen eye on his diet and especially the water he consumed and had, when I visited him, installed a water purification system in the house. Toxins and contaminants are enemies for all aspects of our waterworks—kidneys, bladder and prostate in particular. Again, back to the beginning of this book: It is better and smarter to prevent distress and illness before breakdown happens. Prevention is smarter and better than cure. 'A stitch in time saves nine', as the saying goes.

- The strong love of their country and Beirut, the 'Pearl of the Middle East' of Lebanon, 'The Switzerland of the Middle East' as it is also known.

Once she had listed these points, I said, 'Wow! But, Teta Montaha, that's just about the same as what I teach my clients and students in Norway. And there is real scientific proof confirming what you have known and practised all your life! Amazing!

I wrote down these points as we chatted and Teta Montaha enjoyed her water pipe, or *argyle* as it is called in the Orient. The art of vaporising and smoking flavoured tobacco called shisha, passing the vapour or smoke through a water basin made of glass before inhaling, is practised routinely in the Middle East and other countries. History tells us that these were invented by an Indian physician, Irfan Shaikh, at the court of Mughal Emperor Akbar. But others claim that the idea came from Persia. I must confess I liked the sound of the water chuckling away as the air stirred the water molecules, making them dance and sing for us. Beautiful blends of aromatic herbs, flowers, and the scent from the shisha stimulated the olfactory cells and the limbic areas of my brain, which solidified these happy memories.

One evening, back in the home of Grandmother Teta Montaha in Abdel Wahab El Inglizi, Beirut, I settled down in an old armchair trying to sort out all the impressions after a long day's excursion.

'I hear that you have been to the Monastery of St. Maron, to visit St. Charbel's resting place? How did you like that? Charbel was a Maronite monk and a priest, the first to be canonised, by Pope Paul 2, on 9 October1977,' explained Teta Montaha.

'It was fascinating! How about the documented stories of his ability for miracle healing?' I asked.

'A few months after his death, a bright light was seen surrounding his tomb. The superiors opened it to find his body still intact.'

Experts and medical doctors alike are unable to come up with a medical explanation for the incorrupt body and the fact that a bloodlike fluid flowed from the body. He died on 24 December1898 (70 years old). Both in the year 1950 and 1952, his tomb was opened and his body still had the appearance of a living man. Thousands of pilgrims have since visited his grave.

Through intersession, God blessed many with miraculous healings. My excitement grew as I told the whole family about our personal experience at the monastery. From studies of the Bible and historical documents, I knew for certain that Lebanon, and especially the Cedars, was a holy place and that Yeshua had wandered extensively in the land from south to north. I was curious to find out the route to the Mountain of Transfiguration, as I had figured out it could not be Israel's Tabor or Hebron, as most people believed.

After the whole family went outside and headed to the parking lot, I heard a calling and turned back and walked into the monastery, as I was given the exact directions as to where to find the answer to my pertinent question: 'Where is the Mountain of

Transfiguration?'

I heard the voice of God give the exact direction: 'Turn, go right, bend down by that shelf, in the monastery's bookshop and pick it up! And the first page you open will show you exactly the route Yeshua and his three disciples walked from Caesarea Philippi to the Cedar Mountain, God's Cedar. The book is called *Religious, Cultural and Political History of the Maronites'*, Page 142, by Rev Boutros, Dau. I went back to the parking area where I joined the rest of the family who were happy and flabbergasted when they heard my testimony.

As we shared yet another wholehearted and nutritious Lebanese meal, we bade farewell but not before praying for good health. As I held the hands of the amazingly graceful and healthy Teta Montaha, and received her blessing, we both had tears in our eyes. It was truly a moment to behold. Before our final hugs, kisses and '*au revoir, au revoir*', she revealed the secret to her unique rose-and-orange-blossom water from Damour. A gift of mutual love and respect.

Teach Diligently with Love, and Remember Me in Beirut! 'The Secret is in the Water'—Teta Montaha

'The secret is in the water, Dr. Viktor! And how you treat it: With tender love and care!' (TLC)—which goes to show that the principle of TLC is universal. One of life's many circles completed for a prepared mind and wondrous works of serendipity, don't you think?

Despite Teta Montaha's biblical (and scientifically proven) choices, and being a shining example of how you practise these elegantly, she never forced anybody to follow her examples.

'It's your choice and responsibility!' was her counsel to family members. Some followed it; others did not seem to care and so faced the consequences of disease and shortened lifespan. Teta Montaha had lost her dearly beloved husband, Antoine, who came from the village of Damour; a heavy smoker and champion backgammon player, he had died in his fifties. For Teta Montaha, then 47 years of age, this came as a shock. The grief and devastation of losing the love of her life caused to her to suffer a stroke and loss of speech. However, she recovered rapidly and regained her speech, resuming her daily walks in the neighbourhood of Achrafieh, Beirut.

At the age of 96 years old, she climbed a ladder in order to do some cleaning on top of a cupboard, fell and broke her femur neck. An operation was necessary—and much to the surgeon's amazement, there was no sign of osteoporosis!

This did not come as a surprise to me, as I knew her lifestyle choices in terms of nutrition and water. She avoided all the 'bone robbers' that are present in food, water and the environment. Dr John R. Lee, MD, my mentor and teacher in this field, revealed this to the world about 30 years ago: sadly, the world's highest-ranking country on the osteoporosis scale, Norway, still believes this affliction is some kind of mystery. The treatment and dismal results obtained by the country's 'experts' on osteoporosis are just as poor as they were 30 years ago. But you cannot expect otherwise when you are 'barking up the wrong tree'.

Teta Montaha is a crystal-clear example and inspiration for everybody, not least for her strong faith and admirable attitude despite very unfriendly circumstances: five wars, massacres, shootings, living in shelters for many years during bombings et cetera. One day, I asked her, 'What is your favourite meal or dish, Teta?'

'Tripe,' she answered.

'Tripe!' I exclaimed. 'But isn't that cow's stomach!?'

'Yes—and so? You can also make it without cow's stomach. It's delicious and very nutritious!'

Most people regard animal innards with revulsion, and some won't eat it in any shape or form. This prejudice remains, despite the fact that multitudes of delicious dishes featuring offal are prepared and served by the world's best chefs and consumed by connoisseurs of fine food. Clubs are formed solely for the appreciation and consumption of offal. Sydney Tripe Club is just one.

In France, offal reigns supreme as a delicacy. The French word for it is '*abats*', from the word '*abattoir*'. Is it because 'peasant' food from Gascony has more cachet than 'peasant' food from Northumberland or Leeds? Or is it just better food because of the vastly more sophisticated culinary culture of the places that developed these recipes in the first place? Tripe is a favourite dish in Italy, with a wealth of local versions—for example, '*Trippa alla Fiorentina*', braised with tomato and marjoram and served on a piece of bread called '*Lampredotto*'. It is also served with white beans and grated cheese.

Trippa alla Romana is flavoured with mint. It is served with a cheese sauce.

Conclusion

If your body could talk to you (it can!) what would be its number one question to you? 'Have you remembered your number one body, soul and mind ingredient today?'

'What's that?'

'Joy and gratefulness—expressed and put into action. Spread a little joy!' Look around you! Take a deep breath and be bold. Let go of any self-restraint and inhibition you may have in this area of your life. When was the last time you smiled and complimented the lady at the cash till? Words, actions, time spent, proper attitude, gifts of blessing, and a smile.

'*In the morning sow thy seed, and in the evening withhold not thine hand, for thou knowest not whether shall prosper, either this or that, or whether they shall both be alike good.*' (Ecclesiastes 11:6).

There is no question of both failing—however, both *may* produce fruit.

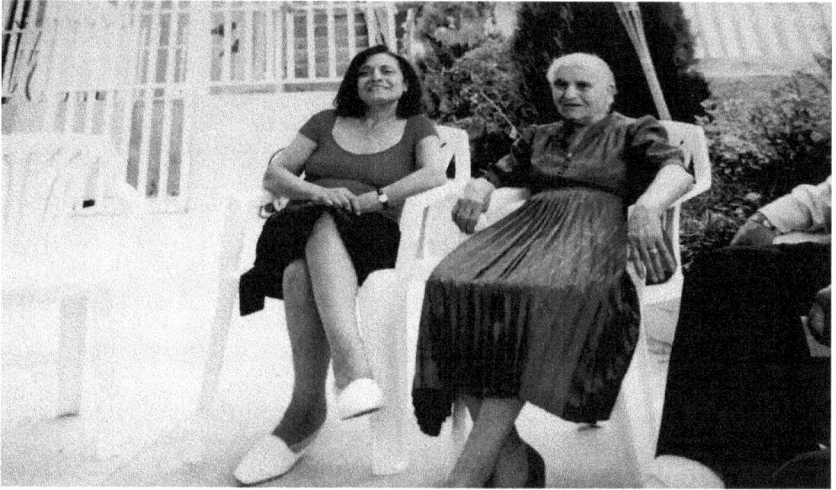

Aunty Laudy,with her mother Teha Montaha Azzi

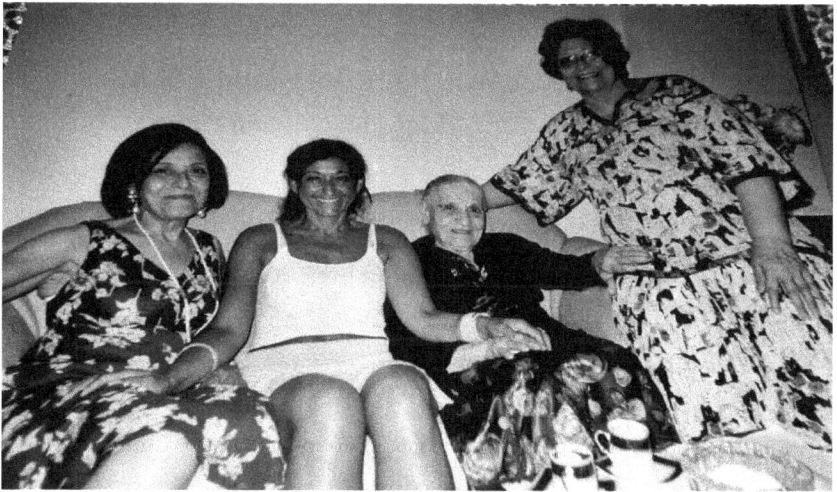

Aunty Laudy, grand daughter Raymonde Karam Fossan and her mother Georgette Karam.

CHAPTER TWELVE

Joy and Gratitude—DNA's Expressive Attitude

'Let us be grateful to the people who makes us happy; they are the charming gardeners who make our souls blossom'. Marcel Proust.

In War and Peace, Leo Tolstoy wrote 'that nothing is so necessary for a young man as the company of an intelligent woman'. All my life I have been surrounded by strong, intelligent and beautiful women and my visit to Lebanon was no exception.

Our Viking Heritage—A World of Exotic Offal and the Unexpected Bond Between Vikings and Phoenicians

The wise old Leo Tolstoy said, 'We are all asleep until we fall in love.' I most certainly had fallen in love with Lebanon and the people I met there.

Question: What does happiness mean to you? And what about luck? How can love change everything?

When I first asked Teta Montaha, at 103 years old, about her favourite dish, her answer, 'Tripe', surprised me a little. Curiosity got the better of me so I decided to do some research and find out why our own ancestors, the fearsome Vikings, relished in exotic dishes which have been completely forgotten by most people today.

Helge Ingstad (1899-2001), a latter-day Viking, was a living link in the mould of the great Norwegian explorers like Roald Amundsen, Fridtjof Nansen and Thor Heyerdahl. H. Ingstad travelled to the Northwest Territories of Canada and lived among the Inuit people, spending four years as a hunter and trapper. When he first arrived in the Canadian Arctic, people in the river communities would bet on the arrival of the river boats. By the time he left, stopping at Fort Resolution on the way out, these bets were on planes.

He proved conclusively that Greenlandic Norsemen had found a way across the Atlantic Ocean to North America roughly 500 years before Christopher Columbus and John Cabot. In his book *Trapper Life*, published in English as *The Land of Feast and Famine*, he describes life with a wandering Indian tribe he called 'wild reindeer-eaters', especially a reindeer hunt, which culminated in a real food orgy. He observed how the Indians did not go for the pure pieces of meat, which they gave to the dogs, but they gorged on liver, kidneys, bone marrow and lots of animal fat (offal). The bone marrow was eaten raw; the head of the reindeer, the brain, the fat behind the ears, the tongue, nose, blood, stomach and intestines were all devoured—glands, sinews and cartilage as well.

This kind of meal is highly nutritious, but to most Western people it seems distasteful, even offensive. The nutritional density and complexity makes this feast fit for a king, and our Viking ancestors were quite used to eating the whole animal, especially organs, fats and bone marrow. But as we have seen earlier in this book, offal is regarded by many connoisseurs of fine food as attractive and desirable from a culinary point of view. There is no doubt about the nutritious value of this kind of food and it would be sad if this knowledge was lost, as the new generation of fast-food lovers do not even know the value of good-quality stock from bones and bone-marrow structures, or the definitive health benefits of such food sources. They contain plentiful amounts of amino acids in balance with fatty acids and other nutrients, vitamins, minerals and trace minerals—preferably offal and organs from ecological farming.

The art of fermentation is well known by ingenious people in the arctic and further south. When the taste buds are not used to or trained to enjoy fermented food, it can be quite an ordeal, as the adventurer Lars Th. Monsen experienced during his trekking through the wilderness of Canada. Fermented reindeer stomach was almost too much to endure, much to the amusement of the tribe.

In Sudan and other countries in Africa, they have a great variety of fermented food, which is impressive and well described by Sue Shephard in the book: *Pickled, Potted, and Canned: How the Art and Science of Food Preserving Changed the World.*

One example is a dish called 'miriss', made from clean fermented fat, which is mixed to a paste and preserved in special barrels. Another product is, 'doddery', produced from fresh bones, which are cut into pieces and put in water in a 'burma' or barrel and left to ferment for three days. Afterwards, the liquid is ground to a mass.

If these food preservation techniques seem a bit strange, an easier and more convenient way is to start with liver and kidneys from lamb or calf. If you ever go to Scotland, do try their national dish, 'haggis'. This consists of minced heart, liver and lungs from sheep or calf, which is seasoned kidneys fat and oatmeal, cooked in the animal's stomach, a little similar to Teta Montaha's tripe in Beirut. Highly nutritious, healthy and tasty!

Growing up, we were served liver regularly—a healthy, plentiful source of Vitamin A, an important antioxidant necessary for good eyesight.

Henriette Schønberg Erken (1866-1953) described in her famous cookbook several dishes of liver and her own liver diet for a special blood condition. In Norway, liver was traditionally prepared by putting it in milk or water a couple of hours before making the dish.

Liver should be prepared with animal fat and a variety of root vegetables. According to Schønberg Erken, it is tastier if one uses white wine and tomatoes in the sauce. Kidneys should be parboiled in vital water and should always be cooled or grilled quickly, to prevent them from becoming hard. Kidneys can be used in stews, pies, casseroles, kidneys bread, kidneys stew, et cetera.

Stomach, tripe: This is quite a common dish and considered a delicatessen in many restaurants. A well-known dish is the French *tripe a la mode de Caen*; i.e., cooked stomach in Calvados. In Eastern Europe, it is quite common; Poland has its flaki, a soup with ox stomach.

Dishes prepared from animal blood (blood pudding, sausage,

blood bread), although forbidden territory for Jews and Muslims, are popular in Nordic countries where they have been a tradition for many years. Also for the Masai people in Kenya, a substantial proportion of their food consists of blood and fresh or sour milk.

'...I'll Grind his Bones to Make my Bread...'

Marrow is the soft gelatinous substance inside the bones. This delicatessen has been relished for centuries and many crushed remnants of bones from thousands of years back have been found on excavation sites.

According to the American sports physiologist Loren Cordain et al., bone marrow has probably been one of the major sources of energy for our ancestors. Bone marrow consists of AA (arachidonic acid) and DHA (docosahexaenoic acid), which are important building blocks for our brains. In addition, bone marrow contains many vitamins, minerals, trace minerals and other vital nutrients. It gives a rich taste to stock and sauces for meat and fish. Hulda Garborg (1862-1934) describes *'mergballer'*, which she made the same way as she makes balls of calf's brain; i.e., 'Marrow in a dough mixed with egg, parsley, salt, civic mace and dipped white bread.'

Time for a little adventure—a little kitchen expedition into the food halls of lore and love for the unknown, yet so healthy, nutritious longevity delicatessen. Bon Appétit! Be adventurous!

The Victorious Healing Story of Viktor

Viktor was a healthy new-born baby when I first saw him. Sparkling eyes, with a very good skin complexion. The pride of his parents, their firstborn child.

At one of the regular visits to the community doctor and nurse, his mother was advised to give him ´extra sustenance´ as they called it. Milk supplement and infant´s porridge were suggested. Even though Viktor was being breast-fed regularly from the day he was born and had achieved ´normal´ weight, his mother thought it wise to follow the advice of the experts. Little did she know of the agony and pain, worry and sleepless nights that were soon to follow.

Viktor started to develop red patches on his legs just two days after his first supplement of milk and porridge (maize). Soon he became very itchy. His face and entire body was covered in red, itchy and now exuding, often infectious sores. He was seen by several doctors, including a dermatologist and an allergy specialist who diagnosed him as a very serious case of eczema, one of the worst cases seen in one of Norway´s major hospitals.

His parents were offered the standard medical treatment: Antibiotics, hydrocortisone and moisturising lotions. The future prospect was dismal. He would most probably develop asthmatic-bronchitis or hay fever in his teens. The offer of treatment was politely declined much to the dismay of the specialist.

Then followed an arduous, long tour to see alternative specialists like several different homoeopaths, naturopath, reflexologist, kinesiologists, laser therapist. In the end all of them gave up their treatment of Viktor, who by then was very restless as his sores were very itchy, exuding and inflamed. His clothes stuck to his body and his mother had to change him up to 13 times a day by soaking him in a solution of Dead Sea water. He would wake up in the morning with his pillow covered in blood, even though his tiny fingers were strapped down with cotton and flannel gloves. Sleepless nights, worry, tears and agony became the pattern. Viktor was about three months old and he was clearly suffering a great deal.

At this stage Viktor´s mother approached me for help. The aim of the treatment which we agreed upon was:

- To remove all known allergens in his food and surroundings.
- Alleviate the skin irritation and reduce the itchiness, as this was a great distressing factor for mother and child.
- Restore the amino-acid balance.
- Supplement vitamins/minerals/others in order to restore his skin.
- To remove infections.
- To restore normal bowel movements.
- To stimulate his thymus gland.

He was immediately taken off the milk supplement and infants´ porridge, the great offenders which started the whole avalanche of symptoms and distress.

An initial improvement resulted, followed by a gradual

worsening of the symptoms. Having noticed that Viktor reacted to his mother's milk, we decided to radically change her diet as well. All the allergy specialists told us that there was no connection between his mother's food intake and Viktor's eczema. But our observation told us a different story. Having changed her diet to omit any suspicious allergens, we noticed an immediate improvement in Viktor's condition.

Then after a few days, Viktor was more or less back to the same stage. The mother still persevered on her basic diet consisting mainly of pure water, natural brown rice, Spirulina, one banana a day, juice from organic fruit and vegetables and homemade gluten-free bread.

On the recommendation of an allergy specialist, a skin prick test was performed on Viktor. The test showed a definite positive reaction of fish and egg, but through our own observation we knew he also reacted immediately if his mother drank cow's milk (pasteurised or non-pasteurised) plus a whole list of other food stuff that we used in the challenging process. What had originally started as an allergy-eczema provocation due to milk powder/porridge supplement had now triggered off a whole chain of allergic reactions. His eczema sores would start to swell and exudate if fish was being prepared, i.e. the smell alone was enough to provoke an immediate skin reaction.

Viktor was clearly hyper allergic, to such an extent that he nearly chocked to death one day at the breakfast table when he inadvertently touched the rim of a jar of herring and put his finger in his mouth.

At this stage Viktor´s mother was clearly suffering a great deal, too, through lack of sleep and the agony and worry of seeing her child, day and night, writhing and rubbing his sore, swollen and itchy skin incessantly.

Considering the fact that conventional medical treatment was out of the question and that the approach of several well qualified natural therapists had failed. I drew up a plan of action, using nutritional methods of treatment.

Having obtained his mother´s approval and full support, I had to establish foremost in my mind that any nutritional intervention would comply with the principle ´nil nocere – no harm´. The therapeutic approach had to be absolutely safe and gentle, yet effective.

I reasoned that Viktor´s delicate biochemical composition of amino-acids, enzyme and co-enzymes etc. was pretty in chaos. I therefore began searching for nutritional supplements that could meet the following criteria:

- Multi-vitamin and mineral, enzyme preparation that contained all the essential amino-acids in their natural balanced state.
- Reduce itchiness and calm the nerve system.
- Aid skin healing.
- Natural antibiotics.
- Natural anti-bacterial, non-allergenic, high bio-availability.

- Buffer or block allergic reactions in the intestines.
- Stimulate the immune system.
- Too quality, assessed by independent laboratories.
- Synergetic in its total effect.
- Easy and pleasing to take for the boy.

After much painstaking research, I opted for high potency royal jelly in citrus honey from Israel; the very best of its kind to be found, a first class nourishment, a mild, absolutely non-toxic preparation even for suckling infants. The rich and varied biochemical composition with its synergistic and therapeutic effect had met all the criteria listed in my plan of action.

I recommended one teaspoonful (at least) of high potency royal jelly a day for Viktor. With its natural sweetness caused by the citrus honey, it was easy and pleasant for min to take, either dissolved in lukewarm, pure water or just a plain teaspoonful. After some days, some improvement was observed, particularly with regard to his restlessness and itchiness.

Viktor´s mother stopped breast feeding him after six months. Even though she had persevered with her own rigid diet, the distress of seeing her own baby´s skin exudate whilst he was being breast-fed became too much of a distress.

Then followed a period where diluted Soya semp (soy milk) was tried. A little improvement was noticed for 10-14 days, before his condition flared up again. Milk of cashew nuts and sesame seeds were suggested, but resulted in the same irritated condition.

This was a period of great frustration for mother and child but still she preserved, giving him high potency royal jelly and strictly following the rules of avoiding anything that would irritate the boy´s skin. (Washing all new clothes to remove formaldehyde, ironing newly washed clothes to remove all bacteria, no softeners used in the washing and using low risk washing powders, double rinsing of washing and no smoking etc.)

A new search for an additional natural supplement/nourishment began that would meet my previously listed criteria. This time I emphasised properties such as: Good skin healing features, buffering/blocking mechanism against allergenic reactions in Viktor´s intestines/immune system. I also envisaged that this new nourishment/supplement would contain proteolytic enzymes and be synergistic in its total appearance.

I spent hours, days and nights searching. When the answer came, it seemed, at least to me, very obvious: Aloe Vera juice and gel, the medicinal plant that had been my treasure and love for many years.

Containing both lignin, saponins, anthraquinones, inorganic ingredients, minerals and vitamins mono and polysaccharides, enzymes (including proteolytic enzymes) amino acids (both essential and secondary) plus, plus. I also knew it contained bromelain, known to buffer or block allergic reactions. Well known for its synergism and its great power of penetration either used on the skin or from within, I recommended Viktor´s mother to give him one teaspoonful of Aloe Vera juice approximately 20 minutes before each feeding to allow the enzymes and other active ingredients to work at maximum potential. The improvement was there to be seen, a great encouragement for all of us!

His upon sores began to close, less frequent skin reaction, less itchiness. This time around, the improvement was stabilised. Again the search of had taken me to far corners of this world, to the USA and Israel again for the same reason. To get hold of the very best in quality, I selected stabilised Aloe Vera gel from Ein Yahav in the Negev desert in Israel. Apart from the stabilised Aloe Vera gel and juice, I recommended bathing Viktor in Dead Sea Salt solution (7-10 per cent strength) as this would also nourish his skin with vital minerals, salts and other micro elements. Both the aloe gel and juice and the Dead Sea Salt baths exhibited great abilities to penetrate the skin, nourishing and cleansing the damaged tissue.

The combination of this treatment worked very well indeed. Viktor's skin regenerated gradually. A stubborn spot on his cheek, however, would not heal until we received a fresh aloe vera leaf from the Negev dessert. Cutting a thin slice of the pulp of the fresh leaf, it was applied to Viktor's only open sore. Literally speaking, within minutes, a thin membrane was formed. The skin was healing!

Considering that most of Viktor's skin had the appearance of a raw hamburger, it was quite amazing to watch the healing in progress. Highly nutritional supplements from within and without and vice-versa.

His skin was completely healed by the time he was nine months old.

Rice and maize porridge were gradually introduced to his diet in addition to Spirulina which was crushed over his plate of porridge.

Spirulina, a plant, being highly nutritious, also came from Israel. My research had shown that many products of Spirulina on the marked contained too many heavy metals. One of the chief objectives with administering Spirulina is to take advantage of its great detoxification abilities. (That is why the Spirulina from Israel exhibited the best quality in this respect. Apart from that, it contained a vast amount of other vital ingredients that were of benefit to Viktor).

During this period, when Viktor was my patient, I kept in close and constant contact with is mother. A mutual trust was established from the beginning and the whole regime of treatment was put in a frame of tenderness, love and care. This principle was first pointed out to me by Miss Hollis, MBE, my former principal when I studied physiotherapy. It has been a major ingredient of all my treatment ever since.

A six-month ordeal had come to an end. The outcome for victorious Viktor was complete and full care of a nasty eczema and a deep rooted allergy for which the doctors and specialists had given him and his mother the bleakest of prospects.

On reaching his first birthday, he had the most glowing and radiant skin one could possibly imagine. Soon after that he proved to all of us that his allergy to fish, egg, milk and much more was something of the past, by eating just that and showing no reaction whatsoever.

According to the experts, they claimed the cure was impossible and the specialist at one of Norway´s major hospitals, where Viktor´s final diagnosis was made, refused to see him because his parents and his natural therapist had refused to follow their scheme of treatment by antibiotics, hydrocortisone and moisturising lotions.

Not only did they not want to hear about this wonderful story of healing of Viktor, but the specialist got away, cursed and threw his mother out of his office.

Later I had the great pleasure to receive numerous patients from all over Norway and abroad, including a family that came all the way from Dubai, United Arab Emirates. Their young boy was also completely healed.

At the same time our Holistic Centre started to use the services of Immunolaboratory in Florida and later York Nutritional laboratory, UK, world leading experts in their field. Their accurate blood analysis produced much faster results when food intolerances were a major issue. Around this time, we started on a long and interesting journey, - a water exploration, beginning with simple filtering solutions, through reverse osmosis, water distillation to water electrolysis.

CHAPTER THIRTEEN

Daniel's Diet and King Nebuchadnezzar

'Beans, beans the musical fruit. The more you eat,
the more you toot.
The more you toot, the better you feel.
So lift up your leg and let one squeal.' Anonymous.

Can ten days of vegetables and water bring about miracles beyond your imagination? If natural solutions of good health and God's blessings are so close and within the grasp of each and every one of us, why are so many falling into sadness and ill health?

You may recall the story from the Hebrew Bible of Daniel and his friends at the court of King Nebuchadnezzar; they refused to eat any of the food offered by the King, and said to the overseer whom the commander of the officials had appointed over them, 'Please test your servants for ten days, and let us be given some vegetables to eat and water to drink.'

The vegetables here are the same as in the Bible Diet— namely pulses, legumes and seeds. Daniel could have chosen to eat clean meat and drink liquids other than water. These were not forbidden according to heretical dietary laws. However, the king's meat did not meet the standards for health. The food was offered to idols.

The king's food was sensual and detrimental, and wines of

the king were likely fermented and also poured out as a tribute to the gods of Babylon. As a captive in a foreign land, Daniel challenged the king, and at the end of the ten days, 'their appearance seemed better and they were fairer and fatter (stronger) in the flesh' than all the children who did eat the king's meals.' (Daniel 1:8)

As for these four youths, God gave them knowledge and intelligence in every branch of literature and wisdom. Daniel even understood all kinds of visions and dreams. At the end of the 10-day challenge, the king admitted that none was found that could match Daniel and his friends; so they entered the king's personal service. 'As for every matter of wisdom and understanding about which the king consulted them, he found them ten times better than all the magicians and conjurers who were all in his realm.' Daniel 1:15-21.

Beans and Vital Water

Pulses, beans and legumes should be viewed as food for ordinary folks and royalty alike, as they are a powerhouse of dense nutrients. Many scientific research papers have been published on the health benefits of beans. The *Archives of Internal Medicine* show in one paper that adding more beans to the diet can help people with diabetes to control their blood sugar levels. Beans contain oestrogen-like compounds and PIs (protease inhibitors). These help prevent the growth of cancer cells by interfering with cancer-producing enzymes.

According to medical anthropologist John Heinemann, 'Pi's

prevent radiation-induced cancer and enhance tissue resistance to invasion by tumour cells.'

Beans reduce cholesterol, as we have seen reported in several medical journals including *The American Journal of Clinical Nutrition* (Oct. 1983). Beans lower serum cholesterol and triglyceride levels, preventing fat from being formed in the blood vessels.

Fava beans are an excellent source of L-dopa, the drug used to treat Parkinson's disease, to control trembling and rigidity. L-dopa from fava beans also stimulates strong, healthy erections in men. 8-16 ounces of fava beans is often enough to relieve male impotence. Amazingly, fava sprouts contain 10 times as much L-dopa as non-sprouted ones.

All beans contain lea thin and choline, which increase acetylcholine in the brain, which can improve memory. People with Alzheimer's have too much heavy metal toxicity, which interferes with nerve-impulse transmission and production of acetylcholine, a neurotransmitter substance.

So if I had diabetes or Alzheimer's, I would certainly eat more beans.

Excellent juices for lowering blood sugar, according to Dr. Paavo Airola, come from beans, nettles, celery, watercress, cucumber, onions, garlic, lettuce.

A recommended, easy and fun read is *The Best Treatment*, by Isadore Rosenfeld H. D. (1992). And of course the only bean you should not eat is the soybean, because it contains neurotoxins and phytoestrogens that are very strong. A baby consuming only soy formula is consuming the equivalent of four birth control pills a day. The high levels of phytic acid in soy inhibit the body's ability to absorb important minerals like zinc, magnesium, copper, calcium and iron.

The goitrogens in soy are potent anti-thyroid compounds that can lead to endocrine disruption. Infants on soy formula have a much higher risk of autoimmune thyroid disorders. Soy also contains protease inhibitors, which can block enzymes that are necessary for the digestion of certain proteins.

Kidneys-bean-pod tea has been used to permanently cure diabetes. This is the *Vital Water* in which the pods, not the beans, have been cooked (Dr Ramm of Preetz Germany). This tea can also bring remarkable permanent cures for kidneys and bladder troubles (Rex Adams in Miracle Medicine Deeds, 1977).

Soy is often promoted as an alternative food for celiac- and gluten-intolerant people, but lecithin can be harmful to the intestines and prevent healing even when gluten is removed. Consumption of soy foods and soy lea thin (in 'health' bars and protein powder) increases the body's need for Vitamin D, B-D calcium and magnesium. In addition, nearly all the soy products on the marked are heavily sprayed with chemicals and gene-modified. 2 chemical compounds in soy have been defined as carcinogen, causing cancer.

Beans are very nutritious, low fat, high fibre and protein, full of vitamins and minerals; however, they come with a major downside: they make you pass wind, big time! Dry beans, when improperly prepared can make give you flatulence. Oh, woe the terrible evenings spent in a 'Dutch oven' with your spouse waking you up with loud joyous gaseous eruptions.

The solution is to soak the beans overnight in *Vital Water*. After they have soaked, you should notice a frothy substance floating on top of the water. This is, among other things, refined sugar, which we are trying to get rid of. Rinse well and clean. Put the beans in *Vital Water*. You can then either cook the beans in a pressure cooker, which will give you nice, tender beans but will take about six hours; or on the stove, which will take four hours. You can also cook the beans in the oven at 250-300 degrees, which will take about four hours. After this you can add good-quality salt.

Good morning Thor of Thunder! Welcome SBD (Silent but Deadly)

If you are still concerned about the issue of passing wind and are afraid the 'fart taxman' may come checking on your methane discharge, take comfort on the following: Be happy and enjoy passing wind! And be happy that our anus is placed at the end of our digestive system. We should be grateful that we are not created like the crinoids, a marine creature with an unshaped gut that has its anus located next to its mouth. And, yes, everybody does it—from kings to presidents, to opera singers, beauty queens, nuns and you and me. See the Britney Spears music video, '*Oops, I did it again*'! Even Emperor Claudius passed a law legalising passing wind, at banquets out of concern for people's health!

Mate-in-a-State shows footage of flatus ignition, and apparently farts burn with a blue flame—and according to Dr. James L.A. Roth, a blue flame indicates the presence of methane in the flatus. All methane producers, an elite group of the population, have founded an exclusive club called The Royal Order of the Blue Flame.

'Are there any books out there on the subject of farting?' you may ask—and, yes, there are several. *'Who Cut the Cheese? A Cultural History of the Fart'* by Jim Dawson. Entertaining, thought-provoking and very funny!

Our friend, dear Ben Franklin, whom you have definitely become acquainted with in this book, wrote the essay, *Fart proudly*, and it is still in print in other forms: *Who Farted Now?* By St. Martin's Press. *The Gas Pass: The Story of Farts* by Shinta Cho and *Good Families Don't,* by Alan Daniel and Robert V. Munsch.

For more information on this fascinating topic, check out *Facts or Farts* by Brenna Lorenz on the Net. Good morning thunder! Or welcome SBD (silent but deadly).

But happy is the man (or woman!) who has an Air Fresh ionisation unit when the morning thunder or the sneaky, silent but deadly ones become too overwhelming!

Conclusion

Knowledge and time-tested health solutions from natural and divine sources are gifts to mankind. It all begins and ends with the proper understanding of living water, the mother and matrix of all life, as Nobel Prize Winner Albert Szent-Györgyi once said.

CHAPTER FOURTEEN

All you Need Is Love, Music and a Cat

'Women and cats will do as they please,
and men and dogs should relax and
get used to the idea'. Robert A. Heinlein.

Leonardo da Vinci expressed his feelings when he said, 'Even the smallest feline is a masterpiece.'

Before heading home for Norway, we went for a stroll through the Achrafieh neighbourhood of Beirut, where Raymonde sometimes played football with Bachir Gemayel, the Christian leader who later became President of Lebanon on 23.8.1982, when the country was torn by civil war and occupied by both Israel and Syria. A much-loved and respected politician and militia commander, he was assassinated on 14.9.1982 along with 26 others, when a bomb exploded in the Beirut Phalange headquarters. It seemed odd that such a peace-loving nation as Lebanon had become a battle arena for many groups and nations. If you would like an in-depth story about Lebanon's desperate travails, I would recommend the explosive *Pity the Nation* by Robert Fisk, a distinguished award-winning author who writes an epic account of the conflicts, carnage, betrayal and political blindness.

It is a well-known fact that many people can suffer from post-traumatic stress disorder (PTSD) often resembling chronic fatigue syndrome (CFS) after travails of war and conflicts of longstanding tension. Stress hormones are released into the bloodstream, affecting all parts of the body, and weakening overall immunity. 'How did you cope in these horrendous circumstances?' I asked Teta Montaha and other family members.

'By loving and nurturing one another.'

'Do you remember, RoRo, when uncle Boulous would surprise us with his newly baked croissants?'

'Of course, Teta!' exclaimed RoRo—and he was around 70 years of age at the time. 'I clearly remember the beautiful aroma and the delicious taste of fresh baking filling the emergency shelter!'

'It made us forget the war for a while', said Teta, smiling, revealing her sparkling eyes with their crow's feet and well-earned lines and wrinkles. 'But boy, oh, boy, did we got a big shock when Maron came running down to our shelter, all covered in concrete dust after a bomb had hit your home, splintered the fine crystal baccarat chandelier, and nearly killed your stubborn dad. Remember, RoRo?'

'Bless him! From that day on, he moved down with the rest of us in the bomb shelter. The man with the big heart, the water carrier who somehow always managed to get us fruit and vegetable throughout those years.'

'By faith and constantly praying' War brings out the worst and the best in people. The loving and caring relationship in this family, which I was fortunate to meet and get to know, gave me a valuable insight into the resilience of the human mind. The family stayed in the emergency shelter on and off for eight years.

Your joy is your sorrow unmasked
And the self-same well from which
Your laughter that rises was oftentimes
Filled with your tears.
And how else can it be?
The deeper that sorrow carves into
Your being, the more joy you can contain.
Is not your cup that holds your wine
The very cup that was burned into
The potter's oven?
And is not the lute that soothes
Your spirit, the very wood that
Was hollowed by knives.
From The Prophet, by Kahlil Gibran

The importance of practising tender loving care (TLC), which had been installed into my heart from childhood, emphasised and taught further by the eminent principal of Bradford School of Physiotherapy, became very apparent as I talked to this family.

To paraphrase a famous line from The Caring Physician, the Harvard terminal physician Francis W. Peabody, 'For the secret of the wounded.'

Everyone has had traumatising experiences during their

lifetime, with all the emotional reactions that follow and the bodily functions that are affected: organ dysfunction, symptoms and diseases. Some researchers and clinicians tell us that all diseases start in the mind, with an emotional imbalance. Scientific proof says that you can heal yourself through the mind. Conventional medicine calls anything that does not outperform placebo 'quackery'—and in doing so implies that all conventional medicine is double-blind, randomised, controlled and hence scientific. Only about 20% of conventional medical treatment fulfils these criteria data from WHO. If most CAM (complementary and alternative medicine) and other medical treatment comes from the placebo effect, it is because the practitioners have understood something vitally important about illness and the relationship between the healer and the wounded (patient) as a caring, nurturing relationship. A well-intended, heart-to-heart relationship of TLC, as I have experienced personally through four decades in the caring and healing profession, and now witnessed through this warm and loving family in Lebanon.

No other factor has a greater impact on our lives than TLC, the healing power of love and care.

Teta Montaha and her family used to have three cats, Minouche, Mimi and Mirzo, who were greatly loved and cared for during the war. Comfort, love and compassion in unison, these cats, one tomcat and two queen cats, were royally treated with sardines and tuna.

When Maron, the head of the family, came home from his long working hours at his garage, he often prepared a favourite meal for his feline friends: cooked chicken wings, the smell of which was quite overpowering for Georgette and the rest of the family. Sometimes boxes of tuna fish and sardines were served as another treat for these compassionate cats. They always seemed to be hungry as they gathered in the kitchen and the trio hit the high notes of meowing! *Meow! Meow!* Afterwards, each of them would clean themselves and jump into somebody's lap for some cuddling, singing the praise of *Hakuna Matata: No worries for the rest of your days, Maron! Do you hear? No worries!*

The three educated cats of Abdel Wahab El Inglizi had picked up some Swahili singing:

Hakuna Matata,
'What a wonderful phrase
Ain't no passing craze
No worries for the rest of your days.'

The tomcat, Mirzo, would sing: 'If my fur and aroma lack a certain appeal, I can clear the bombed neighbourhood for every chicken wing meal!' Onomatopoeias were not foreign territory for them (a word that phonetically imitates or suggests the source of the sound that describes it). But whoever it was who told them that 'hakuna' in Lebanese means 'talk to us' remains a mystery. But talk they did—through their compassion, love and care. A wonderful comfort in the hardship of war.

These marvellous cats were not as well known, however, as

the famous Crimean wartime cats Tom Tiddles, Faith, and Able Seacat Simon and Pfc. Hammer. But the three cats of wartime Beirut all deserve medals for their deep, affectionate love and gallantry.

A Phalangist Leader and a Medical Doctor

Poor Minouche suffered a slow and painful death as a sniper's bullet or a slingshot from some street mugger hit her. She dragged herself home, with some of her intestines hanging out from a gaping and bleeding abdominal wound, and sighed her last *Hakuna Matata* in the garden of K. Maron's home at George Leidan, where Pierre Gemayel, the founder of the Phalangist Party and father of Bachir and Amin, who later became elect Presidents of the country, sometimes came to drink coffee.

Mirzo, the tomcat ruler of the neighbourhood, suddenly disappeared, presumably lost in battle. The whereabouts of the feline cat Mimi, the greatest singer of them all, disappeared during the siege of Achrafieh, never to be found again.

Dr Albert Schweitzer, a Christian doctor who received the Nobel Peace Prize in 1952 for his philosophy on '*Reverence of Life*', put it this way: 'There are two means of refuge from the miseries of life: music and cats.'

Teta Montaha and her family in Abdel Wahab El Inglizi are living proof of just that. The music and dance provided by RoRo at an early age, and the three unique cats soothed and alleviated the constant tension of a war-torn Lebanon.

'Even the smallest feline is a masterpiece,' according to Leonardo da Vinci. From time to time I have treated animals—dogs and cats mostly. Through being with our animals, we induce a calm, relaxed response in our bodies, much needed in our stressful environment. I always recommend that my patients consider getting an animal for mutual care and love. Think about it: 'A meow messages the heart.' A good heart is a form of preventative and palliative medicine of joy, without side effects.

Our cat in Norway is called Sozo, taken from the Greek word, which means *salvation* or *making whole*—implying complete healing and deliverance, just reminding us about Yeshua, Our Lord, the Saviour's name and meaning.

Our four-legged friends deserve the best. I think it was President Barack Obama who expressed it so succinctly when he said, 'How we treat our animals reflects how we treat each other.'

If you put a bowl of alkaline, restructured water and a bowl of ordinary water in front of your dog or cat, they will always choose the one with vital water. By instinct, they know what is best for them—and we, of superior intelligence, should do the same. Pure Energy Norway!

'Give us by Day our Daily Bread' (Luke 11:3)

Grain has been humanity's basic form of nourishment, since the Creation. The ripe gold kernels contain carbohydrates, protein, fats, minerals and vitamins and may be—rightfully—considered the perfect vegetable source. In Isaiah 55:10-11, we read, 'As the rain and snow come down from heaven and do not return to it without watering its earth and making it bud and flourish, so that it yields seed for the sower and bread for the eater, so is my word that goes out from my mouth.'

Wheat and barley are first on the list of the Seven Species in Deuteronomy 8:8, well known in the Holy Land. Botanists refer to emmer wheat as 'the mother of wheat'. This was the name given by pioneering Jewish agronomist Aaron Aaronsohn, who rediscovered it in the mountains of upper Galilee of Israel in the early twentieth century.

It is significant that the word for bread in Egyptian Arabic is *a'ash*, coming from the root word for *life*. But the ancients discovered that, with all its nutrients, grain could not easily be digested in its raw form. But the versatility of this food became apparent when boiled in vital water, becoming or porridge; or bakes, when it became bread. If it gets wet, don't throw it away! The art of fermentation was discovered by a stroke of serendipity—whereby the stored carbohydrates convert into sugar. When the grains are sprouted, grind it and add some water with squeezed fruit and their skins, which contain natural strains of yeast; given the right conditions, this produces beer. It was an ingenious farmer who first discovered this—as chronicled in Egyptian clay models and Mesopotamian text. 'Happy is the man with a mouthful of beer' is an Egyptian saying (Chapter 1).

Grain can be eaten fresh for a short period of time, when it is green and soft, in the spring. This is what Yeshua and the disciples did when they walked through a field on the Sabbath, plucking it and eating it as they walked. The grain at this point is now known as caramel, translated into in English as 'new grain'. Grain can also be eaten roasted, parched or toasted, which converts the starches into sweet-tasting dextrin (Ruth's Book 2:14), a favourite ingredient in macrobiotic cooking.

The original wheat (Triticum durum) and barley (Hordeum vulgare), together with vital, structured, hexagonal water, are all the gifts of health and longevity from our Creator.

'For the Lord your God is bringing you into a good land, a land of streams and pools of water, with springs flowing in the valley and hills, a land with wheat and barley, vines and fig trees, pomegranates, olive oil and honey.' (Deut. 8:7-8)

But watch out for the grim reaper! Healthy bread with unadulterated, all-natural ingredients is rarely found these days when profit, long shelf life and appearance are the name of the game. Modern bread is shockingly full of unnecessary and harmful ingredients such as hydrolysed or hydrogenated fats and oils, gen-modified soy flour, lecithin, emulsifier, additives, bleach, preservatives, and enzymes. These ingredients do not have to be declared. In this way, a Muslim, Jew or vegetarian cannot be guaranteed that the bread does not contain phospholipase, which comes from the pancreas of the pig. Through dishonest and deceitful marketing playing on the look and feel of real baked bread and proper handcrafting, it is nothing but the ugly reaper's recipe to rob us of our health. Another chapter of shame from the food industry. The prophet Isaiah was spot on when he declared, 'Why do you use money for something that is not bread?' (Isaiah 55:2.)

About thirty years ago, a burly baker came to our clinic for treatment, and during one of our conversations I mentioned by chance the name of my favourite bread, the Birkebeiner bread, whereupon he burst out laughing, shaking so much I thought he was going to fall off the plinth. 'You eat that stuff? Ha ha! Some of the secret stuff we put in the breads and do not need to be declared. It is close to rat poison!' he hollered.

I took immediate note—he was, after all, the director of one of the biggest bread producers in the county—and threw away our entire stock of this so-called 'healthy' bread. A little tip for you is to check out Andrew Whitley's book, *Bread Matters*.

A Divine Miracle Healing of Coeliac Disease

Coeliac disease—gluten/gliadin intolerance or allergy—has been steadily increasing over the last decades. There are many reasons for this unhappy state of affairs, but much can be accounted for by looking and investigating the ever-increasing amounts of toxins, chemicals and contaminants of our environment and our disrespectful way of handling nature, water, air and food. Together with toxic vaccination, this explains the epidemic rise of autoimmune diseases—of which coeliac disease is one of many.

Some years ago I got a telephone call from a very concerned

mother who told me about her two boys who had severe coeliac disease—allergic to gluten and confirmed by biopsy, the intestinal walls lacked to a great extent villi and enzymes for proper digestion. Diarrhoea was a constant problem, even though they exercised restrictions in their diets, always trying to avoid gluten. Emergency hospital admission was not unknown for the family. Their mother's request was a straightforward question:

'Mr Espedal, we've heard that you pray for sick people— Can you please pray for our boys and put your hands on them?'

'Of course!' I said.

I will never forget the day when the two boys arrived, 10 and 12 years old, with their mother. Their faith and anticipation of a miracle was clearly evident when I asked them two questions:

'Do you believe in God? Do you think Yeshua can heal you today?'

I got two resounding confirmations. And when they were both lying on the plinth at the same time, I prayed for a divine healing from Yeshua, our great physician, healer and Saviour, as my hands were placed on their tummies.

The mother later told me, 'When we came down to the car, the boys were so excited that they wanted to go home and eat bread and drink coke! Which under normal circumstances would have led to immediate diarrhoea, and possibly hospital admission. I tried to calm them down, but they insisted. The youngest even said, "Mum—when Gunnar removed his hands it was as if there was someone else's hands there!"'

The same day, they feasted on previously 'forbidden food', but this time experienced no pain or diarrhoea. Smiles and a happy family all round. And it stayed that way. They were completely healed of coeliac disease, something the medical doctors at the university hospital confirmed by performing a new biopsy. The insides of the intestinal walls were now covered with normal villi and in perfect functional order. Many years later and they are still healed—a God given miracle!

Conclusion

Are you aware of the pitfalls and deceptions created by the food industry and how to best avoid these? Take one step at a time, by weeding out unnecessary, unnatural and harmful food with additives and contaminants—and instead choose wholesome, nutritional and natural foods.

CHAPTER FIFTEEN

A Little Tour of the Healing Waters

'Would that I were a dry well, and that people tossed stones in me,
for that would be easier than to be a spring of flowing water that
the thirsty pass by, and from which they avoid drinking'.
Khahil Gibran.

Water in all its form and variations, from saunas to spas, from the Dead Sea to *Trinkhallen* have fascinated people all over the world. Embracing the new technology in water purification, ionisation and restructuring has already brought great health benefits worldwide. The thousands of testimonials are as good a proof as the scientific back-up that exists around this health advancement. This is a health blessing that is here to stay.

In various cultures, water has been touted and revered for its curative and pain-relieving features, mainly attributed to the mineral properties, thermal and even miraculous healing qualities.

My first encounter with hydrotherapy, defined as the external and internal use of water for treating disease, happened inadvertently—as you may recall—on a large pond in Manningham Park in Bradford, England on a blisteringly cold late autumn day. The icy-cold water made for an unusual debut into the hydrotherapy world of Yorkshire, which almost ended in shock following hypothermia (abnormally low body temperature). But I was saved by the bell and recuperated in a very hot bathtub, almost deliriously happy, though exhausted, after the strenuous battle to win the boat race. 'Once a Viking, always a Viking!'

The therapeutic use of water, on the other hand, is among the earliest healing practices. Indeed, drinking or bathing in springs, streams or pools for therapeutic purposes predate recorded history. Archaeological evidence points out mineral springs in Asia during the Bronze Age (ca. 3000 BC) and the Bible speaks of it in Joshua 19:35, referring to the city of Hammath (From the Hebrew world for 'hot springs') located at Tiberius in Israel, one of the world's oldest spas. In 2 Kings 5:10, we hear that the prophet Elisha instructed a Syrian to wash seven times in the River Jordan to cure his leprosy.

Whilst in 'the land of milk and honey', it is of course natural to explore the most celebrated and mineral-rich large body of water in the world, The Dead Sea in Israel. As a result of having no outlet and only the River Jordan flowing into the water basin from the north, dissolved minerals are left behind, leading to high concentrations of minerals in the sea, such as sodium, potassium, calcium, bromide and magnesium salts. There are 21 minerals in the Dead Sea, 12 of which are not found in any other body of water. Along the shoreline, there are several thermo-mineral springs containing many minerals, predominantly sulphur, exploiting the health-giving properties of thalassotherapy. It is also the earth's lowest elevation on land, 427 metres below sea level. Biblically, it was the refuge for King David and was a health resort for King Herod. The region produces a wide range of products, from Balms for Egyptian mummification to potash for fertilisers, cosmetics and herbal soaps and sachets.

Dead Sea water has a density of 1.240 kg/l, making swimming more like floating. People come from all over the world to get relief from mainly arthritis, psoriasis, cystic fibrosis and allergy. The stable climate, salt baths, black mudpacks and very low pollen count in the air make it an ideal and unique place. Negev researchers at Ben Gurion University of Negev have discovered that mineral-rich packs can augment conventional medical treatment.

In Genesis 13:13, God destroyed Sodom and Gomorrah, 'the cities of the plain', by an intense conflagration ('fire and brimstone') but not until Abraham's nephew Lot and his family were allowed to flee to safety. According to the Bible, 'the men of Sodom were wicked'. Archaeological evidence located the two cities to the southeast of the Dead Sea or in that vicinity. The cities burnt down with intense heat. The area used to be covered by the Dead Sea before it receded.

A Right Royal Pampering, Cleopatra and I

King Herod the Great built several fortresses and palaces on the Western bank of the Dead Sea, including the fortress of Masada, where John the Baptist was said to have been imprisoned and beheaded.

Cleopatra, the Queen of Sheeba, King Herod, and even the author of this book have all immersed themselves into the Dead Sea, to naturally rejuvenate in this unique hydrotherapy pool—a stark contrast to the freezing cold Manningham Park experience! According to legend, Cleopatra even built the first spa in this area, and celebrities like Julianne Moore and Susan Sarandon have been inspired to relax and rejuvenate in the Dead Sea. When you see the Dead Sea for the first time, as I did in 1987, you become awestruck by the calmness and natural beauty of the place. So it was with some trepidation that I waded into the water, six times saltier than the ocean. The water is warm and feels thick and heavy. The salinity and density make you float like a buoy in the ocean. You can easily read a magazine or newspaper whilst on your back. The Dead Sea and black mud have an astringent effect on the skin: the very natural skin treatment which Cleopatra and the Queen of Sheeba—and I— enjoyed. What fun and frolic, *habibi*, to have shared the same healthy and rejuvenating waters as kings, queens and other royalty.

The Greeks believed that springs and spas had supernatural healing properties because they thought the gods dwelt in these places. Therapeutic centres, often called Asclepieia—after Asclepius, the mythological god of health—were built around the mineral-rich springs throughout Greece. The Romans followed their practice and established spas across their empire, changing their deity name to *Aesculapius*, and built one in Bath, England, so named because of its hot springs, together with a magnificent temple.

During the 18th century, there was a revival in the medical use of spring water among some Italian, German and English physicians. In Karlsbad, for instance, the accepted method for drinking mineral water required sending large barrels to individual boarding houses where patients drank their dosages, prescribed by a physician, in the solitude of their rooms. In 1777, however, Dr David Beecher recommended that patients come to the fountain to drink and do a set of prescribed exercises. This innovation increased the medicinal benefits, and gradually physical activity began to be part of the European bathing regime.

In 1979 Dr. James Currier in England published his book *The Effects of Water, Cold and Warm, as a Remedy in Fever and Other Diseases*, advocating the external and internal use of mineral water as part the holistic curing process. The emphasis on the drinking of the water led to the development of separate structures known as *Trinkhallen* (drinking halls) where those taking part in the cure spent hours drinking water from the springs.

However, by the mid-19th century, the situation had changed dramatically. Visitors to the European spas were now putting the emphasis on bathing as well as drinking the spring water. We now see *trinkhalle*, the bathhouse, the *inhalotorium* (for inhaling the vapours), and the *kurhaus* or conversation halls that became the centre of social activity. Baden-Baden featured golf courses and tennis courses, 'quaint lawns where wild dears are unafraid'. Patients at Baden-Baden were required to see a doctor, as the resort specialised in treating rheumatoid arthritis.

The 19th-century bathing regimen at Karlsbad can serve as a general rule on the daily practice of European spa resorts at the time: 'Visitors arose at 6:00 a.m. to drink the water and be serenaded by a band, followed by a light breakfast, bath and lunch. The doctors at Karlsbad gave advice on nutrition and meals. In the afternoon, visitors went sightseeing or attended concerts. Theatre performances followed the evening meal, which usually ended around 9:00 p.m. with the patients returning to their boarding houses to sleep until 6:00 the next morning, and usually continued for a month, when the patients returned home until next year.

Peter Kesling, a physician and professor in Munich, Germany, has observed approximately 300 spas, all licensed by the federal government, and each having a medical staff, a 'spa doctor' (Badearzt). He saw that people living in and around areas of a spa and drink and use the facilities experienced no goitre, which led to the discovery that the water contained iodine, an essential element needed by the thyroid gland. Elsewhere in Europe and the US, water that included other specific ingredients, such as lithium, used to treat maniac depressive disorder and radon, a radioactive gaseous element reputedly effective in treating rheumatism, began to be in vogue. American spas followed, inspired by the popularity of the European resorts. In the hills of eastern Kentucky was a sort of poor man's spa. In 1911, an advertisement for this spa read, 'Health-Giving Mineral Waters. The water contains 25 grains of solid matter to the gallon, composed mainly of carbonates of calcium, magnesium and sodium, and traces of chlorides and sulphates of sodium and potassium, and a trace amount of strontium.' This water is very wholesome and has great medicinal value,' said Alfred M. Peters, a chemist.

The wealthy and famous came to the baths on a seasonal basis to recuperate and drink the water and to display their opulence. Social activities in Bath, UK, included dances, concerts, cards, lectures, sporting and other leisure activities such as tennis or croquet.

A typical day at Bath might start with an early morning communal bath followed by a private party. Afterwards, one usually drank water from the pump room, a building constructed over the thermal water source, or attended a fashion show. Physicians would encourage the health patrons to bathe and drink the waters with resolution and courage. The rest of the day would be spent on shopping, visiting the library, attending concerts, and stopping at one of the coffeehouses, or simply promenading along the esplanade. The rich and famous participated in this at around 4.00 p.m. Next came dinner, more promenading, and an erupting of dancing or gambling. 'Oh, dear; how strenuous this spa working has become! Must come home to rest, dear', said the water-wise man.

In the English coastal town of Scarborough in 1626, a Mrs Elisabeth Farrow discovered a stream of acidic water running from the cliffs south of the town. This was thought to have medicinal health benefits (see previous chapter on 'acidic water'), and resulted in the birth of Scarborough Spa. Dr White's book about Spa Water and its curing properties was published in 1660 and attracted a flood of visitors to the town. Sea bathing was added to the cure, and Scarborough became Britain's first seaside resort.

In the 17th century, most upper-class Europeans washed their clothes with water and only washed their faces with linen, believing that bathing the whole body was a lower-class activity. But the upper class slowly began to change their attitudes towards bathing as a way to restore their health later that century.

Anne, Queen of Great Britain, travelled to Bath, the former Roman development, to enjoy the benefit of the waters. A short time later, Richard Nash, the arbiter of good taste and manner at the time, came to Bath. Together with financier Ralph Allen and architect John Wood, they transformed Bath from a country spa into the social capital of England. Bath set the tone for other spas in Europe to follow.

The formal architectural development took place in the European spas in the 18th century. The architecture of Bath, developed along Georgian and Neoclassical lines, generally followed Palladian structures. The most important feature was the 'crescent', a semi-elliptical street plan used in many areas of England and which is very characteristic for Bath.

EU Directive: Only Smell, Don't Drink the Water!

In March 2012, the newspapers *The Daily Mail* and *The Daily Express* reported that visitors were told only to smell the healing water of Harrogate, after the bureaucrats at EU declared it a health risk to drink it. Online readers of the news—and the rest of England I presume—reacted with disbelief and anger. The high content of sulphuric acid, the highest in Europe, would not entice anybody to drink vast quantities of it.

Harrogate's healing waters, with the highest concentration of sulphur water in Europe has been drunk by hundreds of thousands including Tsar Nicholas II of Russia and Charles Dickens. The first wells in the town date back to the late 16th century, but it was during the Victorian era that 'taking the waters' became big business. Council officials have now been forced to turn off the taps when the EU rules branded the sulphur water—once said by the Victorians to cure ailments from gout to lumbago—'unwholesome'. Even if the water is turned back on, warning signs will have to be put up encouraging tourists to smell rather than swallow the water. 'You must be joking!

Local Tory MP Andrew Jones said, 'I cannot believe this EU-regulation was meant to apply to water that is part of a one-off historical experience rather than water one would drink on a daily basis for refreshment.'

Historian Malcolm Neesam said, 'Generations of Harrogate's greatest citizens would turn in their graves at the thought that foreign and unelected nosy parkers could ever be in a position to ban the waters of England's first and greatest spa.'

Could this be a 'smoke-screen tactic' to divert the public's attention to the real, toxic cocktail that is actually in every household's water? Heavy minerals such as mercury, cadmium, arsenic, barium, chromium, tin, silver, selenium, which bio-accumulate in the body and act like neuron-toxins, gradually damaging your health. Many of these minerals can cause cancer. Or what about water purification chemicals like chlorine, trihalomethanes, acrylamide from polymers, ethylene chloride, ammonia, formaldehyde, epichlorohydrin. (Check out *National Standards for Drinking Water Treatment Chemicals.*)

Is EU-approved water killing you softly? From one attentive reader, I quote, 'Hartlepool used to have what was probably the best water in Britain. It was hard but lovely to drink and also perfect for making tea. Now, as a result of EU legislation, which demands that certain chemicals must be added to the drinking water, the water has an unpleasant smell and leaves an awful sludge in cups of tea. Another example of EU meddling gone wrong. The purpose of drinking-water regulations is to reduce the concentration of 'nastier', not to introduce further ones. And even more dangerous and bio accumulative ones.'

Yorkshire, 'God's own county', was host to the first stage of the 2014 Tour of France, which went from Leeds to Harrogate—with the result that inspection of the signs warning of the 'unwholesome' sulphurous water in Harrogate was conducted rigorously and thoroughly. A preventative measure so that the cyclists would not end up joining *the pooping friends' network*, or fall off their bikes, biting the dust, so to speak.

Joking and irony (something that I learnt whilst studying physiotherapy in Yorkshire) aside, I personally think the great sporting performance in the wonderful scenery in and around the

Yorkshire Dales won the hearts of millions of viewers. Cheers! A sip of Harrogate's healing water—*A votre santé! Skål!* The Brits are the best! And won the hearts of millions who watched the start of Tour de France, in God's own county!

Sauna, Steam and Vital Water

Did you know that the only Finnish word to make it into everyday English is '*sauna*'? But exactly what is its history, cultural heritage, educative and political support and aid and its proven health benefits? The sauna's function is often misunderstood—and it is definitely not about flirtation and sex.

When you step inside a Finnish sauna, in a dimly lit wood-panelled room, naked men or women sit in silence, sweating. One beats himself with birch branches, *vihta*, which stimulates the skin and its capillary circulation aiding the detoxification process which is one of the most important health aspects of the sauna—not as kinky as it sounds! Whilst this goes on, another takes a ladle of water and carefully pours it over the heated stones of the stove in the corner. There is a hissing sound as the water hits the stone and water vapour rises. You immediately feel the increase in humidity and heat, as a wave of heat envelopes your body from your feet upwards. Your pores open up and sweat pours down your whole body. The cleansing process has started. The muscles of your body relax.

Right from the time the first settlers arrived in Finland thousands of years ago, they dug a ditch in the ground and heated a pile of stones. Water was thrown onto the hot stones to give up a vapour known as 'löyly'. Each sauna is considered to have its own character and its own distinct 'löyly'. The better the 'löyly', the more enjoyable the sauna. When building on a new plot, the first cabin the new settlers put up was the sauna. In cold and harsh climatic conditions, and for cleanliness and hygienic reasons, it was a natural and smart solution, as it provided a welcome relief for sore muscles and aching bodies needed soothing, calmness and relaxation, from the heat. Women gave birth in them because the walls of the traditional smoke sauna were lined with naturally bacteria-resistance soot, making them the most hygienic room in the house.

Saunas were also the place for purification rituals before marriage, and the bodies of the dead were washed and prepared for burial on the wooden benches.

For many Finns, the sauna is a sacred room in a house, closely associated with health and well-being. Finns say that the sauna is a poor man's pharmacy. I would like to add that the sauna is a better, smarter and more intelligent health solution without side effects, provided you follow some basic rules.

Drink plenty of something wetter then water; i.e., vital, restructured water, which cleanses and rehydrates the body much faster, with lower surface tension and altered molecular water structure. You obviously sweat a lot; toxins and waste move out of your body, and if you understand the basic toxicity of ordinary tap water, it is not such a good idea to replenish and rehydrate with toxic, contaminated water with its chemicals and heavy metals (chlorine, chloroform in the ordinary water vapour; lead, mercury, arsenic, fluoride, trihalomethanes from chlorine, a derivate from chlorine and well-known carcinogen). So I would say to all my sauna-loving friends: Don't forget the importance of replenishing your body's fluids with pure, alkaline, restructured water, as this is the only water that will rehydrate at a cellular level and help rebuild your body. An old Finish proverb says that 'if a sick person is not cured by tar, sauna and spirits (strong alcohol), they will die'. (And tar was used historically as an antiseptic.)

Finland is home to 3.3 million saunas. This great health-beneficial institution (minus the chlorine and the nastiness in the water) exists in homes, offices, factories, sports centres, hotels, ships and deep below the ground in mines. 99% of Finns take a sauna at least once a week, and more if they visit their summer cottage in the countryside. Here, the pattern of life tends to revolve around the sauna and a nearby lake used for cooling off. A spokesman from the Finnish Sauna Society, an organisation dedicated to upholding and preserving traditional Finnish sauna culture, proclaims that the sauna is also a place for educating your children as they are taught to behave in a sauna as if they were in a church. No food, drink or mobile phones are allowed in a sauna, which is a meditative, almost sacred place where you talk in a low tone not mentioning your job or religion. No clothes or swimsuits are allowed, for the same reasons as you would not wear anything in the bath or shower; every part of your body needs to be properly cleaned.

The Finnish Parliament has its own sauna chamber for MPs to debate in and all Finnish diplomatic missions around the world have their own sauna.

Former president and Nobel Prize laureate Martti Ahtisaari used sauna diplomacy—diplomatic meetings in the sauna—in the negotiations from Tanzania to Indonesia. During the cold war, Urho Kekkonen, who served as president for 26 years, negotiated with Soviet diplomats in the sauna, at his official residence. Kekkonen believed that all were equal in the sauna, and politics could not be hidden up a sleeve when no sleeve was worn. Finland walked on a diplomatic tightrope during the cold war. Its giant neighbour, the USSR, constantly challenged its neutrality between West and East.

In 1960, Khrushchev attended Kekkonen's sixtieth birthday. The story goes that Kekkonen kept Khrushchev in the sauna until 5:00 a.m., throwing more water on the stones of the stove. Soon after, the Soviet Government issued a communiqué expressing support for Finland's intention to co-operate with the West. It led to Finland joining the European Free Trade Association in 1971. Kekkonen's sauna diplomacy had paid off! The many mysterious healing aspects of water, said the water-wise man.

Khrushchev was criticised at home because a communist should not have gone naked into a sauna with a capitalist and non-socialist. I think we can agree: There would not be a Finland and the famous Finnish sisu, which have fostered so many great long-distance runners and cross-country skiers, without the sauna. It's in their DNA.

But the new science tells us that if water is the only drink for a wise and healthy man, then it follows logically and naturally that the water should be of the highest quality without toxins and contaminants—the very essence you try to detoxify, clean and remove in the sauna. Brother, wake up! Let's rejuvenate and rediscover our newfound health and wisdom—but, hey, let's move into the sauna first!

Wetter than Water

Somebody asked me the following question: 'Is there anything wetter than water?'

As he was feeling severely rough with a hangover of the worst kind, my friend suggested 'a hair-of-the-dog cure', which is the worst advice to give. Dehydration is part of the hangover predicament, and to remedy this problem, you would be wise to follow my advice: Drink plenty of vital water, which is restructured, hexagonal, high redox potential, lower surface tension, high zeta potential (phew, I think we can stop here!).

Suffice it to say this water is wetter; its molecular structure is improved and rehydration takes place at a much greater pace and depth. But since preventative steps are far superior, the following is sound advice: before you decide to 'paint the town red', drink two glasses of vital water with a pinch of Himalayan salt dissolved in it, and a teaspoon of organic honey! Repeat when you come home at night. Works wonderfully! How about that advice from a teetotaller!

If you do have a sauna in the house—wow!—detox and replenish with vital water. Presto! Joy and gratitude.

Conclusion

The conscientious use of water, both externally and internally, works wonders. Still, water
remains a mystery in many ways, a fact which scientists verify. None of nature's substances are shrouded in so many veils of mysteries, secrets and paradoxes as water. We talk about the many healing properties of the water from Lourdes, Tlacote in Mexico or the Hunza of North Pakistan. The hexagonal structure is one of the keys to this mystery.

CHAPTER SIXTEEN

More Good News on Detoxification and Rejuvenation

'Man is a complex being; he makes desserts bloom and lakes die'.
Gil Stern.

In a world of ever-increasing pollution from the air we breathe, the dead and contaminated chemical tap or plastic water we drink and pay for, the artificial, chemical food we ingest, the adulterated fats, the stressful and sedentary lifestyle—ouch! The list seems like a long nightmare!

The massive negative lifestyle changes that we have witnessed during the last 250 years have set our body's self-cleansing system to work on overdrive—overtime. Just to remind ourselves on one little aspect of environmental overload: Our homes are in the red zone; i.e., indoor pollution is, according to World Health Organization guidelines, 4 to100 times worse than outdoor pollution. It affects about one billion people, mostly women and children.

Once a foreign body has entered your body, it has to be detoxified and made water-soluble so that it can be transported and eliminated safely and efficiently. The liver, kidneys, lymphatic system, skin and intestines all play an important role. When this system becomes overloaded, residues of toxins are stored around the body in fatty tissues, organs, the brain, et cetera. Premature aging, cellular breakdown and disease will inevitably be the end result if we don't do anything about it.

Active Detoxification

If you think about the huge amount of toxins in our water, food and environment, it becomes obvious that a regular detoxification is necessary to eliminate most if not all of these—a substantial and efficient investment to prevent and reverse disease, alleviate and reduce pain and bring the body in balance.

A number of research and investigative reports tell us that coronary heart disease, osteoporosis, fibromyalgia, migraine, asthma, allergy and cancer can improve dramatically by chelation—originating from the Greek word *chēlē* meaning *claw*. Negatively charged ions will be attracted to positively charged ions. This occurs by means of EDTA (ethylenediamine acid).

A strong active detoxification protocol should include various factors such as fasting, drinking vegetable and fruit juices (as in juice therapy), alkalising the body through proper nutrition containing all vital ingredients, alkaline ionised, redox water, lymph drainage, vibro-training, trampoline training, Bowen therapy, Rife therapy and oriental belly dance. The latter may come as a surprise to many, but I have seen this work very well in clients for whom I recommend this type of gentle training.

Hand in hand with these therapy interventions goes a positive attitude towards making lifestyle changes on a broader scale. The elimination of toxins from your body and the length of time depends on individual body chemistry. Special care should be taken to stimulate and alleviate the work and function of the liver, gallbladder system and lymphatic system.

Traditional Chelation using Zeolite and Magnetic Clay

Chelation materials will bind to chemical poisonous elements by way of their opposing electrical charges and will be flushed out by the body's own renovation system. The chelation itself can be administered intravenously, intramuscularly or liposomal. Chelation material is taken orally or rectally. Chelation is especially efficient when it comes to heavy metals like mercury, cadmium, lead, arsenic, thallium and iron.

The method is also used in conjunction with coronary heart disease, MS, Alzheimer's, psoriasis and arthritis to remove calcium and fat deposits from the blood vessels.

Let us look at the origin of chelation history. During World War II, the first substance that was chelated was Dimecaprol, also known as British anti-lewisite or BAL, to eliminate lewisite, an arsenic product. This was one of the first chemicals used in biological warfare. The symptoms were skin irritations and sores, lung and liver poisoning. At the same time, health personnel observed an increasing number of people being poisoned by arsenic, which came from pesticides used on farms—the so-called 'Paris Green'.

Today, DMSA (dimercaptosuccinic acid) is the most common chelation ingredient in use, together with DMPS (Dimaval) and ALA (alpha lipoic acid)—first used in the former Soviet Union.

Many people use foods containing high amounts of sulphur as a form of chelation agent: onion, garlic, green algae, chlorella, kelp, coriander, MSM or NAC (N-Acetyl cysteine), even though they are not technically considered chelation agents.

Zeolite: What is zeolite and where does it come from? Zeolite belongs to a family of crystalline minerals that contain aluminium and silica as the main constituents. Zeolite is considered to be an effective chelating agent. The first finding of zeolite was discovered and described by a Swedish metallurgist by the name of Axel F. Cronstedt (1722-1765), who coined the name by putting two Greek words together, meaning boiling stones—referring to the steam rising during volcanic outbreak. In nature, zeolite is found in volcanic formation in the ocean.

Zeolite has many useful properties: ionisation, filtration, removal of odours, gaseous absorption, and chelation of heavy metals and toxins. The most widely used function is in water-filtering systems, but it is also used in air filtration, animal food and fertilisers. Nitrosamines, heavy metals, dichlorobenzene and mycotoxins like Alfa toxin B-1 are absorbed into the zeolite structure. These are all positively charged elements.

Zeolite has structures, pores and canals and can form cage-like structures, similar to a beehive. These structures of zeolite are negatively charged; indeed, it is one of the few negatively charged minerals found in nature. Because of this phenomenon, positively charged elements like heavy metals and other toxic substances are drawn into and captured by the zeolite structures. There are over 50 different zeolite structures in nature and some of these are synthesised and used in industry. The zeolite structure consists of oxides of silica and aluminium with an oxygen atom on either side. Each aluminium oxide is negatively charged whilst the silica oxide remains electrically neutral. This balances the positively charged cations consisting of calcium, magnesium, sodium, potassium and iron. These substances are loosely connected to the structure and can easily be changed and replaced by a heavy metal or other toxins. This cation exchange is characteristic of the zeolite structure.

The chemical composition of zeolite is very much like that of clay—aluminium, silica and oxygen. However, there is a big difference: many types of clay have a layered crystalline structure and contract and expand as the water moves between the layers. In contrast, zeolite has a rigid three-dimensional structure, like in a beehive, consisting of tunnels and cells throughout. The water moves freely in these open canal systems, whilst the framework in the zeolite structure is rigid, acting like a sieve.

There are basically three zeolite structures:

- Clinoptiolite, which is the most common form used in therapy as an alienation agent for detoxification purposes

- Prism-like structures as seen in asbestos
- Chabozite, in which the crystalline structures are more equally ordered

Clinoptiolite: Is there any evidence that zeolite is effective in detoxification processes? Let us focus on the layered type of zeolite, where the size of the canals will determine which molecules will pass and which ones will be trapped. This type, clinoptiolite, has been used for 800 years in traditional medicine in India, Russia, New Zealand and Australia. The substance is used to cleanse drinking water and to improve the quality of animal food. Clinoptiolite is of volcanic origin and is approved by the EU and FDA in the US.

It is a well-known fact that clinoptiolite draws and attaches heavy metals like mercury, cadmium, nickel, arsenic and animal food; the nutritional bio-availability will increase and cadmium is removed—hence the danger of anaemia is reduced. In addition, clinoptiolite strengthens the immune system. The substance was used after the Chernobyl accident in order to absorb radioactive isotopes and heavy metal. The use of zeolite has again come to the rescue in the wake of the Fukushima accident.

Together with iodine, transdermal magnesium and sodium bicarbonate, it should be a home remedy in every household, together with water filtration, an ionisation system and air purification with negative ions. More on this later in the book.

There are several different types of clinoptiolite on the market for therapeutic use. Not only do they have the capacity to remove heavy metals and toxins from the digestive system, but also the ability to stabilise the pH value in the body and alleviate digestive problems like IBS (irritable bowel syndrome), Candida and dysbiosis. Before use, it is important to check that the producers have removed all residues of any possible toxic elements from nature. Just recently, clinoptiolite has been made available through a colloidal solution (the particles are suspended in a solution) of clinoptiolite. Through this process, all pollutants have been removed and the surface area of the zeolite is maximised. Because of all the pores and canals, one gram of activated zeolite contains 90 square metres of activated areal. Activated liquid (AF2) will easily be absorbed through the digestive tract and the bloodstream.

The result is that the chelation agents exert a more direct effect on the toxic substances circulating through the different tissues and organs. AF2 has a special affinity/is drawn to heavy metals, and research show that the smaller diameter of the heavy metal, the greater the electrical charge will be, and this in turn increases the speed at which the chelation takes place. Smaller molecules will penetrate deeper into the structure of the zeolite. *Example*: arsenic, cadmium, aluminium, lead, mercury, bismuth and tin have relatively small molecular diameter and will therefore be drawn more forcefully to the structures of zeolite than larger ones with less ionic charge, like calcium, magnesium, sodium, potassium. These minerals are also necessary for the body. Even organic compounds like VOCs and aluminium will be chelated through AF2. Studies also show that the serum of electrolytes remain unaltered throughout the chelation process as the toxic heavy metals are excreted through the urine, as opposed to BHL and EDTA chelation where electrolytes need to be replaced, especially calcium and magnesium.

Several research studies have shown that AF2 has a stabilising and modulating effect on the immune system. In the presence of heavy metal, cellular metabolism becomes disturbed. The mineral zinc is an important aid in this respect acting in the transfer information between each cell's DNA. The obvious restraint on this activity due to the effect of the heavy metals is lifted throughout the chelation process. In this way, the immune system can operate and healing takes place.

A study conducted by a group of 300 athletes showed that those who used AF2 as part of their training had a much faster recovery time and less muscular pain than a similar placebo control group. The heavy metals will be absorbed by AF2 through a passive process; i.e., the zeolite structure moves freely through the body. When it comes in contact with positively charged particles like heavy metals, viruses, bacteria and fungus, it will attach and 'recapture' these. It will not attack amalgam or artificial joint prostheses because they don't exist in free ionic form. AF2 works without any side effects. You may become dehydrated, but replenish with ionised, alkaline, restructured water with high redox potential and you create the basis for healing. *You're winning on water— wow!*

Conclusion Regarding Chelation

The use of chelation as a detoxification method has been practised for more than 50 years. Yet very few of my patients have heard about it or know what it can achieve. One of the reasons is probably the lack of knowledge among health personnel, from doctors to therapists. With the ever-increasing amount of chemical toxins in the food, air, and water, it should be the number one choice in any detoxification protocol to prevent and reverse disease. You are open to a major threat from the onset of all modern lifestyle diseases if you neglect to incorporate a detoxification programme on a regular basis, de-acidification to change the body's chemistry from acid to alkaline and boost and balance the immune system. These ingredients should be one of the main cornerstones of a holistic health and well-being programme:

- Detoxification
- De-acidification
- Immune boosting—physically, emotionally, mentally, socially, environmentally—and most importantly, spiritually.

If you add to these components oxygenation therapies, bioelectric therapies, exercise and dance, you will live a long, happy and healthy life!

Living Calcium Bentonite Clay

This remedy has been used for several thousands of years in different cultures around the world. All clay originates from volcanic ash. Kaolin clay is mostly known as an anti-diarrhoea product. Most clay products will absorb poisonous material, but illite clay is mostly used by the cosmetic industry as masks or clay mudpacks.

Smectite clay comprises 99% of all clay used for therapeutic purposes. It both absorbs and adsorbs toxins in the body. Explanation: Adsorption is a process whereby a substance will attach itself on the outside of another element (as in a Velcro lock). Absorption takes place when a substance is absorbed into the molecular structure, like a sponge absorbing water. Calcium bentonite clay is part of the smectite family.

These processes take place electrically by ion exchange. Natural calcium bentonite clay has a negative ionic charge. Positively charged particles like microbes, toxins and heavy metals will be drawn towards the negatively charged ions.

The clay works solely on the basis of another element ionic change. Within the smectite family there are hundreds of different types of clay, consisting of 145 minerals.

Montmorillonite clay was named after a French town by the same name. According to Raymond Dextreit, an expert on clay and the author of the book *Our Earth, Our Cure*, this green clay is the most widely used clay for therapeutic purposes.

It is important to assure that the clay is calcium based and not sodium based—the latter being used in industry. A balanced calcium bentonite day should always consist of these three mineral compounds:

- Silicon oxide
- Calcium oxide
- Magnesium oxide

And not more than 2.5% sodium. It is important that the clay is natural. One of the great blessings with the right type of clay is its ability to change the body's pH from a high acidic state to an alkaline state. All clay is alkaline but one in the range of pH 9.3-9.7 is recommended. The clay's efficiency is also important—for instance, 10:1. This ratio will remove 10 times its molecular weight of positively charged ions. There are three types of clay with a higher ratio than 12:1 and a few have a 31:1 ratio.

Alkaline Environment

All food consists of a combination of carbohydrates, protein and fat, further broken down to carbon, nitrogen, hydrogen and oxygen resulting in energy and nutritious building blocks. When the food is metabolised, bi-products are formed including carbolic acid, uric acid, lactic acid, fatty acids and ammonia. All foodstuffs will produce acidic waste products, which have to be removed via urine and sweat. Some types of food like fruit and vegetables contain alkaline minerals like calcium, potassium, magnesium and sodium, acting like a buffering system to neutralise the acidic waste products. Meat, grains, chocolate, coffee and sodas contain certain acidic minerals such as chlorine, phosphors and sulphur.

Our modern diet is lacking in alkaline minerals and has changed dramatically over the last decades. On average, we eat too much acidic-forming foodstuffs and most of us do not have the physiological capacity to neutralise the acidic waste products. The detrimental effect of an acidic nutrition is further reinforced by a mixture of proteins and starches together with drinking fluids containing simple sugars, salt, and in addition the food is cooked or fried. To reach and maintain an alkaline basis, most health experts seem to agree that an 80:20 ratio between alkaline- and acidic-forming foodstuffs is optimal for good health.

Cooked or fried foods lack electrons and enzymes, have a positive ORP and an excess of positive ions, which dehydrates, steals electrons, decreases the energy level and lays the foundation for all kinds of diseases—exactly the opposite of what you would want for a body in balance. Recommended reading: *The Miraculous Properties of Ionised Water*, by Bob McCauley.

Acidic-forming foods:

- Meat, chicken, pork, fish
- Dairy products

- Refined sugars, HFCS (sugar from corn syrup)
- Artificial sugars (aspartame, Splenda, sucralose)
- Fruit juice concentrate
- Chocolate
- Grains, cereals
- Soda
- Mineral water, energy and sports drinks
- Alcohol, beer, wine
- Coffee, tea (black)

Alkaline-forming foods:

- Raw vegetables, early greens
- Avocado
- Grass types, barley, wheat
- Sprouting greens, beans, seeds
- Fresh fruit
- Beans and legumes
- Gluten-free grains, especially sprouted
- Buckwheat, especially sprouted
- Green powder, chlorophyll, spirulina
- Brown rice, hempseed
- Ionised, alkaline water

Our bodies consist of 60% of water more or less. The water content of all muscle tissue is 25%. The water content of all blood is 80%. The water content of the brain is 90%. Almost all biochemical processes in our cells are dependent on water, and normal metabolism can only take place if the cells have at least 65% water content. The water molecules fill the spaces in between the cells themselves (intra and extracellular). As a vital part of the structure of the macromolecules like protein and glycogen, water is all-important and makes vitamins, minerals amino acids, glucose and other nutrients into a solution that can be absorbed. Water has a key role to play in the digestive processes, absorption and transportation of these elements, as well as providing a route for the detoxification processes, and for the body's heat regulation system. Water is vital for general health and well-being, and adequate fluid balance is essential for a swift recovery after surgery, disease or strenuous training / competition. All symptoms are dependent on a pure and high redox potential (ORP).

What about bottled water? All the types of bottled water we have tested came out as slightly acidic. But more disturbing, they had an opposite electrical charge of +100mV or more ORP (oxygen reduction potential), which will steal electrons from your body and cause free radical damage through oxidation. In addition, plastic bottles leach chemicals (phthalates, dioxin) and will cost you an arm and a leg. Approximately 200,000-250,000 NOK over a 15-year period with normal consumption.

An ionised unit will save you money, improve your health and well-being in addition to preventing disease and acting as a source of rejuvenation for you and your family.

Facts About Bottled Water

- Billions of bottles end up as garbage/dumped.
- More than 250 million oil barrels are used annually to produce plastic bottles.
- More than 40% of bottled water sold in the shops as 'pure, healthy water' is filtered, municipal drinking water; i.e., tap water.
- Some bottled water even contain fluoride
- All bottled water has an unhealthy pH—it is acidic.
- All bottled water in plastic bottles contains leached chemicals, among them dioxin, an environment toxin and known carcinogen, as well as other health-damaging chemicals.

Proper water supply is important for energy production, joint lubrication and the reproductive organs. When cells are hydrating, an anabolic phase is triggered which is part of a healing or regenerating mechanism. This phase improves nitrogen balance and protein synthesis and increases growth hormone production. More efficient cell hydration leads to a reduced level of acidity in the cells, improved immune system, increased fat metabolism, more DNA reparation and increased resistance to infections.

When the cells dehydrate, a catabolic phase starts which includes loss of muscle tissue, oxygen deprivation of the cells, damage to DNA and premature aging. As a result, the cells become more vulnerable to free radical damage, more infection and more autoimmune diseases.

In its natural state, water flows over stones, gravel and mountains, cascading down cliffs and falling as rain or snow. This motion is completely different from the motion that occurs in the water pipes transporting our municipal water. Pure natural water is alkaline and carries an abundance of electrons ready to be donated to unstable free radicals. Because of the natural water flow in nature, it carries minerals, which are vital and beneficial for our health.

The new ionisation technology makes this kind of water available for everybody. A great contribution towards renewed energy and health because of greater rehydration properties, minerals, alkaline state, et cetera.

Citius, Altius, Fortius (Faster, Taller and Stronger): Hydration, performance and restitution—the three reasons serious sportspeople and athletes drink or should drink ionised water. Sporty people and athletes know that proper hydration is crucial for optimum performance. As little as 1% dehydration may lead to 2% decreased performance. It does not sound much, but it amounts to two minutes during a competition lasting one hour. In addition, dehydration reduces the body's ability to recover; i.e., it takes a longer time.

Most sporty people and athletes are chronically dehydrated—often without knowing it. And this fact is not because they don't replenish lost fluids, but more that cellular structure remains improperly hydrated. Restructured, alkaline, redox ionised water can rehydrate fast and effectively to reach the cellular structure.

Firstly, it is important to understand that rehydration properly managed at a cellular level cannot be achieved through drinking tea, coffee, sodas, juice or energy drinks. Why? Because these contains sugar, caffeine, phosphor and carbon acids. Since they are acidic and made from water containing chemicals, including aluminium, heavy metals, and other toxins, they are not capable of proper rehydration—in addition to increasing oxidation processes because of free radical damage, opposite electrical charge, becoming an electron thief for the working muscles, stealing minerals and vital nutrients from the body. Sportspeople and athletes are particularly in the danger zone as far as acid and alkaline balance is concerned. Why? Because of physical and mental stress, adrenalin, cortisol and lactic acid lower the body's internal pH.

Not even bottled spring water is capable of rehydrating the body completely, because all the natural properties of the water have been altered or lost. The water has been chemically and structurally altered by chlorination or fluoridation. In addition, it contains heavy metals and toxic poly vinyl chlorides (PVC) from metal and plastic pipes.

Which do you prefer: water that will benefit your body's health and well-being, or water that is ruined, contaminated, toxic and contributes to acidity and early aging? Alkaline, ionised water has regained all of its lost physical properties. Is it not about time you took responsibility for your own health and provided your body with the optimum water—escaping the marketing tricks used by the bottled water industry and the 'sickness industry'?

Just a short recap:

- Ionisation lowers the electrical potential (mV) of the water, creating a negative redox potential (ORP), making it a powerful antioxidant.
- Ionisation changes the structure of the water, making it more easily absorbed by the body, better and more efficient, and therefore rehydrates at the cellular level.
- Ionised water changes cell membranes' electrical potential, which improves fluid exchange and removal of toxins.
- Ionised water increases the amount of free electrons, which assists the body's ability to neutralise and remove toxins.

When I Get Older, Losing My Hair…

When I get older, losing my hair, many years from now is a famous line from the Beatles' song *When I'm Sixty-Four*. Understanding some of the vital aspects of aging and what we can do about it physiologically has been a quest from day immemorial. From the 1400-century conquistador Ponce de Leon's search for the elixir of youth, to the Nobel Prize Winner Henri Coandă's work on the Hunza water and the Hunza people's long and healthy lifestyles. In recent years, scientists have been very much occupied with the study of telomeres and their action and effect on aging.

Water has a crucial role to play in keeping you healthy and younger for longer. Too much acidity results in an acceleration of the aging processes. Your body tries to maintain a blood pH of close to 7.36. If this decreases to 7, it can mean coma and death. Since the pH scale is logarithmic, a little change like this can make conditions four times as acidic; hence the blood pH varies very little from its optimal pH.

To maintain this balance, a mineral buffering system operates, coming from bones and organs. Chronic and prolonged acidity will accelerate the aging process. Even though the blood maybe on the alkaline side, other tissues and their fluids can become acidic. Aggressive microorganisms like parasitic, pathogenic factors can become rampant, disturbing the normal microbic flora. This can lay the grounds for many diseases of the respiratory and digestive systems, the first line of the body's defence.

Free Radicals and Aging

Many decades of research point to the fact that free radical formation is one of the main causes of aging and disease. Through oxidation of cellular structures, the damage extends to the cell membranes, and the cell structures themselves can become inflamed and cause premature cell death.

Our modern lifestyle lays the foundation for many diseases through oxidation and free radical damage. These can be diabetes, coronary heart disease, digestive disorders, asthma, allergy, ME (myalgic encephalitis or chronic fatigue syndrome), cancer, obesity, muscular skeletal disorders, et cetera. The main causes are to be found in toxins and pollutants in the air we breathe, the water, drinks and food we ingest. So here is where our preventative power and effort should be focused.

All of the following can throw your body out of balance:

- Medication, drugs, tobacco and alcohol
- Food lacking in nutrients, but full of preservatives and artificial colourings
- Heavy metals in all kinds of foodstuffs—milk, farmed fish; fluor hidden in various products—medication, food, beverages, tea
- Polyunsaturated oils, hydrolysed, adulterated and rancid, incorrect content on labels; oil mixtures, i.e. olive plus peanut oil
- Chlorinated drinking water; shower or bathing in chlorinated water
- Prolonged stress

- Irregular meals, lacking in vital nutrients
- Lack of sleep and rest
- Sedative, inactive lifestyle
- Lack of Vitamin D (sunshine vitamin)

Lack of water, and especially pure, ionised water, is one of the main reasons behind signs of premature aging. Wrinkles are due to intracellular loss of water content and a gradual loss of skin elasticity caused by diminished collagen and elastin production. The acidic changes seen on the surface of the body are a sure sign of the internal state of affairs. This scenario is very real and is described by Dr. Mu Shik Jhon, the author of the book *The Water Puzzle and the Hexagonal Key*.

A too high level of acidity in the body is like having too little oil. One day it will break down. The same applies to your body.

- 80-90% of people in the Western world are dehydrated, mostly without knowing it
- The main reason for daytime tiredness is lack of water. Remember that coffee and tea act like diuretics.
- One should drink about 0.3 dl pure water per kilo bodyweight per day
- As little as 2% reduction of water to the brain leads to mental confusion, poor short-term memory, decreased focus and concentration

- May confuse hunger with thirst. A study conducted at the University of Washington showed that drinking a glass of water, preferably pure, alkaline water, could alleviate hunger pangs—as part of a weight loss programme
- Research shows that 8-10 glasses of water a day may considerably reduce muscular and skeletal pain. Remember that pure, alkaline water rehydrates deepest, fastest and detoxifies the tissues.
- Chemical research has documented that indigestion and drinking alkaline, restructured water can alleviate constipation.

Alkalinity

As we have seen, ionised water with high ORP will balance the body's pH value and make the inner milieu more alkaline. This process, together with detoxification, will take some time depending on food intake, training status and stress management. If you commit yourself to make a responsible effort in this field, you can considerably accelerate the balancing and healing process.

Detoxification—Revisited

When you drink ionised, alkaline water, several detoxification processes start up. Because you now have an abundance of negatively charged electrons (OH-), these will be donated to cellular structures. The water now being an antioxidant helps to neutralise free radicals, which lack electrons. Numerous scientific studies have shown that ionised water produces significant improvement in these areas:

- Blood sugar balance
- Circulation
- Digestive problems
- Weight problems
- Toxification by heavy metals—reduction due to chelation effect
- Kidney and bladder function
- Pain reduction
- Wound healing
- Function of small and large intestines
- Brain function
- Hormone and immune systems

To summarise, the health benefits/advantages with ionised water are:

- Increased energy levels
- Increased oxygen delivery to the cells
- High ORP, meaning high detoxification factor
- High negative ORP rejuvenated; biological age reversal

- Removes heavy metals
- pH-balancing
- Rehydrates eight times faster than ordinary chemical tap water
- Ionised minerals are easily absorbable

Successful Fasting

Like the law of gravity, God's laws on health issues can't be changed without consequences. Our Creator did not design our bodies to run on junk food, fast food or pre-packed foods prepared in a microwave oven. Due to today's fast-paced lifestyles, some people choose to adopt 'convenience' foods, which lack elemental nutrients and contain ingredients that are detrimental to our health (adulterated, hydrolysed oils and fats, sugars, fructose, MSG, artificial sugar and additives).

Elmer Johnson, an expert health advocate, said, 'There is no portion of the commandments of God in general, or of the Mosaic code in particular, that is not based on a scientific understanding of fundamental physiological laws. The laws of God are enforced and are as sure as the law of gravity.

As we have seen, the healthiest people in the world were generally the most primitive people as well. The common denominator in these cultures is the mineral-rich, alkaline, restructured water as reported by many scientists, including Henry Coandă, the Nobel Prize Winner in physiology or medicine. The natural, nutrient-rich food enjoyed by these cultures is very different from the modern processed food, where food can last for decades on a store shelf. G.M.O., gene manipulated food, Frankenstein food, so-called 'bio-engineered' foods are the norm in an unsuspecting and naïve population. Natural, fresh food as recommended by the Creator is in every respect superior to the 'average Western diet', with plentiful fruits and vegetables, herbs, beans, lentils, wholegrain, along with meat, fish and dairy products. God's dietary recommendation given to the Israelites enabled them to live longer and healthier, at least up until World War I, where both hygiene and food began to slacken among the Israelites.

Sometimes the situation can require that you drop the fork, rest and fast. We know that great Biblical leaders such as David, Daniel the prophet, Yeshua and Paul fasted, and that entire nations have declared fasts during times of crisis or repentance.

Fasting God's way, wholeheartedly, is a tool for cleansing and receiving a breakthrough in body, soul and spirit. People in every culture have an intuitional understanding of fasting. Anyone who has been ill understands that in times of sickness, food cravings come to a standstill. No more hunger means the body's own innate healing system is at work.

Hakuna Matata! Don't Worry, Fast and Be Happy

In the Bible, you will find many fasts that vary in length according to type and purpose:

- A crisis fast, like the 'Esther fast' (Esther 4:16), lasting for three days—a total fast with abstinence from all food and liquids for three days. Due to the general degenerative state of health in the modern world, with poor nutritional status and abundance of toxicity, total fasts like this should not be attempted.

- A modified 10-day fast like the 'Daniel fast' has almost unlimited applications. Daniel and his friends chose to abstain from the king's food and only ate fruit and vegetables and drank vital water, as we have seen, with incredible results. (Daniel 1:5, 14-16.) You may choose to eliminate all sugars, caffeine, soft drinks, sodas, junk foods, pasteurised dairy products, cereals and pork products. It is an excellent way to break addiction to food or habits,—in order to embark on a healthier lifestyle.

- Daniel also completed a serious 21-day water-only fast. But you should confer with a health professional before starting such a fast.

- Moses and Yeshua completed a 40-day total fast without liquids. But this is not recommended for ordinary people, as serious damage can result beyond the three-day point of dehydration.

- Many people have completed 40-day water and juice fasts (using diluted low-acid fruit or vegetable juices with alkaline, restructured vital water). But these fasts should only be done under the supervision of a health professional.

- Intermittent or selective fasting as part of many naturopathic protocols for various diseases where major toxicity is the main problem is very beneficial. Even a one-day fast, complete or partial, can be of great benefit.

The body goes into a healing mode when it is fasting. An important regenerating process takes place when we sleep and have a break from activity and eating. That is why our first meal is called breakfast—we are breaking the fast that heals.

Dr William L. Esser's research on fasting is interesting. He followed 156 people who complained of symptoms from 31 medically diagnosed diseases, including ulcers, tumours, tuberculosis, sinusitis, Parkinson's, heart disease, cancer, arthritis, asthma, bronchitis, insomnia, gallstones, epilepsy and colitis. 156 patients lasted five days; the longest lasted 35 days. Only 20% of the patients lasted as long as Dr. Esser recommended. However, the results showed:

- 113 completely recovered
- 31 partially recovered
- 12 were not helped
- 92% improved or recovered completely!

NB: Make sure you consult with a health professional before you embark on a fast, especially if you have a physical disease.

Finally, it is important that you break the fast gently and don't gorge yourself on bread and pasta. Continue drinking plenty of vital water as your body has now undergone a detoxification process. There are many excellent books out there on the subject of fasting and also healthcare professionals to guide you on this stepping stone to better health and longevity.

From my own experience working on fasting and seeing the beneficial results, and how the scientists are beginning to unravel what the Bible has described as health benefits and spiritual rewards through praying, I highly recommend this practice. From as far back as the 1930s, scientists have shown that mice put on a low-caloric, nutrient-rich diet *live far longer*. There is mounting evidence that the same is true in monkeys, affecting another hormone (IGF-1, growth hormone).

A particular type of mouse that lived an extra 40%, equivalent to 120 human years or longer, holds the world record for extending life expectancy in mammals. Its body seemed to be engineered so as to produce low levels of a growth hormone IGF-1. High levels of this seem to be associated with accelerated aging and age-related diseases, white low levels are protective.

A similar but natural genetic mutation has been found in humans with Laron syndrome. The very low levels of IGF-1 their bodies produce mean that they are short, but this also seems to give them protection from cancer and diabetes, two common diseases which are also age-related.

The IGF-1 hormone (insulin-like growth hormone) is one of

the hormones that keep our bodies alert and on the go, which is fine when you are growing, but not so good later in life. There is increasing evidence that IGF-1 levels can be lowered by what you eat. The restriction of the amount you eat will help, but the clue is to reduce your protein intake so that you switch your body from a 'building mode' to a 'repair mode'. Professor Valter Longo at the University of Southern California has shown this.

Intermittent fasting is an area of current research into a diet called Alternate Day Fasting (ADF), eating what you want one day, followed by a day of restrictive calorie intake, fewer than 600 calories—an easier version is the so-called 5:2 diet where, as the name implies, you eat normally during five days a week, then during two days you eat 500 calories if you are a woman and 600 calories if you are a man. Blood markers like IGF-1, glucose and cholesterol improve significantly and blood pressure will be reduced. As your body weight decreases, the chances of contracting diabetes and cancer diminish. Think what you can achieve if you combine this knowledge with:

- Drinking plenty of restructured water, which detoxifies and supplies antioxidant, tissue-repairing components
- Specific herbal, homeopathic detoxifying substances
- Increased oxygen transportation to the cells' metabolism
- PEMF (pulsed electro-magnetic field) therapies

The IGF-1 reduction can be quite dramatic during the fast, close to

60% or more. Once you start eating again, it will go up, but will still be 20% down. The major inhibitor of IGF-1, called IGF BP-1, is significantly higher during the fasting period. Even when reassuming a normal diet, the IGF BP-1 level is elevated above the baseline value. It is a sign that the body is switched into a mode that is much more conducive to healthy aging. This regime is easier to follow than a complete fast and may be more effective than complete fasting (Ref. to Daniel and his Hebrew friends and their outstanding success, Daniel 1:5, 14-16).

Blood tests also reveal another type of cells, which appear during fasting, which scientists call 'embryonic-like' stem cells that have the ability to regenerate just about anything in the body, triggering it into a repair mode. Scientists are steadily gathering more data, which supports what the Bible tells us about fasting and how it can improve your everyday state of health—living and longevity, improved quality of life, health and wellness, for longer periods of time.

Nothing beats personal experience, though—so why not try it and get some proper advice from a health professional who has personal experience in the art of fasting?

**Just a Little Digression: Politicians on Taking the Mickey
Bliss, Cockney for 'Taking the Piss'—a Euphemism**

A heated dispute between the Norwegian and British Minister of Environment in 1993 on acid rain from the UK and Norway's whale policy ended up with the quick-tempered T. Berntsen calling his colleague John Gummer 'the biggest shitbag he had ever met'. (Norwegian: *Drittsekk*—an inconsequential little creep). Clearly Mr Gummer had angered Mr Berntsen, whose reaction did not come as a surprise to most Norwegians.

Mr Gummer now had another word of insult to add to his list of 'Names the world called me'—having been portrayed in *The Guardian* as a 'pustule' by cartoonist Steve Bell, he was understandably apprehensive about being known in future as John Shitbag Gummer. T. Berntsen said the words he used were no more than an average insult in the British Parliament. He definitely had a point there.

The House of Commons have heard such masterpieces as Clement Attlee calling Winston Churchill 'Fifty per cent genius, fifty per cent fool.' Or what about Tony Blair's comment on Terry Dicks: 'The honourable gentleman is undoubtedly living proof that a pig's bladder on a stick can be elected as a member of parliament.'

A good laugh is wonderful medicine without side effects! I love the Brits!

The Norwegian Prime Minister at the time, Gro Harlem Brundtland, backed her minister and pronounced, 'To dismiss and ridicule the problem of acid rain when a Norwegian minister of environment brings it up with a British colleague is not acceptable.' However, Berntsen later admitted that his choice of words had not been ideal, but stopped short of an apology. 'The lip from Groruddalen' as he is known in Norway, volatile and quick-tempered, was temporarily silenced.

After the Acid Rain Came the Burning Sun

In the seventies, Scandinavia, and the southwest of Norway in particular, experienced the devastating impact of environmental pollution from Europe's coal and oil industry as it came down as acid rain, filled with sulphur—and nitrogen acid. At least 9600 fishers were wiped out in the aftermath and it led to sour bickering between the Norwegian and the English Environmental Ministers, as we saw earlier, culminating in the 'Shitbag' episode.

But since 1980, acid pollution has been reduced by about 60%—unexpectedly creating new challenges. The acidity of the lakes has not changed much, retaining a low pH, with plenty of humus and heavy metals.

Norwegian drinking water is mostly surface water and has not been naturally cleansed by moving through the silt, earth and gravel. More humus is observed in the drinking water and transports mercury, cadmium, lead and arsenic to our drinking water. The heavy metals together with chlorine by-products, the so-called trihalomethanes, are neurotoxins and can cause cancer. The heavy metals accumulate in our bodies, as they do in fish and higher in the food chain.

Professor Rolf Voigt at the University of Oslo is conducting research in this field and is very concerned with the increasing amount of humus in the Norwegian drinking water. The humus has many 'claws' and it is easy for the heavy metals to stick to it. Prof Vogt, together with many other scientists, is concerned that this increasing amount of heavy metal concentration in the drinking water due to the growing amount of humus will lead to more chemicals, including chlorine and other disinfectants, which can lead to health problems. Humus, which is a result of the breakdown of plants, vegetation and animals, will also lead to microorganisms in the water pipes.

In addition to filtration, the waterworks will try to remove some of the humus by adding aluminium ions. Paradoxically, the acid rain from the 1970s had the effect of 'washing' aluminium ions from the soil and attached itself to the humus, with the result that less humus was observed in the water. The conditions are now reversed and more humus with heavy metals is entering the drinking water.

The whole idea of this research came from the observation of the increased concentration of humus in the surface water (Norwegian drinking water) since the 1970-80s.

The increasing amount of chlorine, by-products and other chemicals used in our drinking water is a great health concern. This is just a reminder to take responsibility, clean and restructure the water scientifically. *You* take control over the situation for your own family, rather than leave it up to governmental institution. Remember *educare*: to be drawn out from ignorance. No excuse anymore!

A little post scriptum on the acid reflux of these politicians and others: Maybe it would be worthwhile for them to investigate, and possibly adopt, the practice of the former Indian Prime Minister Morarji Desai, a long-time proponent of urine therapy, as he confessed in 1978 to Dan Rather on *60 Minutes* and during an *ABC News* interview with Barbara Walters. Morarji Desai lived to 99 years of age—a healthy, long life. Although a bit of an oddball, the auto-urine therapy (AUT) he practised is gaining in popularity for combating a host of illnesses and maintaining good health.

Many proponents of AUT like to quote from the book of Proverbs 5:15 in the Bible. 'Drink water from your own cistern, flowing water from your own well. Should your springs be scattered abroad, streams of water in the streets? Let them be for yourself alone, and not for sharing with others.'

Urine therapists often speak of this as the 'water of life', drinking Shivambu, which means drinking the water of auspiciousness. Dr B. V. Khare, an allopathic doctor and Mumbai-based follower of AUT says, 'The Italian surgeon Stanislaw R. Burzynski, now settled in the US, separated neoplastic from human urine and showed remarkable results in the treatment of cancer. Another substance found in the urine is DHEA (dehydroepiandrosterone) a precursor to testosterone and other sex hormones, and melatonin. Research has shown this to have anti-cancer, anti-obesity and anti-aging properties. It has also been found that when ingesting recycled urea, it is converted into amino acids. But somehow I don't think that the Oriental philosophy of drinking a cup of your own urine would mitigate or balance the attitudes of the two politicians mentioned earlier. It is, after all, very difficult to teach an old dog new tricks! Maybe somebody should tell them to drink *vital water*, to restructure their cortical connections!

Amazing miracle

One day a young mother came to our clinic certainly did not need any cortical re-structuring, but detoxification and balancing using the infinitely effective Bowen technique. An eminent practitioner, Alistair McLoughlin from Lancashire in England, first introduced me to this brilliant healing modality. Later I had the privilege to study Bowen therapy under Mr and Mrs Rentsch, some of the first who were taught by Tom Bowen himself. The subtle "moves" across muscular-tendinous and nervous junction help the body to heal itself by de-stressing and retuning the body to healing modus retuning the nerve signals in the body´s connective tissue.

Kirsten the young mother was on heavy medication for severe asthma and used to take 30 cortisone tablets a day. From being petite and normal weight she was 120 kg and experiencing muscular and joint pain when I first saw her at the clinic. During a short stay at the hospital, she learnt that her condition could be fatal. The grave situation spurred her on to take responsibility for her own life.

Many side effects of the medicine had caused overgrowth of fungus, especially in the intestines, throat area and the blood was heavily toxified. Clearly an acidic state needed to be cleared. In

Kirsten´s case the Bowen therapy aimed at clearing blockages in the blood and lymphatic system, and drainage of the lungs. During the first 7 weeks she lost 30 kg muscular and joint pain had vanished and she could live without medication. As a result of this happy ending, Kristen started to study Bowen therapy, the life-saving technique. She now devoutly treats her dearly beloved horses in the district and have already experienced amazing results

Conclusion

Without the many self-regulatory detoxification systems at work, we would see an even greater breakdown of body systems, and an increase in illness as a consequence. But being aware of the toxins, especially the heavy metals, avoiding these and detoxifying on a regular basis, you are on the stepping stones to better health.

Creating an alkaline, oxygen-rich supply to the body environment is such an important daily routine—one that should be naturally incorporated for the whole family.

CHAPTER SEVENTEEN

You Are What You Drink, Eat, Digest, Think and Breathe!

'We forget that the water cycle and the life cycle are one'. - Jacques Cousteau.

Every year, Norwegians celebrate on 17th May, and 2014 is the 200th anniversary for our Constitution. What follows is a nutritious 'hip hip hooray 17th of May Celebration Salad' fit for a King, and a healthy power-lift for people from all walks of life. The food and drink consumed by the representatives during the discussions prior to the Norwegian Constitution was quite unhealthy by any standard of the imagination.

A typical breakfast consists of cold food, lots of meat, accompanied by Madeira, beer and a wee dram! There is no doubt that the representatives drank a lot of alcohol during these sessions. Madeira was known as the 'wine of liberty', the favourite drink of George Washington and Thomas Jefferson, and also the chosen drink when the Declaration of Independence was signed in 1776, and later when George Washington was elected as President.

Benjamin Franklin enjoyed Madeira and mentioned the drink several times in his autobiography. Not a very wise choice, considering that he suffered from painful gout. Punch was also a popular drink at the time, according to Peter Thompson's *Rum, Punch and Revolution*. The drink supposedly stimulated political discussions. Punch soon became the favourite drink of authors and journalists who probably needed courage to write their bold commentaries. The original drink consisted fruit juice, sugar, syrup and water with wine or brandy, which was brought to Europe from the West Indies by British sailors at the beginning of the 16th century. Around 1650, rum was the chosen tipple rather than brandy, and in 1671 a Rum House was first opened. The Norwegians, who admired all things British, adopted rum punch. Together with Madeira, punch and other lubricants of mind and matter, tight tongues and inhibitions where loosened, and the Norwegian Constitution of 1814 emerged.

200th Anniversary!

Power to the People's Constitution

Salad of 1814-2014

A VICTORY SALAD FIT FOR A KING!

This is what you need:

1 big bunch of parsley, either curly or flat (oriental parsley)

2 cups of cucumber, diced

1 cup of tomatoes

1 cup of red pepper

¼ onion

½ cup of organic hempseed

½ cup of lemon juice, freshly squeezed

2 cloves of garlic, minced

7 tbsp. of organic hemp seed oil

1 cup of celery, sliced

½ cup of grenadine

This is how you do it:

Soak all the vegetables in alkaline water with a pH of 10 for about 10-12 minutes. This will clean and remove containments and residues of pesticides. Rinse well.

Chop the parsley and throw it into a large bowl, along with the

cucumber, tomato, red pepper, onion and hempseed and grenadine.
In a blender, combine the lemon, garlic, hempseed oil and Himalaya salt until you have a smooth consistency.

Pour over the salad and mix well.

Powerful nutrition in every delicious mouthful of heavenly gratitude. Enjoy!

Some useful information of this gem of a seed, the little hempseed: This is the most nutritionally complete food source in the world. This little seed contains all the essential amino acids and fatty acids necessary to maintain healthy human life. No other single plant source has all the essential amino acids in such an easily digestible form. The essential oils are in perfect balance for meeting human nutritional needs. The organic hempseed and its hempseed oil are perfect for nourishing the bi-lipid cell membranes with 'oxygen-magnets' so that maximum oxygen can be delivered to the cells. Together with restructured water, which alkalinises, oxygenates and detoxifies your cells, this is by far the most important step you can take to prevent lifestyle diseases like cancer, heart disease, diabetes, Alzheimer's, dementia, and anti-immune diseases. At the same time, use the knowledge from this book to avoid the adulterated, hydrogenated (hydrolysed) oils and 'lite' products that will gradually erode and destroy cellular membranes and therefore the availability of oxygen.

Trans fat from oils and margarine, soft or liquid plant fat

from corn, soy, rapeseed oil (flax), and sunflower oil should be shunned. Use organic coconut and butter for cooking.

On salads: Organic hempseed oil, or organic virgin olive oil. Make sure it's certified and tested by an independent source, because more than 70 % of olive oils are mixed with cheap soy or peanut oil!

Viktorklinikken's Supercalifragilisticexpialidocious I.S.A.Y.

This is what you need:
½ cup of chopped Brazil nuts

1 bunch of parsley, finely chopped

Juice of one lemon, 350 gr. beans, turned

2 gloves of garlic, finely chopped

Freshly ground pepper. ½ tsp. of Himalaya salt, a pinch of turmeric spice

3 bunches of broccolini (or broccoli)

3 tsp. hempseed oil

½ cup of cottage cheese

Soak vegetables for 10-12 minutes in water with a pH Of 10 to cleanse and make them crisp.

This is how you do it:
Steam broccoli and beans 3-4 minutes until they are just tender.

Add to the other ingredients and mix well.

Will serve 8 as an accompaniment.

Great Chieftain to the Pudding Race

Robert Burns was not the first to pay tribute in verse to the haggis—the super-sausage from Scotland. The ancient Greeks had their own version of haggis and, according to Aristophanes' in *The Clouds*, they had to approach the cutting of it with extreme caution. In the play, Strepsiades relates his own personal experience:

Why, now the murder's out!
So was I served with a stuffed sheep paunch I broiled.
On Jovesday last, just such a scurvy trick;
Because, forsooth, not dreaming of your thunder,
I never thought to give the rascal rent,
Bounce go the bag, and covers me all over
With its rich content of such varied sorts.

Thanks to a fellow student at the college of physiotherapy, Fred Masson, from Aberdeen, I was initiated into the fine art of preparing and devouring Haggis, the National Dish of Scotland, beloved and reviled by natives. It sometimes horrifies even native Scots when they hear it described for the first time.

Ready and Ripe for a Trifle of Tripe?

The ritual of initiation took place in 1971 at Salt Hospital, Victoria Road, in the lovely community of Saltaire, built by Sir Titus Salt. A wee dram afore we went into devouring this delicatessen of sheep's lung, heart, liver, stomach, suet, oatmeal (ground type), onions, salt, freshly ground pepper, cayenne, nutmeg and stock.

As we obviously did not have a piper playing, I improvised by pinching my nose tightly with one hand, whilst tapping my windpipe with the other, making a piper-like sound. It works! Fred and Alfred, my co-students, and Hazel and Emily from the kitchen hospital staff were in stitches as I proceeded to prance around in the kitchen and hospital corridor, doing my 'crazy clan performance'.

The cockroaches, often to be seen in the hospital kitchen, enjoyed the beat of the music so much that they suddenly appeared from every nook and cranny and lined up for an impromptu dance. How weird and hilarious! If you go to www.youtube.com/watch?v=Yfka9m6NhzE and watch La Cucaracha (The Dancing Cockroach video), you'll see what I mean. A good laugh will extend your life!

As soon as their performance ended, the cockroaches disappeared again. Later, the *Daily Mirror* reported they'd been found in a Cadbury Chocolate Factory, but that's another sweet story for another time. For those of you with a more scientific mind, you can learn a little neuroscience by following Greg Cage and the Cockroaches Beat Box on YouTube (Talk Video/TED.com).

I believe, as did James A. Michener, (1907-1997), the famous and prolific American author, that the master of living draws no sharp distinction between his labour and his leisure, his mind and his body, his work and his play. He hardly knows which is which, because education, creativity and play go hand in hand, in pursuing a vision of excellence. We are both *Homo sapiens* (thinking man) and *Homo ludens* (playing man),—Maybe we need to make more room for the Playful Man in our society? For an in-depth study of this phenomenon, you may like to read *Homo Ludens, A study of the play-element in culture*, by J. Huizinga (1872-1945), first published in Germany and Switzerland (1944).

'A wee dram for the soul of Rrrobbie Burrns!' Salts Hospital was never the same after this show and I think even Sir Titus Salt would have appreciated the convivial atmosphere at the hospital he had built in Saltaire, my residence for my first year of studies. In line with a cheerful ceremony in the hospital's kitchen, we finished the evening off singing *Auld Lang Syne*, accompanied by the self-appointed, original bag-piping Viking, hoping to escape *katzenjammer* (caterwaul) the morning after.

Conclusion

The sound of roaring laughter is more contagious than any cough, sniffle or sneeze. Sharing is caring, and nothing is better than sharing a good laugh. It binds people together and increases happiness and intimacy. Humour and laughter strengthen your immune system, boost your energy, diminish pain and protect you from the health-damaging effects of stress. Best of all, it's fun, free and easy to spark off ripples of laughter, as you make your endorphins dance and really move into the feel-good zone of well-being.

CHAPTER EIGHTEEN

RECIPES:

Teta Montaha's Tabbouleh—The Queen of the Table

'From the bitterness of disease, man learns the sweetness of health'. - Catalan Proverb.

Lebanese cuisine, with its world-famous mezze, is delicious, tasteful and healthy—and combining it with pure restructured water, it's even better.

There are so many ways your health can benefit from the use of living, restructured water, as you will see from this chapter. Hopefully, the following pages will whet your appetite in more ways than one!

¾ cup burghur (cracked wheat)—rinsed in vital water

3 cups of parsley, finely chopped after rinsed in alkaline vital water

3 medium-sized tomatoes, finely chopped

1 small onion, finely chopped

2 tbs. olive oil, finest quality

1/3 cup of lemon juice

Place burghur in a bowl. Cover with boiling water.

Stand for 15-20 minutes, dependent on the coarseness of the burghur—until softened.

Drain and rinse in cold vital water.

Press water out with a spoon.

Place burghur, parsley, onion and tomatoes in a bowl

Stir to combine.

Place oil and lemon juice in a screw-top jar. Secure lid. Shake to mix. Drizzle over the tabbouleh. Season with salt and pepper and toss to combine. Ready to serve. Enjoy!

Some families prefer to add mint, cucumber, garlic, paprika and other ingredients. But that is not the traditional way in Lebanon, as Teta Montaha points out.

Ripe and ready for some Tripe?

Teta Montaha's Fabulous Ghammeh (Tripe)

In Lebanon, you can buy both tripe and intestines cleaned. To serve 6-8, you will need the following for stuffing:

200 gr. chickpeas soaked overnight in plenty of vital water with 1 tsp. sodium bicarbonate.

450 short grain Egyptian or calasparra rice.

2x800 gr. freshly cooked tomatoes

500 gr. minced lamb meat.

2 tsp. of allspice (7 pepper mixture)

½ tsp. finely ground black pepper

½ tsp. ground cinnamon and/or 2-3 tsp. of cumin.

4 lamb's trotters

2 cinnamon sticks

1 medium-sized lamb's stomach, washed and rinsed.

Ghammeh is always cooked with raw lamb's feet for a rich broth. Drain and rinse the chickpeas and rub them with sodium bicarbonate and leave for 15-20 minutes before you rinse them. The purpose of this operation is to soften the peas and reduce the cooking time.

Rinse the rice, drain and put in a large mixing bowl. Add the remainder of the stuffing and mix well.

Put the trotters in a large bowl. Cover well with vital water and put on medium heat; as the vital water is about to boil, skin it clean with all the cinnamon sticks, cover and cook for 1½ hours.

You should have cut the tripe into pieces half the size of an A4 sheet of paper and should have 6-7 pieces. Sew 1½ of the sides of each piece of tripe to create a pouch.

Fill these with stuffing, making sure that they are only three-quarters full. The rice will expand during cooking and you need space for it to fill the pouches. Sew up the open ends and set aside.

Add the stuffed tripe to the trotters. More vital water is added to cover if necessary, and salt to cook for 2½ hrs. or until tender. Serve very hot with some broth on the side.

Before serving, take the gelatinous bits of meat off the bone and cut them into small pieces to add to the broth. Season with a little garlic and lemon juice just before serving. Absolutely delicious!

Enjoy Teta Montaha's dessert

From the heart's kitchen in Abdel Wahab El Inglizi comes a gorgeous recipe of Lebanese baklava. This is an authentic Lebanese dish. Meghli is served on special occasions, such as the birth of a child.

Ingredients:

1½ cups of pounded rice

8 cups of vital water

2½ cups of sugar /or 1 tsp. of Stevia, a safe and healthy herb

1 tbsp. caraway seed

1 tbsp. aniseed seed

¼ tsp. powdered ginger

Preparation

Pound rice in a mortar until fine and powdery. Pound spices separately. Mix rice with two cups of Vital Water.

Add sugar or Stevia, caraway and anise. Add it to the remaining 6 cups of vital water, which should be boiling. Add ginger. Boil, stirring occasionally, until mixture coats the spoon. About one hour of cooking is needed, at least.

Pour into individual dishes. Decorate with blanched almonds, walnuts, pine nuts, pistachios and coconut.

This is what you need:

500 grams of filo pastry sheets

500 grams of butter melted

500 grams walnuts and/or pistachios coarsely chopped

200 grams sugar powdered

¼ tsp. freshly ground allspice

¼ powdered cinnamon

For syrup:

300 grams sugar

¾ cup of vital water

1 tbsp. milk

A few drops of orange-blossom essence

This is how you do it:

Mix together sugar, spices and nuts.

Use a flat baking tray and fit the pastry sheet into it.

Brush with melted butter (ghee).

Repeat for half the sheets, piling up.

Spread out mixture evenly over piled sheets.

Repeat alternating sheets and ghee.

Brush uppermost sheet and remaining ghee.

Cut in squares or diamonds, using a pizza cutter.

Bake in preheated oven for 30 minutes at 180*C.

If using hot syrup, keep aside to grow cold first.

Alternatively, use hot if using cold syrup.

Do not do both or the dish will go soggy.

To proceed:

Use milk to clarify syrup.

Make syrup with sugar and vital water, till just under one-thread consistency.

Add essence and stir.

Strain, pour over cold baklava or cool and pour over hot baklava.

It takes about 1 ½ hr. to make

Makes: 20-24 pieces approx.

Bon Appétit! Best fresh. Will last 3 weeks or more if refrigerated.

Aunty Laudy's Moghrabieh

Moghrabieh is a Lebanese couscous, a traditional dish much loved in the Middle East. The name means 'dish of the Maghreb'. Lebanese couscous is larger than traditional couscous and made of semolina flour rolled into pearl-sized balls. Traditionally, a rich chicken and onion broth is served with it, with pieces of chicken, onions and chickpeas.

How to Make the Chicken Stock

First step:

Prepare the chicken and onion stock up to a day in advance. Season the whole chicken with Himalaya or Maldon salt, pepper, cumin and cinnamon or allspice. Brown it in oil in a heavy stockpot over medium heat with the onions until they become evenly golden, approximately 10 minutes.

Second step:

Add enough vital water to completely cover the chicken, plus several bay leaves, and simmer until the chicken is completely cooked. This takes about 1 hour. Remove the chicken and onions and put aside. Discard the bay leaves.

Third step:

Remove bones and skin from the chicken and cut the meat into large chunks.

Heat olive oil over a medium to high heat in a large, heavy sauté pan until shimmering, and then add the drained Moghrabieh and sauté for several minutes, stirring frequently. Add the reserved stock, cumin and cinnamon (or allspice) and simmer over medium heat until the couscous is cooked thoroughly, approximately 15 minutes.

Add the chicken meat, onions and one can of cooked chickpeas, which you have rinsed well,
and simmer until heated through, about 5 minutes. Season to taste and serve immediately.

A little word of warning:

Use caution when heating oil, and never leave the stove unattended. Keep an eye on the children at all times. Ensure that the chicken is cooked thoroughly before serving.

Tips:

Clarified butter can be used instead of olive oil to sauté the Moghrabieh, if desired.

The finished dish can be kept, tightly covered, in the refrigerator for up to 48 hours.

Music and dance: Enjoy the wonderful Fairuz and do a little improvised belly dancing. *A votre santé!*

Raymonde's Traditional Ashta—Clotted Cream
Made with Rose Water and Orange-blossom Water from Damour.

Do you remember the rose-and-orange-blossom water which Teta Montaha collected and prepared with such tender, loving and caring hands? Remember she said, 'The secret is in the water and how you treat it!'

'Ashta', the king of fillers, is a slang word for 'Kashte', which refers to clotted cream prepared with rose-and-orange-blossom water. Ashta is used as filler in desserts such as Knafeh (kungafa), Znoud el Sett. Atayef (Katayif), and many others. Also used on top of fruit cocktails.

Original Versus Modern Ashta

There is more than one method for making Ashta. The modern way is to use boiled milk, corn flour and bread. But compared to Raymonde's recipe, it doesn't compare at all.

Traditionally, this dish should be prepared with preferably raw milk. Depending on the milk's fat content, you may get only one tablespoon of Ashta for one cup of milk.

Using raw milk or whole milk mixed with cream (half and half), bring to boil while you stir, lower the heat and squeeze in a few drops of lemon juice. As soon as the milk starts to clot, add the rose water and the orange-blossom water, and start scooping up the Ashta (clotted cream) from the surface into a strainer. *Voila*!

Once the Ashta cools down, you can use it as filler in Arabic sweets, or you can serve it with fruit cocktails garnished with honey and nuts.

Raymonde's Royal Baba Ghanouj
Inspired by Teta Montaha's TLC

(Raymonde's music choice: Wael Kfoury from Zahle)

A study conducted at the Institute of Biology of Sao Paulo State University, Brazil, found that eggplant juice significantly reduced body weight, plasma cholesterol levels and aortic content of cholesterol in rabbits with high levels of cholesterol. Baba Ghanouj is made by mashing roasted eggplants or aubergines with tahini paste, some garlic and a bit of white vinegar to lighten the colour. It is a wonderful cold appetiser along with pita bread and some salted Lebanese pickles such as turnips, chilli peppers and cucumber.

What you need:

3-5 eggplants, medium size

5 tbsp. of tahini paste

Juice from one freshly squeezed lemon

3 garlic cloves, crushed

1 tbsp. of white vinegar

1 tsp. of Maldon or Himalaya salt

This is how you do it:

Roast the eggplants in the oven on medium heat, for about 30 minutes. Peel them whilst still warm.

Strain the water from the eggplants by placing them in a colander or kitchen sieve, so that you don't end up with a watery Baba Ghanouj.

Place the eggplants and all the ingredients in a food processor and run 2-3 minutes until you get a paste.

Place Baba Ghanouj paste on a serving plate and garnish according to your taste with chopped parsley, olive oil, sumac spice, chilli, salted pickles, et cetera.

Serve cold as an appetiser with pita bread. *Bon appétit!*

Accompanied by Raymonde's choice of music, Nawal Al Zoghbi, and a little improvised oriental belly dancing, this makes for a perfect dining experience.

Most people don't think of tahini or sesame seed paste as a lifesaver, but new research has shown that it is capable of reducing blood markers of cardiovascular disease risk by 39% within only 6 weeks.

It is a sad fact that most people resort to statin drugs or aspirin and not to exercise and improved eating habits, eating nutritious food. Through decades of intense marketing and deceptive education, millions have been manipulated to think of the number one killer as an inevitable unhappy occurrence, with patented medicine being the first choice for 'minimising risks', instead of exploring the core, and the real cause of the problem.

Cholesterol is not the main problem. The damage happens long before that, through a series of wrong lifestyle choices. Through a little investment and persistence in terms of preventative, therapeutic and goal-oriented lifestyle changes, a lot can be achieved. Often it is a question of adding something therapeutic, in terms of what we eat, and taking away something detrimental, like polluted, unhealthy water, changing the body's acidity, and not eating chemical and contaminated dead food.

In the Archives of Iranian Medicine, you can educate yourself on the great health benefits of eating tahini on a regular basis. A research study was conducted with patients with type 2 diabetes, a group with increased risk of developing cardio vascular disease. After six, weeks the researchers noticed a significant improvement in the group that ate tahini every day, compared to the group that continued with their 'normal' diet. There was a 39% decrease in the so-called atherogenic index plasma (AIP)—a significant and positive change for such a small change in diet. It should be noted that the tahini brand used in this research had no additional oil or additives. It was ground sesame seeds, plain and simple. If this had been a drug trial, it would have been broadcast in all the media worldwide as the next life-saving blockbuster drug. Did you know that sesame seeds contain four times as much calcium as milk? And that great milk-drinking nations like Norway have the highest incidence of osteoporosis and fractures? And that the Norwegian dairy industry is one of the main sponsors of our Olympic competitors? Another form of deceptive marketing. And the medical 'experts' keep on advising osteoporotic patients to drink more milk! Sending 'the dog barking up the wrong tree'.

Sesame seeds are truly a superstar among medicinal foods. Eating just 40 grams of sesame seeds, or the equivalent of 2 tablespoons of tahini is far superior to Tylenol in reducing pain from knee arthritis. About 40 health benefits have been confirmed by using sesame seeds, the remarkable healing food.

The unique properties of the lignans found in sesame seeds have been proven to fight inflammation and cancer, boost the body's antioxidant capacity and enhance vitamin E bio-availability. These two lignans, sesamol and sesamin, are also proven to reduce cholesterol levels. The synergy between the lignans and the vitamin E is a possible explanation for the lipid level improvements.

Research has shown that the sesame lignan can be converted by the micro flora of the intestines in humans into the mammalian lignans, enterolactone and enterodiol, which have positive effects against hormone-related diseases such as breast cancer. In 2003, Jacklin et al found that sesamol induces growth arrest and apoptosis (cell death) of cancer and cardiovascular cells. A further study with 220 premenopausal woman reported that the risk of breast cancer fell with increasing levels of enterolactone concentration from lignans in sesame seeds. (Piller, Chang-Claude, Linseisen, Cancer 2006.)

Human clinical research from previewed publications has revealed that simple dietary changes, as simple as eating tahini every day, can have huge impacts on risk factors for the number one killer in our society. Is it not time to wake up and re-evaluate what is going on in the field of medicine? Drugs don't cure diseases any more that bullets cure wars. Foods, on the other hand...

How Mama Pure Energy Norway makes her Tahini paste

This is what you need:

Sesame seeds

Olive oil

And this is how you make it:

Use 2-3 tablespoons of olive oil for every cup of sesame seeds. Make a little or a lot by adding or removing ingredients.

Toast sesame gently over low heat, stirring often, for about 10 minutes and you will see how they change in colour. Remove from heat and let it cool.

Add the sesame seeds to the bowl of a food processor along with ¼ cup of olive oil for every cup of seeds, mix until a thick paste forms, scrape down the sides, and add more olive oil if needed until it reaches the consistency you prefer. Store in a glass jar tightly covered in the refrigerator.

Your homemade tahini will have a rougher texture than the store-bought version and may even have a stronger flavour. The reason for this is that the store-bought variety uses hulled sesame seeds, which makes for a smoother tahini. It is also possible to buy seeds that are not hulled, as they are more nutritious. *Voila!* So easy! Now you have a fabulous homemade super-food ready to be made into hummus, dressings, sauces, baba Ghanouj, mixed into soups or made into sweet treats—whatever your heart desires.

Pure Energy Norway Dr. Viktor Hummus recipe

Use the Prof. Kiss Principle: Keep it simple, silly! Between lovers of hummus, there are two recipes. Some love the zest and deep flavour of tahini; others prefer to go without it, but for a smooth hummus, it beats the store-bought variety any time.

Is there a secret?

Quite simply, the secret lies in the order in which you add ingredients to your food processor. Seriously, it's that simple, according to Prof. Kiss.

This is what you need:

425 grams of chick peas, also called garbanzo beans.

¼ cup of lemon juice, about one large lemon

¼ cup tahini

Half of a large clove of garlic, minced

2 tbsp. of olive oil and a little more for serving

½ tsp. of Maldon or Himalaya salt.

2-3 tbsp. of vital water

A dash of ground paprika for serving

This is how you do it:

Combine tahini and lemon juice in the bowl of the food processor. Mix for 1 min. Scrape sides and bottom of bowl and mix for 30 seconds. This extra time helps to whip or cream the tahini, making it smooth.

Add the olive oil, minced garlic, cumin and salt to the whipped tahini and lemon juice. Mix for 3 seconds and scrape sides and bottom of the bowl and mix another 30 seconds.

Open a can of chickpeas or packet (ecological), drain and rinse properly with vital water. Add half of the chickpeas to the food processor and mix for 1 minute. Scrape sides and bottom of bowl. Add remaining chickpeas until thick and smooth.

Scrape hummus into a bowl and drizzle about 1tbsp. of olive oil over the top and sprinkle with paprika. *Voila! Bon appétit!*

You can store homemade hummus in an airtight container and refrigerate for up to one week.

A Note from Dr. Viktor, the Pure Energy Norway Man

If you are concerned about toxins and nutrition, as you probably are, it is actually very easy to cook the beans, plus they are healthier than those out of a can, because of the BPA in can liners. Also, when food is prepared for canning, the temperature kills many of the nutrients. You are further removing nutrients and fibre when you peel them. Also, you should avoid using the water in the can at all costs (hence the rinsing in vital water). The water in a can contains, in addition to BPAs, preservatives, such as but not limited to citric acid. Don't be fooled: this citric acid does not come from oranges or any other citrus fruit, but from genetically modified corn. Therefore, I recommend soaking the dry peas in vital water overnight, rinsing them well and cooking them with a bit of baking soda, which helps them cook better, quicker, and will help you digest them better, too.

Serve with some Kalmia olives, carrot sticks, pepper, celery, artichokes or whatever you prefer, usually served with pita bread. If you don't have a food processor, you can use a mortar and pestle. While the peas are still in the cooking water, stir them gently with your hand, rubbing them softly between your fingers. The skins slip right off and float above the peas, where they can be scooped up. The peas can then be ground using your mortar and pestle to a silky smoothness.

The slow approach of gently using your hands, and the rhythmic movements of grinding gives you time to relax and contemplate, and the whole process becomes almost therapeutic! Afterwards, you will realise that we all need to slow down occasionally and be more of an observant and active participant in the things we do. *Mindfulness.* Life is full of these precious moments. Enjoy! Engage your whole family in teaching your kids the love and the skill of cooking. As the saying goes, 'The kitchen is the heart of the home. And from it springs all life!'

Dr. Viktor Pure Energy Norway Man—Homemade Ode to the Sesame Seed

Oh, for the love of the tough little powerhouse called the sesame seed;
Oh for the little giant of joy!

A spoonful of tahini or hummus a day will keep the doctor away.
How delicious and yummy-yummy.
A vibrant, long life and a happy tummy!
Good health, good luck and God bless you!

Mama Pure Energy Norway RoRo's Lentil Soup

For thousands of years, the unassuming lentil has been considered a poor man's food. Although they may be cheap, they are very nutritious, filling and the most flavourful of all the legumes.

Lentils, with the botanical name *lens culinaris esculenta*, have been a source of sustenance for our ancestors since prehistoric times. The word *lentil* comes from the Latin lenis, and indeed, this bean cousin is shaped like a double-convex optic lens, which took its name from the lentils. In *Parashat Toldot* we read the history of how Esau sold his birth right to Jacob for some delicious lentil soup. Esau returns from his long day of hunting and demands some of 'that red stuff', but Jacob won't give it to his brother unless Esau agrees to give up his birth right. Esau forfeits his birth right, and the text tells us, 'Jacob then gave Esau bread and lentil stew; he ate what he calls ha-adom ha-adom hazeh, and drank, then he rose and went away.

Lentil soup is thought to have originated in the Middle East and lentils are known in India as dal or dhal. There are hundreds of varieties of lentils, with as many as fifty or more cultivated for food in many colours, with red, green and brown being the most popular.

Lentils have an earthy, nutty flavour, and some varieties lend a slightly peppery touch to the palate.

This is what you need for 8 servings:

6 cups of chicken or vegetable stock, organic

1 pound red lentils

3 tbsp. olive oil

1 tbsp. of minced garlic

1 large onion, chopped

1 tbsp. of ground cumin

½ tsp. of cayenne pepper

½ cup chopped cilantro

¾ cup fresh lemon juice

This is how you prepare it:

Bring chicken or vegetable stock and lentils to the boil in a large saucepan, then reduce to simmer for 20 minutes, medium-low, and cover.

Meanwhile, heat olive oil on a saucepan over medium heat. Stir in garlic and onion, and cook until onion has become translucent, about 3 minutes.

Stir onions into lentils and season with cumin and cayenne. Continue to simmer until the lentils are tender, about 10 minutes. Carefully puree the soup in a standing blender or with a stick blender until smooth. Stir in cilantro and lemon juice before serving

There are many variations of this nutritious and delicious soup. You can, for instance, sauté celery and carrots with the onion and garlic. But the above is a traditional recipe passed down from Teta Montaha, Teta Georgette and Raymonde (RoRo).

Pure Energy Norway!

Conclusion

By following the recommendations in this book, you will live a healthy and long life, well blessed with fun and well-being, beginning with living water…

One world famous person who followed much of the health advice given in this book but lacked a few very vital pointers, is the witty, wise and ingenious writer, inventor and politician, Benjamin Franklin.

CHAPTER NINETEEN

Benjamin Franklin, A Most Remarkable Man

'Early to bed and early to rise, makes a man healthy, wealthy and wise'. Benjamin Franklin.

On a visit to London at the age of nineteen, Ben went on a boating excursion with his printer friends. During the trip, he leaped into the 'Thames River and swam from Chelsea to Blackfriars', performing every kind of feat, underwater and over. The story does not tell whether Sir Richard had taken off his 'Considering Cap', an expression borrowed from *The Drinker's Dictionary*, originally printed in Benjamin Franklin's *The Pennsylvania Gazette*.

Having swum in the River Thames myself a little too freely with the Creator, I don't think either Ben or I were aware of the many deceptive and devious undercurrents and eddies that exist on certain stretches of the River Thames, where many people have drowned. I think we both should have been grateful to wake up the next morning and not find our names on the obituary page.

Benjamin Franklin was endowed with so many talents and his often humorous outlook on life is well worth remembering: 'I wake up every morning at nine and grab for the morning paper. Then I look at the obituary page. If my name is not on it, I get up!'

Benjamin Franklin was 'the first' in many areas: He started the first circulating library in the colonies at 21 years of age;

organised the first volunteer fire company in 1736; the first insurance company in the colonies; invented the famous Franklin Stove, which was actually called the Pennsylvania Fireplace. Ben could have made a fortune selling the stove, but gave the marketing to his friend, Robert Grace, and refused to accept any personal profits from the enterprise. His satisfaction came from the fact that his stove warmed the houses of America more safely and effectively than ever before. He was also very happy that his stove would allow for better ventilation and greater fuel efficiency. In this respect, he showed great insight regarding the importance of the indoor climate for people's health and well-being—a visionary and great preventative explorer of environmental factors' influence on health.

In 1751, Benjamin Franklin was instrumental in the founding of the first hospital in America, as he was a great fundraiser. James Parton, an early Franklin biographer, called Ben 'The first effective preacher of the blessed gospel of ventilation. He spoke and the windows of hospitals were lowered; consumption, the white scourge, TB ceased to gasp and fever to inhale poison.'

Perhaps Benjamin Franklin is best known for his many inventions and experiments in electricity. Since he wasn't very good at mathematics, he experimented by trial and error with simple objects including wax plates, iron rods, tubes of resin, a gun barrel. The lightning rod is one of his many inventions.

His 'single fluid theory' led to the electron theory, with Nobel Prize winner in physics Robert A. Millikan calling Ben's experiment that led to his theory, 'Probably the most fundamental thing ever done in the field of electricity.'

He was also instrumental in officially starting the University of Pennsylvania, in 1791. Ben, who had had less than two years of schooling himself, was the clear and unchallenged ancestor of a major university. As a young man, he taught himself to read French, Spanish, Italian and Latin and had a great passion for self-improvement. He certainly was what we'd call an autodidact: a person who has learned a subject without the benefit of a teacher or a formal education. Ben enjoyed the simple life, though he could have made a fortune.

The following are some of the more curious inventions from the genius mind of Benjamin Franklin:

The rocking chair: In the seventies, I suggested that the elderly in healthcare should use this invention, to stimulate and maintain good circulation as they would rock back and forth.

A library step stool which could be lifted and folded.

A Mechanical Arm for reaching books on high shelves.

A Writing chair (still used).

An Odometer: to measure distance walked or travelled, originally used by the postal service.

Further inventions by this amazing man included a new kind of anchor, a pulley system, improved street lighting, and bifocal spectacles. In 1761, he created a musical instrument, a *harmonica,* as Ben would call it. It became wildly popular in the eighteenth century, and even some of the great luminaries such as Beethoven and Mozart have composed music for this instrument. Franklin also taught himself guitar, violin and harp. He even composed a string quartet, '*Simplicity*' that stressed easy playing.

On the Game of Chess, Ladies, Distraction and Inspiration

The World Champion of Chess, Norwegian Magnus Carlsen, who outplayed Viswanathan Anand from India, is also keen on working out, playing football and skiing. With a good sense of humour, he is a little like Benjamin Franklin.

The game of chess was especially important to the latter. In his *Morals of Chess* (1779), he states, 'For life is a kind of chess, in which we often have points to gain and competitors or adversaries to contend with, and in which there is a vast variety of good and ill events, that are, in some degree, the effects of produce or the want of it. For, by playing, we may learn foresight, circumspection and caution.

Benjamin Franklin helped to draft the Declaration of Independence in 1776, the Treaty of Paris in 1783, and the Constitution of the United States in 1787. In addition, he negotiated and signed the Treaty Amity with France in 1778, which secured

France's financial and military support, without which the American Revolution would likely have fallen apart.

One evening in Paris, Franklin played late into the night with Madame Brillion de Jouy, a much younger woman with whom he was close friends. Later, while she lay in the bath, Franklin wrote to her: 'Upon returning home, I was astonished to find that it was almost eleven o'clock. I fear that we were so overly engrossed in the game of chess as to forget everything else; we caused great inconvenience to you, by detaining you so long in the bath. Tell me, my dear friend, how are you feeling this morning? Never again will I consent to start a game in your bathroom. Can you forgive me this indiscretion?'

A relaxing bath, spa or hydrotherapy par excellence, combined with cerebral gymnastics and an elegant and eloquent Benjamin Franklin by one's side would definitely make for body-mind-soul therapy of the highest magnitude.

Thomas Jefferson (1743-1826) and America's third President recorded the exchange when Franklin was in Paris:

'When Dr. Franklin went to France on his revolutionary mission, his eminence as a philosopher, his venerable appearance, and the cause on which he was sent, rendered him extremely popular. For all ranks and conditions of men there entered warmly into the American interest. He was therefore feasted and invited to all court parties. At these he sometimes met the old Duchess of Bourbon, who, by being a chess player of about his force, they very generally played together. Happening once to put her king into prise, the doctor took it.'

'Ah,' she says, 'we do not take kings so.'

'We do in America,' says Doctor Franklin.

The great statesman, doctor and inventor certainly had charisma, charm and humour. The latter he used eloquently in the 'dialogue with his big toe' in *Dialogue Between the Gout and Mr Franklin*. Despite his vigorous physical workouts, adherence to nutritious food and temperance in drink, a virtue he tried to stick to throughout his life, life in Paris, with its many temptations in this field, must at least have made his gout worse.

An article in the *New York Times* in 2009, titled 'Disease of Rich Extends Its Pain to Middleclass', announced a comeback of the painful disease, which afflicts the big toe, caused by a build-up of uric acid due to the breakdown of purines in the food. Purines are found in abundance in many meats, fish, seafood and sugary drinks with high-fructose corn syrup (HFCS), alcohol, cocktails and beers. Certain vegetables also contain purines—such as asparagus, cauliflower, spinach and mushrooms, organ meats, bread, turkey, tuna, goose, pate. The increased acidity and lack of oxygenation in the tissues leads to accumulations of waste products that, together with a possible insidious lead poisoning, would have been contributing factors towards B. Franklin's gout, gallbladder and kidney stones. Remember, he worked for many years as a printer, and lead poisonings and other heavy metal accumulation s not uncommon in such a working environment.

Gout and arthritis are successfully treated if the patient is:

- Willing to alkalise by drinking vital water, eating alkalising food, and avoiding food that produces acidity in the tissues. A study of Franklin's favourite foods, especially during the period he spent in France, showed they were definitely on the acidic side.
- Detoxify using herbs, minerals, chlorophyll, zeolite, et cetera.
- Strengthen and balance immunity.
- Royal Rife treatment.

We follow this protocol regularly, with great success, at the Viktorklinikken. While he was suffering from an attack in October 1780, Franklin wrote the *Dialogue Between the Gout and Mr Franklin*. The humorous outlook on this condition and how he relates this story makes for a good laugh and longstanding joyful medicine which we should all take daily.

Happy Herbal Remedies

I could tell you about many unsung heroes in the herbal family. Take, for example, mint, rosemary and balm—associated with longevity and clarity of mind. The Englishman John Hussey lived till he was 116 and drank balm tea every morning—as did Loewe, Prince of Glamorgan, who lived to 108.

In Spain, rosemary is called *the pilgrims flower,* and Queen Elizabeth of Hungary used it regularly when she was 72, for her gout and crippling rheumatism. She regained her health and vigour to such an extent that the King of Poland asked her for her hand in marriage.

A popular herb from the many herbs in the garden of King Solomon, a very wise and rich man, was thyme. In the 39 *Books of Talmud* dating back to the first century, thyme with its volatile oils is mentioned alongside cumin, caraway, clove, rosemary, mint and many others as great remedies against many maladies, including gout, gallstones and kidney stones.

Thyme was found in the tomb of Tutankhamen and grows in Egypt today. Maurice Mességué, the famous French herbalist, mentioned the volatile oil thyme from the Louis plant as an excellent weapon against infections, from boils to typhoid fever and TB to gout.

Just before I finish off, for all folks suffering from inflammation, pain and swelling, let me draw your affection to a miracle herb from the Last Supper: parsley. This unassuming herb is a powerhouse of healing properties. At the Passover table, parsley symbolises a new beginning, since it's one of the first herbs to peep up from the ground in the spring. Parsley is a well-known remedy, prepared properly, which removes poisons from the body, and waste products that contain uric acid. It acts on the tubules of the kidneys by virtue of two substances, apiol and myristicin. Parsley acts like a natural diuretic, draining excess swelling and fluid from the body.

The famous herbalist Culpeper wrote that the seed of parsley was effective in dissolving kidney stones and easing pain. Boil in vital water and simmer parsley for 10-12 seconds to prepare your daily tea—perfectly wonderful! Cheers my friend, Ben! You're my holistic hero!

Indeed, with so many contaminants and toxins in water, food and environments these days, a tea, for example, rosemary and sage, works wonders at keeping the chemical substance acetyl-choline (a nerve transmission agent) in good working order. 'Sage is effective for quickening the senses and memory!' wrote John Gerard (1545-1612) in his journal. 450 years later, British researchers discovered why and how this remedy worked: by inhibiting the enzyme that breaks down acetylcholine. Today, it is considered useful in helping to prevent Alzheimer's.

On a Boat Trip Across the Atlantic

Even on the boat trip home, Benjamin Franklin continued his experiments, and when he returned to Philadelphia in 1785 from his services in France, guns fired and church bells rang to welcome him home. This brainy, humorous, charming and kind man, a celebrity, albeit a little gout-ridden, returned in style. He became president of Pennsylvania's Supreme Council, equivalent to governor today, a call he could not resist in spite of his health problems.

'My country's folk,' he joked, 'have taken the prime of my life. They have eaten my flesh and seem to have resolved to pick my bones!'

Benjamin: 'son of my sorrows' in Hebrew—so named Rachel her youngest son of Jacob, who later changed the son's name to 'son of the south' or 'son of the right hand'.

Well, Ben, oh, Ben, you created so much light and joy around your creative, versatile, original lifestyle. Unknown to most people, B. Franklin loved turkey and wished it had been chosen as the US's national bird, rather than the Bald Eagle. He states, 'For the truth, the Turkey is in comparison a much more respectable Bird and a true Native of America... He is besides, though a little vain and silly, a Bird of Courage, and would not hesitate to attack a Grenadier of the British Guards who should presume to invade his Farm Yard with a red Coat on.'

Experimentations in the field of electricity led to him killing animals by electrocution, because it was more humane than the existing slaughter methods, and made them 'uncommonly tender'. More human, certainly, but also risky: 'Two nights ago, being about to kill a Turkey from the shock of two large Glass Jars (Leyden Jars), containing as much electric fire as forty common Phials, I inadvertently took the whole thro' my own Arm and Body.' Benjamin Franklin.

'Dizzy Person + Turkey = Wobble, wobble! Corn + Turkey = Cobble, Cob-ble!'

Dear Ben (Benjamin Franklin): I concur with your statement on the turkey! You are my holistic hero and I raise to you my glass of vital water, the only drink for a wise man! *Cheers*! Had I been around, I would have given you the following pieces of advice:

- Water is the *only* drink for a wise man! (Henry David Thoreau 1817-1862)
- Check your diet and curb your sweet tooth tendency!
- Let's go and swim in the River Thames for some fun and frolic! Or a freshwater lake in Norway? How about a dip in the famous Lysefjorden, 'the most dreadful place on earth', according to Victor Hugo?

Come to think about it, I might have shown you how celery juice, with its 20 or so different anti-inflammatory properties, lowers uric acid. And the immediate cause of gout is accumulation of uric acid in the joints from eating too many sweet and starchy foods, thus forming chard-like crystals in the joints which give rise to sharp, excruciating pain, and sometimes kidney stones.

Herbs and Spices

Herbs and spices are an incredible source of antioxidants with great antimicrobial and anti-inflammatory properties. The powerful chemicals they contain can be used in the treatment of many conditions and, with their synergistic effect, they are more balanced and have a greater advantage over isolated drugs and their toxic side effects.

The Bible mentions 128 plants that were in everyday use in ancient Israel, Lebanon and neighbouring regions. Medicinal herbalist James Duke, Ph.D., former chief of the USDA Medicinal Plant Laboratory and author of *Herbs of the Bible: 2000 years of Plant Medicine,* describes a detailed list of fifty of the most important healing herbs, spices and essential oils from the Scripture.

If you go Ezekiel 47:12, you will catch a fascinating glimpse into the divine healing properties of leaves and refreshing fruits. 'Along the bank of the river, on this side and that, will grow all kinds of trees used for food. Their leaves will not wither, and their fruit will not fail. They will bear fruit every month, because their water flows from the sanctuary. Their fruit will be for good, and their leaves for medicine.'

A herb is defined as a seed-bearing annual, biennial or perennial that does not develop a persistent woody tissue but dies down at the end of a growing season (unlike a tree). It is valued as a plant for its medicinal, savoury or aromatic qualities. In our Western cultures, this heritage is almost forgotten, but there has been a renewal of interest in herbal medicine over the past years, as shown by the work of Dr. David Daron who identified and photographed 80 different plants mentioned in the Bible that still grow in Israel today.

Did you know that murder plots and national atrocities were spawned by vegetable gardens? King Ahab's wife, the infamous Jezebel, got furious and took matters into her own hands when Naboth refused to sell his vineyard. (Some versions, like The New

International and New American versions translate it 'vegetable garden'). Naboth was wrongfully stoned, and King Ahab suddenly became the unlawful owner of the garden he wanted.

In the kingdom of plants, herbs and seeds, God offers us healing medicines for preserving and enhancing life. (I. Kings 21:2-13)

Under the emerging new global government, which allows global domination to take root, biotech and big agricultural corporations control the world's food supply at the expense of personal liberty. According to a proposed new law, it will be illegal to grow, reproduce or trade any vegetable seed or tree that has not been tested and approved by the 'EU Plant Variety Agency'. The new law basically puts the government in charge of all plants and seeds in Europe, and prevents home gardeners from growing their own plants from non-regulated seeds. If they do, they will now be considered criminals. A community petition on Avaaz.org titled 'We don't accept this' is nearing 100,000 signatures and may have a worthwhile influence in convincing Europe's unelected bureaucrats to drop the law.

It reminds me of the Codex Alimentarius laws, the single greatest threat to our access to natural health products and the right to control our food supply, GMO food, organic food, food additives, pesticide residues, food supplements. The development of the Codex laws is not good for people or the environment, as they greatly favour the pharmaceutical industry, which will profit from the increasing chronic disease burden that results. The increasing use of GMOs, which are endorsed by the Codex, is a huge problem for human health and the environment alike. The nutritional content of food is a low priority.

Are you willing to let governments and corporations control what you put into your body? On the basis of ample scientific evidence, it is the micronutrient deficiencies associated with modern Western diets and the toxicity of the water and the environment that are responsible for the epidemic of chronic disease, including the 'Big 5': heart disease, cancer, diabetes, obesity and osteoporosis which contribute to the greatest burden on our healthcare system, as Dr. Bruce Adams, Professor of Biochemistry and Molecular Biology, University of California, Berkley, and many scientists with him, proclaim.

Thomas Jefferson (1762-1821), the Third President of the US, and author of the Declaration of Independence, said, 'If people let governments decide what foods they eat and what medicines they take, their bodies will soon be in as sorry a state as the souls of those who live under tyranny.'

Do you see the parallel between Jezebel's unlawful robbery of Naboth's garden and the Codex/EU laws to 'perfect' us, and rob us of our own choice of nutritious food including vital water and food supplements to prevent and even reverse the 'Big 5'? We must not only protect our lifeblood but that of future generations.

Conclusion

The change that you want to see in the world today begins with the change you are willing to make in your personal life today. Choose wisely.

CHAPTER TWENTY

Healing Herbs, From the Garden of God

*'Whoever believes in me, as the Scripture said; out of his heart will
flow rivers of living water'. John. 7:38.*

Herbs and spices have been around since time immemorial in
folklore and ancient cultures. A substantial part of this folklore is
centred on the supernatural healing powers added to the food from
herbs and spices, with their many remarkable qualities. A romantic
cook would understand the symbolism associated with different
herbs and spices. For example, rosemary symbolises remembrance,
and bay leaves represent fidelity, while cardamom and cinnamon are
said to inspire 'passionately wild abandon'.

From the marvellous variety of herbs, these are some of my
favourites:

Aloes. Aloe vera barbedensis, miller, aloe ferox (cape aloe):
Nicodemus used aloe and myrrh before he wrapped the body of
Yeshua (John 19:39-40). The Aloe sailed the ocean blue to America
and is now a household remedy, especially in the treatment of burns
and skin irritation, as it aids in the healing of open sores. It has
anaesthetic and antibacterial properties. It increases blood flow to
the affected area and acts as an astringent when applied topically
(see the *Story of Viktor*). Aloe Vera also works remarkably well with

sports injuries, contusions, bruises, inflammation and swelling in conjunction with traumatic sprains and much more. Aloe was my first love in the field of herbal plant medicine, and standing in the Negev desert in 1987 with a baby Aloe in my hand in the Moshav, Ein Yahav, was an unforgettable experience.

Coriander (coriander sativum): Both an herb and a spice. In much of the world, coriander is used in reference to cilantro leaves. In America, it generally refers to the dried cilantro seeds, which are used as a spice both in whole and ground form. Coriander seeds have a bit of a spicy, citrus flavour. Its name is derived from the Greek work *koriandron*, meaning a cultivated 'buggy'-smelling plant. Coriander seeds have been found in ruins dating back to 5000 BC. Also known as Chinese parsley, has been used traditionally as a remedy against indigestion, neuralgia, rheumatism and toothache, and was also a well-known culinary herb used in salsa and ceviche, as well as Indian and Asian specialities such as garam masala. When adding fresh cilantro to a hot dish, make sure to do it at the last minute to get the full benefit of the aroma. According to scientific research, cilantro is a heavy metal chelator for mercury, lead, cadmium and aluminium, removing these from the body. Coriander contains about 20 natural chemicals possessing antibacterial properties that help to cleanse the body, and its essential oil treats indigestion and excess gas. Cilantro root may substitute garlic, but wash the root thoroughly before mincing or crushing.

Remember to put all herbs, fruits and vegetables in water

with a pH of 10 for 10-12 minutes to cleanse and remove pesticides (the negative electrical charge in the alkaline water that attracts the positively charged chemicals).

Black Cumin (nigella sativa): Originally, this herb was used to purge the body of worms and parasites. According to an Arab proverb, black cumin is 'the herb for every disease except death'.

In Europe, these seeds are often mixed with peppercorns and taste hot to the tongue. Thymoquinone and nigellone, the chief ingredients in black cumin oil, relieve bronchial spasms and are used for asthma, bronchitis, emphysema and coughs. They also boost the immune system. Abscesses and tumours of the abdomen, eyes and liver were treated with cumin oil, due to the fact that the oil contains anti-tumour sterol and beta-sitosterol.

Black cumin or '*Habbal ul Sawda*' as it is known in Arabic is considered a super-food and is mentioned in the Old Testament when the prophet Isaiah talks of 'harvesting the black seed'. The seed is a significant source of fatty acids, proteins, carbohydrates, vitamins and minerals B-1, B-2, B-3, calcium and iron, phosphors et cetera. Black cumin has been proved scientifically to have strong antibacterial, antiviral, anti-inflammatory and antioxidant properties. Black cumin is enjoying a revival across the Muslim world and in the West. It is even an ingredient in Evoca Cola or 'Islam Cola'. Black Cumin is called a panacea ('a cure-all').

Dandelion (taraxacum officinal): This tenacious plant, for some an annoying weed, is a powerful healing plant, which among other things contains boron, 130 parts per million of boron, running a close second to cabbage, which has 150. Boron together with silicon (also in cabbage) is an important building mineral for strong bone structure.

Dandelion is one of the bitter herbs eaten at Passover. Traditionally, it has been used as a remedy for cancer, diabetes, hepatitis, osteoporosis and rheumatism. It is an excellent diuretic and is used in weight loss and to get rid of oedema (swelling). Rather than depleting the body of potassium like synthetic diuretic drugs do, dandelion provides extra potassium.

The leaves are rich in Vitamin C and contain more beta-carotene than carrots, and its roots acts as a diuretic and purgative for treating kidney and liver disorders.

Some believe that the Greek words for *lion* and *tooth* led to the first part of the dandelions botanical name, '*Leontadon*'. It is also believed that the French word '*dent-de-lion*' ('tooth of the lion') led to the name *dandelion*.

As a poultice, dandelion has been used in the treatment of breast cancer. European herbalists consider dandelion to be one of the best herbs for building blood and helping anaemia, and use the herb for diabetes and liver diseases. It is used in salads and in cooking (root).

One patient reported the following:' I had little energy and abdominal pain on the right side and assumed it was due to liver congestion or infection. I stopped taking all vitamin and mineral supplements and started dandelion in capsule form. It was simply amazing! I was re-energised; my whole body felt renewed. It was as if all the toxins had been flushed out and the pain vanished. A miracle!'

Dandelion has been used to stimulate the flow of bile from the liver. It works so well that, with long-term use, it can expel the first stages of liver cirrhosis. This herbal flower is much cursed and looked down upon, as it has a tendency to crop up on the lawns—when in fact it should be revered for all its powerful healing properties, which can restore your health and balance.

Dandelion juice is a remarkable remedy in fighting rheumatoid arthritis and other chronic joint diseases. In stubborn cases, a mixture of dandelion and watercress, both bitter herbs from the Last Supper, has been described as having great success. Together with a restricted diet, avoidance of foods that cause intolerance symptoms and plentiful vital, restructured water, this is a great recipe for joint pain, swelling and reduced mobility.

Dandelion is regarded as God's gift for the relief of liver and kidney problems, Bright's disease, gallstones and kidney stones, arteriole-sclerosis, obesity and high blood pressure—and there are many testimonials to prove it.

Some of dandelion's uses are listed hereafter.

Night blindness: According to *Deutsche Medisinishe Wochenschift* (16.2.19.51), Dr. Niedemeier is treating night blindness with great success, most probably because of a substance called helemin in dandelion, together with vitamins A and B, which is also found in abundance in this plant.

Amazing energy boost: from two bitter herbs from the Last Supper. If you drink one cup of dandelion juice with the same amount of watercress, a 'natural high' or an intense surge of energy will hit you once the liquid reaches the liver. In some older, people it may be a little overwhelming so it may be wise to dilute it with vital water or carrot juice.

A healing remedy for breast pain: in China, dandelion is used in inflammatory cancers, mastitis (breast inflammation), lack of milk flow, et cetera. The whole plant is used, both externally as a topical poultice and internally as a juice. All parts of the plant contain a somewhat bitter, milky juice. But the juice of the root, as this is most potent, is the part most often used for medicinal purposes.

To remove warts: An old folk remedy is to squeeze the dandelion stem and then apply the whitish milk over the warts. Within a week or so, the wart shrivels and disappears. I can vouch for that—it works.

Liver congestion: A soup of dandelion roots, sliced and boiled in vital water with some leaves of sheep sorrel, also one of the bitter herbs from the Last Supper, and the yolk of an egg taken daily for one month can cure obstinate cases of liver congestion.

Respiratory infections: Numerous clinical studies have shown dandelion to be effective against pneumonia, bronchitis and respiratory infections, as well as stomach problems, improving digestion and alleviating and removing stones or gravel from the gallbladder or kidneys.

The young leaves may be used in salads. Rinse well and let the leaves and other parts of the salad soak in pH 10 water. Rinse well. Some grated garlic, Himalaya salt, hempseed oil, a few tomatoes and spring onions and a grated lemon peel together with lemon juice—and *voila*, a nutritious and tasty salad!

Dandelion wine and beer are common refreshments in the US, Canada and England.

The rousted roots are used to make dandelion coffee, almost indistinguishable from ordinary coffee in taste. It stimulates the whole digestive system, assisting the liver and the kidneys to do their function and helping the bowels to work efficiently, preventing formation of gallstones, hepatitis or liver inflammation.

Sheep sorrel (rumex acetocella): is a perennial weed that has been used in multiple roles for centuries, including:

- Anti-cancer therapy
- Anti-inflammatory agent
- Antibacterial agent

- Immune system booster
- Antioxidant
- Vitamin deficiency
- Food preparation

The entire plant, including the roots, is used as the main ingredient in Essiac tea, René Caisse's famous anti-cancer recipe. It contains an abundance of disease-fighting substances such as Vitamins A, B-complex, C, D, E and K, and natural molecules used to make many drugs, including anti-cancer medications. Sheep sorrel works very well in sinusitis as it reduces pain, inflammation and swelling, mainly due to the tannins in the plant, which help to decrease mucus formation. There is a lot of clinical evidence for its effectiveness in treating sinusitis. Due to the presence of oxalic acid, people with a history of kidney stones should avoid this herbal plant.

According to René Caisse, sheep sorrel has the greatest liver detoxification properties of the four ingredients in the Essiac preparation. Outside of health uses, sheep sorrel has been used extensively in the culinary world for hundreds of years. It is known for its sour taste, and it is even called '*azeda*' in Portugal, which means 'sour'. A common weed and a powerful herbal plant, which we ate a lot of when we were playing in the fields.

Nikoline Broccolini! Yummy! Yummy! Sauteed

This is what you need:

1 bunch of broccolini

Kosher salt or Himalaya salt

2 tbsp. of Virgin Coconut oil

½ lemon, zested

1 tsp. of lemon juice

¼ tsp. freshly ground pepper

This is how you do it:

Blanch the broccolini in a large pot of boiling vital water with salt, for 2 minutes. Drain immediately and immerse in ice-cold vital water.

Melt the coconut butter in a large sauté pan. Add the lemon zest and garlic and stir. Drain the broccolini and add to the garlic mixture and heat for 2 minutes. Add the lemon juice. ½ tsp. of salt and pepper. Toss well before serving. *Bon Appétit!*

The granddaddy spice of 'em all—Turmeric (curcuma longa):
This herb and spice possesses great anti-inflammatory and antioxidant properties. According to Sayer Ji, founder of Green Med Info, this herb has an unparalleled record in its proven scientific value to our health and well-being. Unlike any other herb, turmeric has many hundreds of positive side effects with its exceptionally

high margin of safety, compared to hydrocortisone, ibuprofen and chemotherapy drugs. This remarkable Ayurvedic medical herb, with its primary polyphenol known as curcumin, has many amazing properties, among them:

- Destroys multi-drug-resistant cancer
- Protects against radiation-induced damage
- Protects against heavy metal toxicity
- Prevents and reverses Alzheimer's-associated pathology
- Reduces inflammation.

Currently 580 conditions react favourably to the use of turmeric. This is a non-patentable medicine and its very existence is a threat to the trillion-dollar pharmaceutical industry.

Turmeric is widely used in cooking and gives Indian curry its yellow colour. Make sure to use organic and unprocessed turmeric to get the maximum benefit from this herb. Don't waste your time and health with synthetically processed herbs and spices.

The ancient Polynesians carried turmeric with them on their incredible voyage across the Pacific Ocean to Hawaii. Today, the Hawaiians still use this spice, known to them as olena.

While Marco Polo was in China in 1280 AD, he recorded in his diary, 'There is also a vegetable which has all the properties of true saffron, as well as the smell and colour, and yet it is not saffron.' For this very reason turmeric, has been used as a culinary substitute for saffron in Europe for over 700 years.

Turmeric can even promote skin health by cleansing and maintaining good elasticity, providing nourishment for the skin and balancing the effects of skin flora. It has anti-aging properties due to its antioxidant properties. Turmeric acts like an adaptogen, helping to support your body's immune system against stress. Turmeric is one of the principle herbs in Ayurveda—India's ancient holistic health system. Ayurveda means 'knowledge of life'. Herbs lie at the very heart of Ayurvedic medicine.

In Ayurvedic terminology, turmeric's properties include:

- Verdana sthapana: Promotes a healthy nervous system and alleviates discomfort
- Sangrahani: Helps to absorb vitamins and minerals.
- Anulomana: Helps through a purging action. Removes waste and rebuilds healthy blood.
- Rakta stambhaka: Promotes circulatory system wellness.

An estimated 500 million Indians still use the spice today.

Mint (mentha longifolia): Mint is a sweet-scented historical plant and is mentioned in two of the Gospels (Matt. 23:23, Luke 11:42), Yeshua said, 'Woe to you hypocritical Torah-teachers and P'rushim! You pay your tithes (1/10) of mint, dill and cumin, but you have neglected the weightier matters of the Torah-justice, mercury, trust. These are the things you should have attended to—

without neglecting the others.' Complete Jewish Bible. (*Hypocrite* in Greek means '*one who wears a mask*'.)

Mint used to be part of Greek mythology and, according to legend, 'Menthe', originally a nymph and Pluto's lover, made Pluto's wife, Persephone, angry who, in a fit of rage, turned Menthe into a lowly plant to be trod upon. Pluto who could not manage to undo the spell but softened it by delivering Menthe a sweet scent, which would perfume the air when her leaves were stepped upon—thus the aromatic herb mint. I guess that is why I have an abundance of these beguiling aromatic plants in my garden, as the invigorating scent fills the air on sweet summer days as I brush past them. The scent recalls many happy memories!

Traditionally, mint is used for digestive relief. Peppermint oil is anti-allergic, anti-spasmodic and is used in aromatherapy to stimulate brain activity. It is also used to remove the smell from stale rooms that need refreshing, or the old Hagar the Horrible who's been bar-hopping and zooted and needs to retrieve a bunch of parsley or a twig of mint to refresh before facing Helga, his large and bossy housewife (Kari was his second wife, in case you wondered).

Frequently used in salads, as garnish on food, in tea, or ice tea. If you soak mint and other herbs in alkaline vital water 10 minutes, pH 8-10, it cleanses the herbs and the flavour and aroma becomes noticeably stronger. Great in smoothies. Very alkaline.

Nettle (urtica dioica): 'Stinging nettles' get their name from the Latin word *urtica*, meaning to burn, because of the tiny hairs on the leaves that cause a burning sensation when touched. Nettles are mentioned in the Book of Job.

There is virtually nothing this versatile plant can't be used, and today it features in a wealth of products, from hair conditioners to beer. They are storehouses of health, are rich in vitamin A, G, E, K as well as other antioxidants, minerals (boron), may relieve arthritis, and can be used in stews, soups, mashed with potatoes and blended into smoothies.

In 18th-century England, nettles were sold as a vegetable at the market and traditional English country gardens always contained a nettle bed as 'The first green vegetable to appear after the long winter's diet of salted meat.' (Isabell Shipard: '*How Can I use Herbs in my Daily Life?*')

In short, this herb is diuretic, astringent, tonic, nutritive, antispasmodic, antihistamine, herpetic, nephritic and anti-rheumatic. Very much an alkalinising herb. Anti-parasitic and antibacterial. Used for: T. B. bronchitis, cough, weight reduction, gout, rheumatism, arthritis, tendonitis, bursitis, allergies, hay fever, asthma, neuralgia, MS, skin complaints, PMS, external and internal bleeding (astringent function).

To fall into a bunch of stinging nettles as a kid, running around in his shorts one fine summer, is no joke. That's what happened to my beloved little brother. Oh, the screams and pain are still vividly ingrained in my mind. We rushed him to Mum who knew a thing or two about first-aid healing remedies. Baking soda to the rescue! (vinegar also works). Soon the pain and skin blisters subsided. What a relief—phew!

Dill (anethum graveolens): Dill's unique health benefits come from two types of healing components: Monoterpenes, including carvone, limonene and anethofuran. It also contains flavonoids including kaempferol and vicemi.

The monoterpene components have the ability to activate the enzyme glutathione-S-transferase, which helps attack the antioxidant molecules glutathione to radicals, which could otherwise do damage in the body. We speak of dill's volatile oils, which act as 'chemo protective' food, much like parsley. This can help to neutralise particular types of carcinogens, for instance benzopyrenes, which are part of pollution from trash incinerators. Dill also has an antibacterial and anti-Candida role to play together with garlic and other herbs. Dill contains calcium, magnesium, manganese, iron and dietary fibre and is good as part of an osteoporosis prevention programme. Also a whole range of vitamins.

Dill's name came from the Old Norse word '*dilla*', which means 'to lull', a name that reflects its calming effect as a stomach soother and insomnia reliever. Dill, as we have seen, is mentioned in the Bible (Matt 23:23, Luke 11:42) and was popular in the ancient Greek and Roman cultures, where it was considered a sign of wealth and was revered for its many healing properties. The Conqueror Charlemagne even made it available to his guests at banquet tables, so his guests who had indulged too much could benefit from its carminative properties. Today, dill is used in the cuisines of Scandinavia (fish, salmon, 'gravlax', egg, salads) as well as in Central Europe, North Africa and Russia. It is also mixed with potatoes, green beans, and plain yogurt.

Cumin (cuminum cyminum): Many seeds, including cumin, look rather unassuming, but you can't judge a book by its cover, as the saying goes, for cumin has made it into the stellar ranks of Indian, Middle Eastern and Mexican cuisine, and health-wise it is anything but ordinary.

Not surprisingly, cumin seeds resemble caraway seeds, as well as parsley and dill, which belong to the same family (umbelliferae). Cumin is an excellent source of iron. In addition to playing an integral part as a component of haemoglobin, which transports oxygen from the lungs to all body cells and is also part of key enzyme systems for energy production and metabolism and essential for keeping the immune system healthy. Iron is particularly important for menstruating women, growing children, adolescents and pregnant women.

Research has shown cumin to be of benefit for the digestive system, as it stimulates the release of pancreatic enzymes, compounds that are necessary for proper digestion and nutrient assimilation.

Cumin is known for its anti-carcinogenic properties because of its radical scavenging abilities and its ability to enhance the liver detoxification enzymes.

Cumin, together with mint and dill, is also mentioned in the Bible (Matt 23:23, Luke 11:42), not only as a seasoning for soup and bread, but also as a currency to pay tithes to the priests. In ancient Egypt, cumin was not only used as a culinary spice but was also used to mummify pharaohs.

Cumin was well known for its culinary, cosmetic and medicinal properties but became a symbol of frugality and greed in ancient Rome. Both Marcus Aurelius and Antoninus Pius, emperors with a reputation for the avarice, were nicknames that included a reference to cumin.

During the Middle Ages in Europe, cumin was at its most popular, becoming recognised as a symbol of love and fidelity. People carried cumin in their pockets at weddings, and married soldiers were sent away to war with a loaf of cumin bread baked by their wives. Cumin acts as a natural preservative, making the bread stay fresher for longer.

In Arabic traditions, a concoction of cumin, pepper and honey is thought to have aphrodisiac properties. It's certainly tasty, but whether it will actually inspire cupid's arrows in these days of Viagra and other love poisons is uncertain. But as a flavour in vegetable, chicken, lamb and fish dishes, together with legumes, lentils, garbanzo beans and black beans, it certainly adds extra punch and power!

Tips:

- Take organic plain brown rice and magically give it extra zest and pizzazz by adding cumin seeds, dried apricots, almonds and a dollop of coconut oil.
- Seasoning healthy sautéed vegetables with cumin will give them a North African flair.

Garlic: (allium sativúm): Garlic has the power to transform almost any meal into a bold, aromatic, healthy statement of culinary excellence. It provides you with a wide array of health-promoting benefits, such as reducing the risk of heart disease and lowering cholesterol.

You can increase garlic's health benefits by letting it rest after you have sliced or crushed it, which will give the alliinase enzymes in garlic an opportunity to be released and work on behalf of your health. Never use microwaves for any type of cooking; with garlic in particular you will destroy all of the cancer-protecting substances, and will in fact induce and promote cancer in your body if you continue using a microwave oven. Some of the most valuable components of garlic remain effective for only 2-16 hours at room temperature when it is present in extracted form, but when still inside of the crushed garlic, allicin will stay viable for 2-2½ days.

Garlic may improve your iron metabolism. The reason for this is diallyl sulphides in garlic can help increase the production of a protein called ferroprotin. This is a protein that runs across the cell membranes and forms a passageway that allows stored iron to leave the cells and become available where it is needed.

In addition to being a good source of selenium, garlic is what scientists call a 'seleniferous' plant, meaning it can absorb selenium from the soil even when conditions are unfavourable for uptake because of low selenium concentration of the soil.

The cardio-protective effect may be due to hydrogen sulphide gas. Our red cells can take up sulphur-containing molecules in garlic, called polysulphides, and use them to produce hydrogen sulphide, which in turn can help keep pressure in check.

The anti-inflammatory properties of garlic have been known for a long time and may even extend into the areas of obesity.

Garlic is an excellent source of vitamins, minerals and trace minerals, manganese, selenium, B-6, Vitamin C. Oxidative, free radical damage to the endothelium, the inner lining cells of the arteries, is counteracted and reduced by the regular use of garlic, which stops unwanted inflammation, plaque formation and clogging (atherosclerosis), and lowering levels of homocystein and other biomarkers of cardiovascular disease. Selenium and manganese are important factors in the body's natural antioxidant defence system through strengthening the glutathione peroxidase and superoxide dismutase system.

Garlic also has antibacterial and antiviral properties, which is very important for fighting Candida overgrowth and other parasites, and pseudomonas aeruginosa in burn patients. Garlic was also used as a disinfectant for wounds during World War I, and for treating antibiotic-resistant bacteria and excess growth of Helicobacter pylori in the stomach,—a key risk factor for stomach ulcers.

Cruciferous vegetables such as broccoli, broccolini, sprouts, cauliflower, cabbage et cetera, and garlic have important anti-cancer properties, especially for colorectal and renal cancer.

Garlic is a member of the Lily family and is a cousin to onions, leeks and chives. For a small vegetable, garlic has a huge and well-deserved reputation. Although garlic may not always bring good luck, protect against evil, or ward off vampires, it will transform almost any meal to a feast fit for kings and queens.

Ancient Egyptians seem to be the first to have cultivated the plant and it played an important role in their culture. Garlic was not only bestowed with sacred qualities and placed in the tomb of Pharaohs, but was given to the slaves to improve their strength and endurance when they built the pyramids. The Greeks and the Romans, who gave their athletes garlic to eat before competition and before going to war, also knew this.

Tips:
- Puree fresh garlic, garbanzo beans, tahini, olive oil and lemon juice to make a quick and easy hummus dip.
- Sautee steamed spinach, garlic and fresh lemon juice for a healthy dish.
- Add garlic to soups and sauces.
- Purée roasted garlic, cooked potatoes, organic coconut oil

together to make delicious garlic mashed potatoes. Season to taste.

Lack of knowledge about the most effective ways and means of detoxification protocols will obviously reduce the chances to obtain balance, good health and vitality.

As you will remember, the Last Supper took place the night before the death of Yahve. The Lord's Supper and the Passover, which is to commemorate the Angel of Death sat by Yahve, to pass over all Jewish homes that had the blood of a killed lamb on their doorposts, and kill every first-born in the land of Egypt, to punish the Pharaoh for refusing to release them from bondage.

The lamb was roasted and served (Exodus 12:8) with seven bitter herbs, unleavened bread with four cups of wine, thus reminding them about Jehu's four promises:

'I will bring you out,' 'I will deliver you,' 'I will redeem you,' 'I will take you to me for a people.' (Exodus 6:6) It was also served with an egg, to symbolise rebirth and spicing.

Yeshua instituted the Lord's Supper at the close of the Passover Supper, with Himself as a sacrificial lamb. Why the bitter herbs? This was to remind them of the bitterness of bondage away from home, prisoners in a foreign country?

The bitter herbs could be horseradish, green onions, sow thistles, dandelion, sheep sorrel.

Saltwater: Complement bitter herbs with dishes of saltwater, into which greens are dipped (karpas). Salt represents the tears of slavery. Millions of Jewish families sing hymns reflecting on the Saviour's redemption from physical and spiritual death:

> *Therefore, let us rejoice,*
> *At the wonder of our deliverance.*
> *From bondage to freedom,*
> *From agony to joy,*
> *From mourning to festivity,*
> *From darkness to light,*
> *Before God let us ever sing a new song.*

What if a Plant is Worth its Weight in Gold?

The mysterious history of **horseradish** goes back 3000 years and has been used as an aphrodisiac, a treatment for rheumatism and sinusitis. It was one of the seven bitter herbs used for the Passover Seder, as a culinary zestful accompaniment for beef, chicken or seafood.

Legend tells us that the Delphic Oracle told Apollo, 'The radish is worth its weight in lead, the beet its weight in silver, the horseradish its weight in gold.'

Why the name 'horseradish'? In German it is called '*meerrettich*', meaning 'sea radish' because it grows by the sea. Many believe the English mispronounced word '*mareradish*'.

Eventually, it began known as horseradish. The word 'horse' as applied in 'horseradish' is believed to denote large size and coarseness. 'Radish' comes from the Latin word 'radix', meaning root.

During the Renaissance, the use of horseradish spread from Central Europe to Scandinavia and England. It was not until 1640 that the British ate horseradish—and then it was only consumed by labourers and country folk. By the late 1600s, horseradish was the standard accompaniment for beef and oysters. In fact, the English grew the pungent root at inns and coach stations, to make cordials to revive exhausted travellers.

My first encounter with horseradish was in the early seventies when Christine served her delicious Sunday roast of lamb and Yorkshire pudding, and among the traditional trimmings was the horseradish. Oh, what a delightful combination of tastes—an instant love affair was born with this pungent, powerful root! Talking about reaching parts of your body those other accompaniments could barely touch—'the cobra, flame, fantomas' talked about in Russia, with something extra on top! 'Oh, for the love of horseradish!' James Herriot and I would declare unambiguously!

After Saturday's, training and partying, a poor student, almost exhausted, was instantly revived by a scrumptious Sunday roast of lamb with all the trimmings—and to me, the unknown yet so powerful medicinal herb called horseradish was an energy booster and aphrodisiac, which gave sustenance and perseverance for many hardworking days of studying… and more partying!

Did you know that horseradish contains a special enzyme called horseradish peroxidase, which has the ability to remove toxins and pollutants from wastewater? It has a longstanding tradition for being a 'mucokinetic'; that is, it has the ability to thin mucus and phlegm, thereby making it easy to remove the mucus out of the system.

As the medical botanist Dr. James Duke and medical anthropologist Dr. John Heinemann point out, there is nothing like a teaspoonful of fresh horseradish to clear the sinuses. Another endorsement comes from two surgeons, Glenn W. Geelhoed, MD and Robert D. Willix, MD who recommend a Japanese horseradish wasabi in their book *Natural Health Secrets from Around the World*. They say that a daily dose of horseradish is necessary only until the symptoms of your allergy subside. After that, only a few teaspoons of horseradish are needed each month to prevent an allergy attack.

Horseradish has only two calories per teaspoon, is low in sodium and provides dietary fibre. Great to use in soups and stews, in mashed potatoes or in a Bloody Mary drink. Horseradish is added to some pickles to add firmness and 'nip'.

How about this recipe, which is very popular in Siberia: Mix tomatoes, horseradish, garlic, sea salt, ground pepper, paprika, red pepper, vinegar, a little sugar in a blender. Serve with main meal, including dumplings (*komler* in Norwegian). This side dish has many names: Khrenoving sauce, khrenoder (Radish throttle), Vyrviglaz (Yank out the eye), cobra, flame, fantomas. So, yes, it is strong!

In South America, horseradish was rubbed on the forehead to relieve headaches, and some folks still swear by it. Before being named horseradish, it was known in England as 'redcole' and 'stingnose'. Germans still brew horseradish schnapps and some add it to their beer. Wise. The most widely recognised horseradish fan in the world might be Dagwood Bumstead, who consumed it regularly in the popular comic strip *Blondie* by Dean Young and Stan Drake.

'To a worm in horseradish, the world is horseradish' (Yiddish expression). Love it!

Two Noble Herbs—Almost Forgotten

Chicory and endive, the one a dusty roadside herb and the other its only relative—a vagrant. But these two herbs, today almost forgotten, were among the seven bitter herbs of the Last Supper, both attributed to having miracle healing properties.

The first mention of chicory as a healing remedy is from the first century AD when, and together with endive, it was respected by all the great sages of Western medicine, because chicory juice is a known remedy for tumours and cancers of the liver, stomach and the uterus. The juice from the crushed and macerated leaves works as a sedative and is very soothing, relieving oedema (swelling from water retention). It has also been used as a remedy for asthma, dysmenorrhoea (irregular menstrual cycle), and dyspepsia. Its seed, would you believe it, is regarded as an aphrodisiac.

The milky substance of endive has been used for cancer of the uterus, liver, and spleen. Endive is used to increase bile flow, and with chicory it can dissolve gallstones.

Osteoporosis

There are many ways to cure osteoporosis. The pioneering work of the late Dr. John R. Lee, MD who used natural progesterone cream transdermally, together with vitamins, minerals and food/lifestyle changes, is one road I have guided many patients along, to full recovery, shown on BMD (bone mineral density)—from full-blown osteoporosis with fractures to a non-existing, cured state.

Through various herbal extracts, alkaline, restructured water, oxygen therapy and herbal juice from three Bible plants, chicory, endive and escarole, the bitter herbal plants from the Last Supper. Suggestion: Drink one cupful of juice a day from these three plants for six months; there's good chance your osteoporosis will have disappeared. Because of the bitter taste, it is fine to mix it with carrot or beet juice.

These herbs contain vitamin A, B, C, E, K, riboflavin (B-2), folic acid, B-9, B-5 (pantothenic acid), pyridoxine (B-6), thiamine (vitamin B-1), niacin (B-3). The vitamins are essential; i.e., the body requires them from external sources to replenish and require for fat, protein and carbohydrate metabolism.

Additionally, escarole is a good source of calcium, magnesium, phosphorus, selenium, manganese, copper, iron and potassium. Manganese is used as a co-factor for the antioxidant enzyme, superoxide dismutase. Potassium is an important intracellular electrolyte, which helps to balance the effects of sodium.

Egyptian researchers have proved that chicory root has two heart benefits. It slows a rapid heartbeat (tachycardia) and has also a mild heart-stimulating effect, a bit like digitalis. A cup or two of chicory coffee acts like a liver tonic and a heart protector.

Chicory tea and extracts of endive has been used successfully against liver congestion, liver jaundice and gallstones and protects against chemical pollutants and toxins. Chicory-root coffee has been shown by Indian scientists to have promise as a male birth control; those who had been drinking chicory tea had high cu fertile sperm counts.

Watercress Against TB and Sexually Transmitted Diseases

The fifth bitter herb from the Last Supper has been used favourably against tuberculosis (TB), which is still a major problem in many third-world countries and recently re-emerging in Western countries. **Watercress** is also used as a remedy against sexually transmitted disease. The high sulphur content in this herb helps to kill the viruses that cause Chlamydia. Mixing it with turnip or carrot juice makes it more pleasant to drink. Within about seven weeks of drinking two cups a day of watercress, a cure is usually seen.

An effective recipe against TB is watercress juice combined with turnip juice with liquid Kyolic garlic. The sulphur content from both the watercress and the garlic give the TB a double-whammy and it has been documented to do the trick in stubborn cases of drug-resistant TB.

The Chinese have known for years the many great healing properties of watercress for treating TB and gingivitis, an inflammatory condition of the gums. In southern China, the people simply chew watercress to get rid of the symptoms of periodontal disease.

A Bible-Food Remedy for Shingles

A dosage of 500 mg. of the amino acid lysine twice a day is often enough to combat this painful and distressing disease, Herpes 20 Zooster. Watercress contains a high amount of lysine. Many types of beans also contain a lot of lysine: black-bean sprouts, lentils and sprouts, fava beans and even parsley.

A Multipurpose Miracle Remedy from the Bible

The famous French herbalist Maurice Mességué said that watercress has a purifying action. He recommends taking 'a glass in the morning and the poison will vanish!' Watercress is effective at getting rid of intestinal parasites and is recommended for chronic bronchitis, for neuralgia and toothache, hair loss and diabetes. For external application, I use it as I do cabbage, in poultices and compresses for gout and rheumatism. For skin complaints like acne or dermatitis, it is excellent.

Among the many microorganisms the Jews were exposed to was venereal disease—a major punishment from the worship of Baal, a widespread practice at the time of Moses involving extremely licentious rites. Of course, the Jews of antiquity knew nothing of viruses and bacteria, but by following the Bible and the Mosaic laws, which required them to eat certain foods rich in the amino acid lysine, which stops the growth and spread of the herpes virus in the cells of the body, a preventative cure was at hand. Lysine seems to wrap protective coating around each cell, preventing the virus from getting in. Two Biblical foods high in lysine are raw milk and meat.

Conclusion

Enjoy, explore and experience. Remember: Curiosity is the perfect antidote to boredom. And for curiosity, there is no cure!

CHAPTER TWENTY-ONE

Questions and Answers

'Music and love. 528Hz to your DNA. In the Spirit of Revelation:
You are the artistic rendering of mathematics and physics in a
quantum field. You are dancing in a cosmic sound and light show'.
Dr. Leonard G. Horowitz.

Question: How can you drop a raw egg onto a concrete floor without cracking it?

Answer: Concrete floors are very hard to crack!

Question: With the increasing numbers of men (44%) and women (39%) being diagnosed with cancer, which foods would you recommend in order to nourish and detoxify your body?

Answer: Cruciferous vegetables like broccoli, cauliflower, cabbage, Brussels sprouts and others have the ability to prevent and halt certain types of cancer of the breast, lung, colon, uterus, liver, and cervix. It is thought that this is due to the phytochemical substance called sulforaphane, indole 3-carbinols and crambene, which are able to stimulate enzymes working to detoxify the cells.

I would also add garlic with the allium, which stimulates the enzyme alliinase, which produces anti-cancer compounds. It is important to let the crushed garlic rest 15 minutes before the active ingredients are released.

In a double blind, randomised study with more than 3000 subjects over seven years, it was shown that the cancer risk for those who had the highest allium score was cut by 60%.

Turmeric: Hundreds of studies have showed that curcumin is a very potent anti-inflammatory herb and a potent anti-cancer compound, which works in many unique ways. (Ref: The Life Extension Foundation).

Hemp: The seeds and the oil from this plant contain the most balanced and richest sources of parent essential oil (80%) and a 3:1 ratio for omega 6 to omega-3. As you know by now, essential fatty acid is of prime importance to ensure optimal oxygen to the cells and their membranes.

Aloe Vera: Research has shown that this plant has unique properties: Anti-tumour, immunomodulator, macrophage (killer cells) activates as well as increases the production of nitric oxide, another anti-tumour property.

Medicinal Herbal Compounds: Reishi, cordyceps, astralgus, et cetera have anti-tumour properties, containing alkaloids, tocopherols, phenolics, carotenoids, folates, and organic acids.

Reishi prevents tumour proliferation and growth, increasing

the level of antioxidants and boosting the immune system.

Iodine: Is a substance lacking in the average diet and can be implicated in breast and ovarian cancer. You find iodine in sea vegetables such as kelp, kombu and nori. They also contain calcium and potassium and many other trace minerals, and help to promote an alkaline environment, which is a deterrent for cancer to survive. Chlorella and spirulina are two proven cancer fighters, which have the ability to bind to and eliminate heavy metals, promoting a balanced intestinal micro flora fighting Candida and other pathogens.

Frequently Asked Questions

Question: What are the main causes of disease as you see it, and how can we eliminate those causes?

Answer: Toxins and heavy metals that have built up in your system. These cause acidic conditions in your body, and the breakdown of cellular membranes because of the processed and adulterated food that cannot supply the parent essential fatty acids (The EFA-magnets) to supply adequate oxygen for your aerobic cellular metabolism.

That's why it is of paramount importance to detoxify using alkaline, vital restructured water with high redox potential, and to eliminate toxins with herbal preparations, and detoxify using sauna, electromagnetic procedures PEMF, and rebounding to mention just a few. Basic cleansing of colon, gall bladder and liver, kidneys/bladder, heavy metal cleanse, parasite cleanse, Candida cleanse, full body fatty tissue/lymphatic cleanse.

Reduce intake of toxic elements by using purification and alkalinisation of water and air purification / ionisation.

Take vitamins, minerals and enzymes on a regular basis in a bio-available form. It is a well-known fact that our soil is depleted in minerals and thus our food lacks proper nutrition. Reduce and neutralise all electromagnetic pollution from mobile phones, Internet, microwave ovens (these should be banned).

Reduce stress. Pray. Fast. Meditate. Dancing with water. Celebrate! Change DNA structure, epigenetic receiving and broadcasting ability into a harmonious signalling system—through mind, words and action.

Increase cellular oxygen uptake by proper EFA saturation of the cellular wall structure and restructured water, which has the ability to oxygenate the cells of your body.

Train—but don't strain. Try to smile a little whilst you jog. Move and dance and sing as if nobody's watching or listening.

Question: What is the main difference between traditional medical treatment and the holistic natural approach?

Answer: Drugs and medical intervention treat the symptoms, not the cause, of illness. Drugs suppress symptoms and were not created to cure anything. Serious side effects often occur. Drugs cause imbalance and symptoms that require more drugs to suppress these, and so you are nowhere near solving your health problem; you are creating new ones. The drug companies know this very well. Good for business—bad for you. They are blatantly lying when they say they are looking for a cure. 'War on Cancer' is an example. It is like throwing dust into people's eyes.

All research is about finding new patentable medicine. All money donated to charities and foundations are funds to patent new medicine and create some social function within the charities. All government funds go the same way, to patent new drugs. What about funds for preventing, treating and curing disease with natural methods? They exist, but are suppressed so that the chances are quite slim that you have heard about them before, as they are far away from the public eye. You see, the natural methods are not patentable methods to prevent, treat and cure disease. If you look at the basic causes for all diseases outlined above, it is fairly easy to treat and cure disease. And it is inexpensive compared to the exorbitantly high price on drugs and medical intervention such as chemotherapy radiation and surgery. The results: Abysmal! No better than 60 years ago, with few exceptions. Because the 'dog is barking up the wrong tree' and the drug industry knows it!

There is no doctor or drug company that can come forward and say that every disease is not caused by: Too many toxins in the body, nutritional deficiency, electromagnetic pollution, acidity and lack of oxygen in the cells. It takes a paradigm shift for this to take place, and the official health system as we know it today will be changed dramatically.

Question: If the drug companies know this, does it mean that our government and politicians know this, too?

Answer: Absolutely. This truth will put the drug companies out of business. If exposed, it will cost the government millions. Those influential people behind the scenes know and speculate on this, as their wealth and power is built on a sick, manipulative and lying industry as millions are getting sicker and more impoverished, as cancer, diabetes, and heart diseases are epidemic and increasing. Do you know that diseases caused by hospital errors or medication are the number three cause of death worldwide? When you increase your knowledge in this area, you take responsibility to prevent and escape the sickness industry.

Question: Where do I start to heal? And how?

Answer: Start with one of the items above, and do it at your own comfortable pace. As you have learnt from reading this book, water is by far the most important matter for your cleansing, rehydration, rebuilding, strengthening, alkalisation (remember pH—potential hydrogen—and that viruses, bacteria and parasites cannot thrive and live in an alkaline body), and oxygenation.

'Water is the mother and matrix of all life,' said Albert Szent-Györgyi (Nobel Prize Winner).

You can choose to drink ordinary tap water, which is full of contaminants, fluoride (depending on where you live), heavy metals, chlorine and trihalomethanes, et cetera. All tap water is poisonous, as it is loaded with health-degrading chemicals. Chlorine scars your arteries and, together with hydrogenated oils and homogenised dairy products, causes heart disease because of lack of parent essential oils in the cell membranes. Trihalomethanes, a by-product of chlorine, is a carcinogen (causing cancer). Most water contains fluoride, a horrible and poisonous chemical derivate from the aluminium industry. Tap water is only useful for washing your floor. If you love your pets, don't even think of giving it to them. It gradually bio-accumulates in your body, weakens your immune system and breaks down your body.

Those in charge of your domestic water, food industry's processed junk food and the drug industry have one overriding goal: Profit. And more profit. Keep people confused and ignorant. Duped and doped. Divide and rule.

Vital water is purified and alkaline with antioxidant properties, and restructured to rehydrate all your cells and revitalise your body. Remember, it is your own body's innate healing system that is set in motion towards better health and well-being.

Talking about acidity as opposed to alkalinity, what is turning your body from acidic pH to alkaline pH? There may be several reasons that your body composition and chemistry has turned on to the acidic side. The cause could be: nutritional deficiency, heavy metal toxicity, parasites, allergy/intolerance of food, infection, stress, emotional trauma or vaccination. The cause must of course be addressed. But drinking vital water will work on many levels at the same time to bring your body into balance. Thousands of happy testimonials show us just that.

As you know, you need to drink water, pure and vital water with the ability to cleanse your body and give you extra antioxidants to combat free radical destroyers and ensure more oxygen to the cell tissues, and maintain a proper pH balance.

The next small—but very important—step is to use a rebounder or a mini-trampoline. Start slowly, about 5-10 minutes a day. Enjoy and dance, improvise steps and routines to music. A rebounder, like no other exercise instrument, stimulates all of your body's cells—simultaneously. It strengthens and tones muscles, tendons, ligaments, joints and all the connective tissues as well as improving lung and heart capacity. A truly effective and joyful form of exercise.

Question: Now that you have done your exercise and replenished your fluids with pure vital water with all its wonderful properties, what would be the next important step?

Answer: Nutritional supplements. A mineral supplement and parent essential oil to rebuild and maintain proper cellular oxygenation.

Cells need oxygen for their metabolism and the right kind of essential oil, a balance between omega-3 and 6, of parent oil, is essential. They will act as oxygen magnets in the cell membranes, the double-layered cell wall, ensuring that adequate oxygen is passed into the cell to make sure that the mitochondria (the energy power workstation) can work properly. Remember: adequate oxygen to the cells prevents you from all cancer!

Congratulations! You have now taken your first three fundamental new steps towards a healthier, wiser and better life. You have co-operated with your body's own wisdom on how it likes to run!

Question: In your lectures, I have noticed that you talk less about calories, fats proteins and carbohydrates, even when it comes to weight loss. Why is that?

Answer: Almost every year a new diet plan appears on the scene promising an easy way to lose weight. Right now, it is the 5:2 plan. Knowing what kind of fat is unhealthy, which proteins and sugar to avoid is important but not nearly as important as your knowledge of the poisons, toxins and addictive chemicals that are in your food and water. More important than calories, fats, proteins and carbohydrates is the chemical fertilisers, pesticides, the irradiation of the food, the processing that is being carried out, the genetically modified 'Frankenstein foods', the sickening fast food, et cetera.

How to avoid these, detoxify and rebuild your body's

immune system: If you follow the advice outlined in this book and take to the vital waters and all the health this can bring you, your body weight will come down naturally. I have seen this countless times with my patients. Vital water with its antioxidant and alkaline properties will most certainly aid in your goal to lose weight.

Question: Can't I ever eat a cheeseburger again?

Answer: You can eat cheeseburger, French fries, ice cream and cakes, as long as you make them at home, preferably with organic ingredients. Fast-food restaurants I don't recommend as they use chemicals and contaminants that are very unhealthy, including hydrogenated oils, to make their 'food'. The chemicals in their 'food' make you addicted and sick and are deficient in essential nutrients. They contain an outrageous amount of free radicals, which makes your body more acidic and prone to infections and disease.

Make sure to drink Vital Water to detoxify after a fast-food meal, as the toxins, many of which are neurotoxins that interfere with brain and nervous system functions, tend to bio-accumulate in the body.

Question: Can we really be sick and get a disease just by breathing the air?

Answer: Absolutely. Indoor climates are highly toxic with various chemicals from household cleaners, sprays, air conditioners, fans, frying pans, et cetera. Most people spend almost 90% of their time indoors. In a study conducted by the EFA it was shown that the indoor air was 30 times more polluted than downtown Los Angeles! Airborne bacteria, viruses, moulds, dust, smoke, detergents, radon, carbon monoxide and hundreds of other pollutants are constantly in the air at your home and in your workplace.

It is time to take responsibility and purify the air by installing an air ioniser. When you know that these substances are harmful to your immune, respiratory, cardiovascular and reproductive systems, it is about time to take action, especially when you think about infants and children, who are very vulnerable. Air pollutants are one of the major causes of allergy, asthma and respiratory illness in children. Another point is that for every exhalation, 55 gallons of air becomes polluted.

Vital air capacity or pulmonary function measurement can predict life span better than any biomarker of aging. The best air to breathe deeply is highly energised air, which is rich in oxygen—as found in a room with a negative air ioniser or outdoors in the forest, at the sea, or in the mountains. The reason for a negative air ioniser is that all pollutants in the air have a positive charge, which, like free radicals, lack electrons and become oxidative, causing cellular breakdown. Placing lots of green plants in your home is also a good thing as plants absorb carbon dioxide and give off oxygen.

Oxygen, as we know, is crucial in the energy production of the body's ATP. The body creates almost 20 times more energy with oxygen than without (38 molecules of ATP during aerobic respiration compared to two molecules of ATP during anaerobic respiration.) Oxygen is not only the key to good health and well-being, but it is also essential to prevent disease. Science has shown that cancer, Candida, cardiovascular heart disease and many other diseases are due to lack of oxygen (apoxia). As we have seen, it has been indisputably proven that cancer cells cannot survive in an alkaline- and oxygen-rich environment. And the opposite is true: They thrive in an anaerobic, oxygen-depleted environment. High-quality air is a must for anyone wanting to be healthy and full of energy.

Question: Is there any therapy that can improve oxygen uptake?

Answer: Absolutely! Negative air ionisation will increase oxygen capacity. Negative ions are the vitamins of the air. Oxygen uptake increases (up to 6 times higher) when the red blood cells are activated, in addition to cleaning the air. Medical research has shown that on over-supply of positive ions can adversely affect physical and emotional health. A negative, portable ioniser should also be with you when you travel, stay in hotel rooms, airplane cabins, crowded rooms, et cetera. Especially for athletes: Check out HEZ (hydrogen efficiency zone) *ad modum* John O'Neill, an Australian Decathlon Champion and author of *Breaking the Sound Barrier of Human Energy Production*.

Remember the EPO 'magnets' for oxygen transportation into the cells (Prof. Brian Peskin) and PEMF therapy (pulsed electromagnetic field therapy), which improves oxygen uptake? This will help oxygen to bind to haemoglobin, transferring it into the cells and assisting directly in ATP production. Along with deep breathing of fresh air, natural earth-based PEMF is the best oxygen therapy there is, and this method also improves circulation to and from the lungs, which we can attest to at Viktorklinikken where we have used it for over thirty years for many ailments and trauma— for example, observing 50% reduction in growth time for fractures.

No need to explore the Russians' use of the noble gas xenon in the 2014 Sotchi Winter Olympics. This is in the grey zone of blood doping, as it stimulates a transcription factor (like a switch), a protein Hif-1 alpha, which causes the body to produce other hormones including testosterone and will increase erythropoietin (EPO) in the body.

With the knowledge from this book, you are now able to prevent diseases effectively, reverse ailments and supercharge your immune system.

'You are what you eat, drink, breathe, think and do.' Patricia Bragg (Author and Health Consultant).

Question: Is there a difference between fitness and health?

Answer: Oh, yes! As we have seen in the example with Jim Fixx, the well-known celebrity runner who started the popular running wave with his book *The Complete Book on Running,* you can be very fit, but unhealthy: Jim Fixx dropped dead of a heart attack whilst out jogging.

Other people are unfit, slightly overweight and yet strong, flexible, and very healthy, and live a long and happy life. A moderate level of fitness is desirable. It is more important to be healthy than fit, but striking a balance between the two is essential. If *healthy* is your number one priority, you have most likely invested some time in achieving a level of fitness, and should be better than the vast majority of the population. Remember, in every endeavour, one small step at a time: A journey of 1000 miles always starts with one step first—your attitude, not your aptitude, determines your altitude.

Question: What about the research being done on the cure and prevention of disease? The war on cancer? Aren't governments spending millions on this research?

Answer: This is probably the biggest deceptive lie out there; a fraud that has been passed on to the public throughout many years. In 1971, Nixon started the 'War on Cancer' campaign, intending to 'research' to find a cure. In 2014, the French President, François Hollande, decided to spend huge amount of money on the same cancer issue. The money is used to find another patentable drug or patentable medical procedure and not the real cause, as they are not looking at the preventative aspect, as there is no money to be made in this way.

All the research is conducted so that the drug companies can own a patent on a product, sell it and make an inordinate amount of money. There are absolutely no funds available for non-patentable natural methods to prevent, treat and cure disease. These are ridiculed, suppressed, hidden and buried from the public, often branded as 'dangerous quackery'. Yet they exist, underground so to speak, and are very effective.

But first things first! Begin with vital water and vital, nutritious food. Make sure you de-acidify, detoxify and re-oxygenate your body.

The slogan from Nixon from 1971 and the same procedure followed up by President Hollande in 2014 are an efficient and deceptive way of funnelling more money to the drug industry—intentionally sending 'the dog to bark up the wrong tree'.

Question: Do you say that the pharmaceutical industry is not setting out to find a cure for diseases?

Answer: No drug has ever been invented to cure a disease and never will be, as they are only intended to cure symptoms, not address the cause of disease. The pioneers who find the cause of a disease are regarded as a threat to the industry's hunger for profit, are threatened, harassed, arrested, destroyed and eliminated. The history is full of such examples: Hoxsey, Rife, Galileo, Naesens, Burzynski, Semmelweis and others.

Question: What is, in your opinion, the cause of cancer?

Answer: The real root cause of cancer was discovered by Dr. Otto Warburg, the Nobel Prize winner, 1931. His discovery still stands today. All normal cells have an absolute requirement for oxygen, but cancer cells can live without oxygen; i.e., anaerobic cells. This is a rule without exceptions. Deprive a cell 35% of its oxygen for 48 hours and it may become cancerous.

Dr Warburg made it absolutely clear that the root cause of cancer is oxygen deficiency, which creates an acidic state in the human body. Dr Warburg also discovered that cancer cells are anaerobic (do not utilise oxygen) and cannot survive in the presence of high levels of oxygen, as is found in an alkaline state. Too much acidity in the body, meaning that the pH, potential hydrogen, in the body is below 7.365, constitutes an 'acidic' state.

Dr. Warburg, Director of Kart Wilhelm Institute (now Max Planck Institute), one of the world's leading cell biologists, investigated the metabolism of tumours and the respiration of the cells and found that cancer cells thrive in an environment of acidity, of low pH 6, due to lactic acid production, elevated carbon dioxide and lack of oxygen. There are many secondary causes of cancer such as toxins, heavy metals, radiation, viruses, emotional trauma, but there is only one primary cause of cancer—impaired cellular respiration.

Question: Tell me more. Can you expand on Dr. Warburg's discovery?

Answer: Sure. If you take away cells' ability to breathe—mechanically, chemically or energetically—cancer, which is anaerobic (living and thriving without oxygen) will result. Cells are constantly dividing and dynamically changing, and when newly formed (embryonic) cells are denied 35% or more of the oxygen they need, their respiratory enzymes are no longer saturated with oxygen. When the oxygen-transferring systems are no longer saturated with oxygen, the cells are damaged severely, as respiration decreases dramatically.

Respiratory enzymes that are not saturated with oxygen end up breaking down—like driving your car without oil. As respiration falls, the cells struggle and find it difficult to keep up the high-energy production levels, which are normally sustained by converting oxygen into ATP energy (ATP—adenosine triphosphate). As the high energy complex of the cell fails, the cell loses its higher functions and becomes primitive, losing its ability to differentiate, and becomes a plant-like cell, seen as green under proper magnification, just like a plant.

The conversion to plant cell function is the only option left because the cell has been starved of its natural oxygen supply. Plant cells use fermentation, a much simpler and more inefficient form of energy creation common to simple organisms. Fermentation is a simple process that converts sugars (glucose) into a weak form of energy, producing a lot of acidity and lactic acid, allowing the cells to grow and grow as the fermentation proceeds, without any cell differentiation. In other words, life is sustained and confirmed in the form of a plant.

Question: How does chemotherapy (cellular poison) and radiation (burn) work at the cellular level?

Answer: Without reversing the cells, the conventional 'war on cancer' with its 'burn and poison' strategy is useless and doomed to fail—and when you think about it, it is not intended to cure and irradiate cancer. After all, the cancer industry is one of the most profitable of the drug industries.

You may remove small tumours surgically, but the surgery may release fermenting cells into the body. If the body is not clean and saturated with oxygen and enzymes, the germinating cells may find a new house in which to settle. Cancer caused by x-rays or radiation is nothing other than destruction of cellular respiration. You can kill cancer cells by radiation and chemotherapy, but at the same time you damage the normal cells' respiratory enzyme-dependent system.

To maintain or improve the oxygen delivery system of the cell, you need to get the unadulterated essential fatty acids into the bi-lipid cell membranes—the parent omega 6. These will act as oxygen magnets for the transportation of oxygen into the cells. Dr Warburg's conclusion proved that just 35% oxygen deprivation to the cells results in cancer developing automatically! Lack of parent essential fatty acids (EFA), which must be supplied by foods and certain oils because your body cannot manufacture them on ITS own, is a crucial factor. It is very important that these foods are grown and processed organically, with low heat and no artificial preservatives; if not, EFA will be ruined just like the trans-fat and hydrogenated cancer-causing oils that you have in processed food.

Question: Where do I get the EFAs and how?

Answer: It is essential that you distinguish between parent and derivative EFA. There are two types of parent EFA: parent omega-3 or ALA (Alpha linoleic acid) and parent omega-6 or LA (linoleic acid). They have a complementary function. The body uses a much greater quality of parent EFAs than derivatives (up to 20 times more).

EFA oils are found mostly in plant- and seed-based sources. Seeds such as sunflower, sesame, hemp, pumpkin and flax, as well as raw milk, cheese and eggs—organic; and organic, beef, lamb, chicken. But in order to protect yourself from cancer, cardiovascular disease, diabetes and Alzheimer's, you need to supply parent EFA oils like hempseed oil, sesame seed, pumpkin, sunflower oil, safflower.

Parent omega-3 is mainly used for energy and not incorporated in the cell membranes or used for derivatives. The body only needs a little of it and will attempt to remove any excess.

Only a very little parent omega-3 is required for adequate cell membrane structure. Too much omega-3 and its derivatives ruin the cell membrane structure and reduce your anti-cancer protection.

Question: What is your opinion on fish oil? There seem to be a consensus that Omega-3 from fish and fish oil (cod liver oil) is healthy.

Answer: This is based on opinion, not science. The fish oil industry has convinced the public about the necessity to take omega-3, and this has become the number one bestselling supplement. But it is not backed by science; in fact, I have for almost 30 years recommended that it is best to stay away from fish oil and supplements in this field, including krill. Fish oil comes from rotten or discarded fish products. It is about 200 times more rancid inside your body as oxidation takes place, which leaves you very vulnerable to inflammatory conditions, cardiovascular and heart disease, arthritis, cancer, diabetes, Alzheimer's and osteoporosis. If you are on the fish oil omega-3 bandwagon, heaven help you! You are heading for disaster.

In 2013, the medical establishment embraced a fundamental scientific discovery when it was reported in one of the world's most prestigious medical publication, *The New England Journal of Medicine,* that fish oil was completely ineffective in preventing heart disease for a very large section of high-risk patients. Dr Eric Topol, the editor-in chief of *Medscape,* recommended stopping fish oil supplementation for the prevention of heart disease. For in-depth knowledge on this subject please go to:

http://brianpeskin.com/peskinMDCTscan.pdf and

http://brianpeskin.com/BP.com/studies.html

Question: Do you have any scientific studies to refer to when it comes to fish oil and omega-3 supplements from this industry?

Answer: In 1995, Harvard School of Public Health conducted a two-year study to see whether there was any difference between one group who consumed olive oil and the other fish oil. The latter group failed and became less fit and healthy.

A scientific study conducted in Norway on osteoporosis patients had to be stopped after a few months because the bone scans showed that those on omega-3 from cod liver oil showed a worsening of the osteoporotic condition. This came as an embarrassment to the medical community and the results were quietly hushed up and forgotten by most people.

The IOWA (investing oils with respect to arterial blockage) experiment was run by Professor Brian Peskin of Houston, Texas. If you are not familiar with Professor Peskin's work, I can assure you that the results of his experiment are both staggering and shocking. This was the first time one could observe the arterial flexibility between subjects taking parent essential oil and those taking fish oil, using photoplethysmography. There was a stunning 73% effectiveness (absolute, not relative). The median duration was

24 months and those taking PEO showed on average 11 years lower than their physical age.

Several other experiments along these lines were performed and each time with the same conclusion: compared to parent essential oil, fish oil is worse for the cardiovascular system.

The claims of success regarding fish oil and krill oil are simply built on advertisement deception, masquerading as science, and in this case it can join the long rank of misguided and wrong advice on people's health. The *Nil nocere* ('First do no harm') is completely forgotten. Professor B. Peskin's landmark studies have proven this once and for all.

Meanwhile, people are being declined by the industry and tricked to believe that fish oil is safe, when it is clearly the opposite: people are hurt and die prematurely due to error in medical research. A very interesting article by Sharon Begley in *Newsweek*, 'Why almost everything you hear about medicine is wrong', cites world-renowned physician, mathematician and statistician John P.A. Ioannidis, MD, BSc on the manipulation of data and 'massaging the pharmaceutical statistics. Another example from Scandinavia: In an experiment, researchers found that people using cod liver oil had three times more melanoma (skin cancer) than the control group.

Question: What is the science behind statins like Lipitor?

Answer: There is only a one per cent difference in effectiveness between the results with Lipitor and the results with a placebo. Termed absolute risk.

Question: What about farmed fish?

Answer: I would not recommend it, because of heavy metals, contaminants and the feed, which consists of corn, soy and other adulterated omega-6, which changes the essential fatty acid profile.

Question: What kind of oil do you use?

Answer: For frying, virgin coconut oil; baking sometimes ghee, proper organic butter, and virgin olive oil.

Question: Why did the elephant paint himself in different colours?

Answer: So he could hide in the crayon box.

There are more than 80 organizations working on water and sanitation issues in many countries around the world. Clear water has become the most precious resource in the 21st century. Clean water is not a privilege, but a right.

Some of these organizations are:

MIYA, a good doing company, which provides urban water efficiency solutions, focusing on reducing non-revenue water. Millions of cubic metres of clean water is lost daily because of poorly maintained water system.

Colombia water centre (CWC) is part of the Earth Institute works to finance and address sustainable water use and allocation.

Three Avocados is a social enterprise that generates fluids for clean water in Africa through the sale of coffee.

Water is life is a non-profit organization that works to provide clean water to those in need through short and long term solutions. Water is life produced a water filtration system called The Straw, which provides clean drinking water when immersed into a water source. The innovative device last up to a year and removes water borne diseases with each sip.

Puremadi is a non-profit organization from the faculty and students of University of Virginia who create water filter technologies that improve human health and quality of life. Their first project was a ceramic filter using local materials, partnering with the University of Venda in Thohoyandon in South Africa.

Charity: Water is a non-profit organization based in New York which brings clean and safe drinking water to people in developing countries. The founder and CEO is Scott Harrison, a former nightclub promoter who found his Christian faith and mission after he left the hedonistic partying lifestyle to focus on charity (from the Greek word caritas, which means love). With its dedication to transparency funds are raised using the social media.

H2OPE

Always looking at the bright side of life is more fun and amazing, it rewards your cells with energy to tackle, seemingly impossible and life threatening situation. Epigenetic expression, as the scientist tells us. Love is the catalyst by which all good things happen. Letting go is the effortless way to achieve your heart's desire.

Maybe the old man in the following history knew a thing or two about energy and Quantum Physics:

A group of Chinese men were walking through the woods beside a rushing river. Suddenly they caught a glimpse of an old man bobbing up and down in the roaring rapids. Scared that the old man was dead, they ran to the edge of the river trying to fish the old man out of the water so that he would not be swept out to the sea. Their effort came to an abrupt halt when the old man emerged out of the water, dried himself and started to walk away. The willing rescue team ran after the old man and asked: "How did you survive in that water? No one could swim in that water without being killed".

"It is really easy", the old man replied. "I just went up when the water went up, and down when the water went down". Lesson?

Don't resist the flow. (Flom. The Greatest Manifestation Principle in the World by Carnelian Sage)

I am reminded of the famous ad poignant words of Winston Churchill "Never, never, never give in, in anything great or small", a saying that his grandchild Winston, Member of Parliament, had printed on top of his notepads as a daily reminder.

If Not You, Then Who...

In conjunction with Happy World Water Day, 22nd March, which has been celebrated and initiated by the UN since 1993, I have received a lot of questions concerning water, which I have compiled and answered hereunder.

The Academy-Award-winning actor Matt Damon, co-founder of water.org, announced in February 2014 that he would go on strike from using toilets, creating headlines around the world and raising awareness around the global water and sanitation crisis. Many people seem to think that water is just water—two hydrogen molecules and one oxygen molecule bound together. But in reality, it is the lifeblood and energy system of our bodies. It affects nations, economies and is a life-or-death question that everybody should be able to respond to (*'Show me your responsibility, and I'll show you who you are.'*).

Many aspects of our lives have suffered due to disregard and lack of respect, and the heaviest cost is going to be held up against

493

us if you and I continue to neglect water as *the most important ingredient in anyone's life*. 'It is the mother and matrix of all life' (Nobel Prize Winner Albert Szent-Györgyi). There is no life without water.

Question: Why is this important to me?

Answer: 1 in 3 people in the world do not have access to clean, safe and private toilet.

- 780 million people don't have access to clean water, but 6 billion people have cell phones.
- 2.5 billion people still lack access to a private toilet or basic sanitation.
- 3.4 million people die of water-related diseases each year.
- Every 20 seconds, a child dies of water-related diseases (3 children a minute).
- Women spend 200 million hours collecting water every day.

We're all in the same boat. 'Am I my brother's keeper?' asked Cain when he'd murdered his brother Abel and God asked him, 'Where is your brother?'

Question: So what has Matt Damon got to do with toilets?

Answer: Health and hygiene have improved with the use of toilets and better sanitation. Can you imagine how it is to go to the toilet in a muddy ditch, by the river, fields, railway tracks or the wilderness in general? In participating in a series of videos using comedy, taking the stigma or 'mickey bliss' out of this subject not discussed in the public, Matt Damon aims to raise awareness of the water and sanitation crisis. Going down this rather unusual road, he has been able to generate millions of views on YouTube 'for something ridiculous' (going to the bathroom to poo or pee), to show the importance and gravity of the global water and sanitation crisis. Well done, Matt!

What can you do? Join Matt Damon and http://www.water.org and visit http://www.StrikeWithMe.org.

Question: Is the water crisis and sanitation problem something that belongs only to third-world countries?

Answer: No. Water shortage has also begun to hit many other countries and has become a security issue, with conflict already breaking out in several countries. More violence will break out as the situation escalates, reaching a culmination point where water-dependent power grids will falter, and more forest fires and closures of business will ensue. Once an environmental issue only, the world's water crisis is now a security threat.

Question: Which countries are we talking about?

Answer:

Brazil: The main water system that supplies Sao Paulo is 75% empty. An abnormally high-pressure weather system over southeast Brazil is the main cause.

Iran: Lake Urmia, the single largest lake in the Middle East, has dried up. Severe drought has sucked up the massive saltwater body. Ships are rusting in the mud. President Hassan Roubani calls the condition 'a national security issue'. He is promising to 'bring the water back'. Other lakes and major rivers have also been drying up, leading to disputes over water rights, demonstrations and riots.

India: Residents of Bicholim and neighbouring towns in west India can no longer get water from their taps.

US: A scorching drought across much of the western United States has dried up water reservoirs and sparked several wildfires. Whole hordes of cattle livestock are starving. Many rural communities could lose access to drinking water in the nearest future.

China: Huge amounts of China's wetlands have drained up since 2003: about 340,000 square kilometres of wetlands—about the size of the Netherlands. Much of China's electrical power is run by water, and the repercussions could mean 'lights out' for the country.

Jordan: A massive water shortage and power cuts have resulted in eruptions and Jordan's Prince Hassan recently warned that the lack of water in the Middle East could spark violent conflict.

South Africa: The national water shortage could rehash the apartheid period, where only certain communities had access to basic resources.

Libya: This country ranks as one of the most water-insecure places in the world. The supply of water for Benghazi could run dry in the nearest future.

Kosovo: The government has put out restrictions on water usage. The landlocked country of 2 million citizens is struggling to supply water and is facing its worst drought in three decades.

The willingness to accept responsibility for the welfare of our fellow human beings is a call of love for humanity—empathy set in motion. Responsibility in Action!

CHAPTER TWENTY-TWO

Alpha and Omega, the Living Water

'Happy World Water Day 22nd of March'

'Water is Mother and Matrix of all life.' - *Albert Szent-Györgyi*

Artesian Water, the Lake of Light and Theobroma, the Drink of the Gods

A few days after the UN's World Water Day on 22.03.2014, I revisited Lysefjorden, 'the mysterious long and dark corridor', as Victor Hugo described it.

This is the place where the initiation and inspiration came to me to embark on an exciting life journey in the landscape of the healing arts. The exploration of vital water, the mother and life provider for us and the planet we live on, and the natural solutions that originate from the proper use of vital water as the most important gift given to mankind.

H_2O. A molecule unlike any other. A bit like the fairly-tale trolls at the beginning of the book, *The Three Billy Goats Gruff*, there are plenty of *real* trolls, beasts, liars and deceivers in the world system, who manipulate the masses to accept the accumulating toxins in our municipal water systems (fluoride, mercury, lead, cadmium and much more), in our environment, and the food we eat.

The strategy is killing you softly. Will the real and honest change makers—that is, you and I—unite and stand up, protest and never give up until clean, revitalised water, our most precious God-given gift, is reclaimed in its true and healthy form?

Meanwhile, we can initiate this change by starting to take responsibility to drink vibrant, vital, restructured water, eat just natural, unadulterated food, keep moving—and smiling!

'When you look into the Water, you Measure the Depth of Your Own Soul.'

Following in the footsteps of the famous Norwegian author Bjørnstjerne Bjørnson (Nobel Prize in Literature in 1903), I chose April to return to Eidane, the start and the end of this book. April is the month during which all the old falls away and the new is rooted; the month where the last strong winds sweep down the valley, the snow and ice are melting, new life springs forth, and the seed of summer is planted.

So it was on a sunny Sunday in April that I returned to my childhood's Eldorado with my daughter Nikoline Florentyna, on the hillside by the farm, where I had clutched my father's hand 60 years ago, seeing nature for the first time through his eyes.

Nikoline and I were both standing at the same spot looking down on the 'vital water from the earth's innermost cathedral', as my dad had once said. Out of nowhere appeared a happy, purring black cat communicating with us! Probably a far-distant relative of the old farmhouse cat!

The water-wise, grey old man receiving ancient wisdom from nature and a loving cat. In my mind's eye came our father and uncle, smiling, sweating and quenching their thirst on the homebrewed beer made by tender, loving hands from the vital water of an artesian aquifer.

Before returning to the farm, my daughter and I rowed out across the sunlit lake, in a rowing boat with old-fashioned oars kindly lent to us by the farmer at Eidane, Kjetil.

The lake of light, a great shimmering crystal on the surface of the earth, embraced us as we headed towards one end of the lake. Nikoline Florentyna was sitting at the stern of the boat. From the steep hillside, we heard the sound of clinging bells and saw a flock of sheep baaing.

'What is a sheep's favourite dessert, Nikoline?' I asked.

'Dunno, Dad.'

'Baaa-klava!' (Remember the recipe from Lebanon, earlier in the book?)

'Or how about this one, Florentyna: What did the sheep say to his sheep friend? "I love ewe!"'

As medicine goes, a good laugh enriches and enlivens your life. At least that's what the old man tried to convey, having failed to impress his daughter, 'The blooming victory of the people' (the original meaning of her name, *Nikoline Florentyna*), by reciting the famous poem Terje Vigen by Henrik Ibsen (1861):

'there lived a remarkably grizzled man
on the uttermost barren isle,
he never harmed, in the wide world's span,
a soul by deceit or by guile;
his eyes, though, sometimes would blaze and fret,
most when a storm was nigh.
and then people sensed he was troubled yet,
and then there were few that felt no threat.'

The poem recounts dramatic saga of Terje Vigen, who in 1809 tried to cross the English blockade of Norway's southern coast in a small rowing boat in a last desperate attempt to smuggle food from Denmark back to his starving wife and daughter. He was captured and imprisoned, and not released until 1814 (the year of Norway's Constitution), after the Napoleonic War was over—only to find that his small family had starved to death. He later became a pilot, and years later rescued an English lord who turned out to be the commander of the ship that had captured him.

As I rowed towards the end of the lake, only ruins of a farm existed at a place called 'The end of the water' (*Vassbotn*). A cascading stream kissed the lake, throwing up diamonds into the sky in the sharp light of the April sun.

The dancing water and the light serenade of the reflection of trillions of exuberant molecules in motion brought to my mind the tune of Dean Martin's *That's Amore* (1952) as we touched the river's mouth.

'When the moon hits your eye like a big pizza pie,

That's amore.

When the world seems to shine like you've had too much wine,

That's amore.

Bells will ring ting-a-ling-a-ling, ting-a-ling-a-ling.

And you'll sing "Vita Bella".

Hearts will play tippy-tippy-tay, tippy-tippy-tay, like a gay tarantella!'

As the reflection of bubbling water multiplied the heavens above, the dancing water molecules resonated a happy, healing melody, enchanting us both, as if trillions of never-ending water molecules were singing:

'Thank you! Thank you for sharing some of the water's secrets with the world! But there is yet more to be revealed!'

'God bless!' I turned the boat around and headed to the other side of the glittering lake where a new surprise waited for us. A playful, exuberant final celebration unfolded as I heard the last little matryoshka presenting herself.

The old farm, now completely new with a beautiful house, outbuildings, cottage and—a surprise—a chocolate factory building producing delicious homemade chocolates! Using the vital water of an aquifer 'from the innermost water cathedral', the young, innovative, June Kristine and her husband Mads-Ove had just started a new adventure, a chocolate fairy tale!

Wow! A brand new assortment with names of characters, including: *Pilt-Ola*, who walked through the whole of the Soviet Union to the east coast (Vladivostok) and back again with a dream of going to America, a well-known entrepreneur of his days. Apparently a distant relative of mine; *Skrøylå, Preikestolen* (Pulpit Rock), the world-famous tourist spot Gruden, from a farm in Eidane, where people walked a whole day from the neighbouring village to collect used coffee grounds. They returned happily home to enjoy 'newly brewed' coffee for many days; *The Bear*: In memory of a bear that was killed in 1885 by 18 people on the way to a baptism in a church in Lysebotn. The bear was killed with stones, rope and oars. It was named 'Ingerbjørnen' after the girl who was being baptised— and can be viewed at Stavanger Museum. The assembly of 18 people rowed all the way to Forsand, about 50 km, with the bear in tow!

Chocolate doesn't make the world go around, but it sure makes the ride worthwhile! And remember, in Cuba, real men do not eat strawberry ice cream—they eat chocolate.

And from the mouth of a wise old man I once heard these words: 'If it makes you happy… eat it. But if it doesn't… give it to me! Good Health, Good Luck, God Bless You!'

As a connoisseur and lover of chocolate, the Lysefjorden Sjokolade at Eidane had tickled me pink and made a perfectly divine ending for one true fairy tale—and hopefully the beginning of a new one.

As the sun reflected the granite mountains on the lake, the crystal eye of the water, I could hear the voice of aunty Helene: 'Coffee and cakes!' which always included some chocolates, homemade bread and farmer's butter. I remember the smell so clearly. Happy memories. Every afternoon was a delightful healing experience to behold, when the whole family was gathered in the farmhouse kitchen, and sometimes a warm cup of cacao with a dollop of whipped cream on top was served. A drink revered by the ancient Mayan culture as 'the drink of the gods' (Theobroma). I pondered on the fact that only the elite of Mayan society could afford to drink it as the cacao seeds were used as currency; how only the rich could afford to 'drink their money', and how the colonists discovered the cacao drink and brought it back to Europe where it became a fashionable drink among the high society.

In the old kitchen, I often felt a touch of heaven. Chocolate cake and cacao—always with a big jug of vital water from the artesian well on the table.

The Blooming Victory of the People

A rowing trip to 'the end of the water' and back again. Theobroma, delicious chocolates from Lysefjorden Sjokolade, a world-class product from magic Eidane. The aroma from the farmhouse kitchen still tickles my olfactory epithelium cells and Bowman's glands— triggering 'the Proust effect', a memory recall, like a mnemonic device. The image of the remembrance of happy memories from the past is crystal clear. Over and over again I taste the fresh homemade bread with the farmhouse butter made from raw milk, and hear the characteristic *pling! pling!* sound of the milk separator ushering in a new adventure, Pling! Pling! A true fairy story.

A NEW GENERATION OF WATER
Are you ready to unshackle your chains?

Many people are dehydrated without knowing it and still more are unaware of the fact that one water molecule at a time passes through small openings in the cell membrane, the so called aqua-porins, first detected by Peter Agre who received the Nobel Prize for this discovery. Ordinary tap -water molecules are too big, slow moving and clustered and need to be broken up before it can reach the inside of your cells which require extra energy. When you attach a Pure Energy Norway water generator on the outside of your cold water pipe, the clustered water molecules start breaking up into smaller, faster moving, hexagonal water molecules, slipping easily through the cell membrane without wasted energy expenditure.

The newly formed water molecules move faster, rehydrates more efficiently and carries more energy into the cells mitochondria, the energy powerhouse of your cells. As more oxygen, hydrogen and nutrients are carried into all your 600 trillion cells, the body`s metabolism and function is drastically improved. In addition, the water is now purified with a great ability to remove heavy metals from the body as the liver and kidney reservoirs of hydrogen is replenished, making their part of the detoxification process more efficient. The density of the water with 0 degrees Celsius is 1.00 g pr cm3, the restructured and hexagonal water from Pure Energy Norway has a density of 0.96 g pr. cm3 which reflects the more open molecular structure of the new and living water.

For more information, or to purchase a Pure Energy Norway water device email: gunnar.espedal@gmail.com or go to our website: http://www.gunnarespedal.com

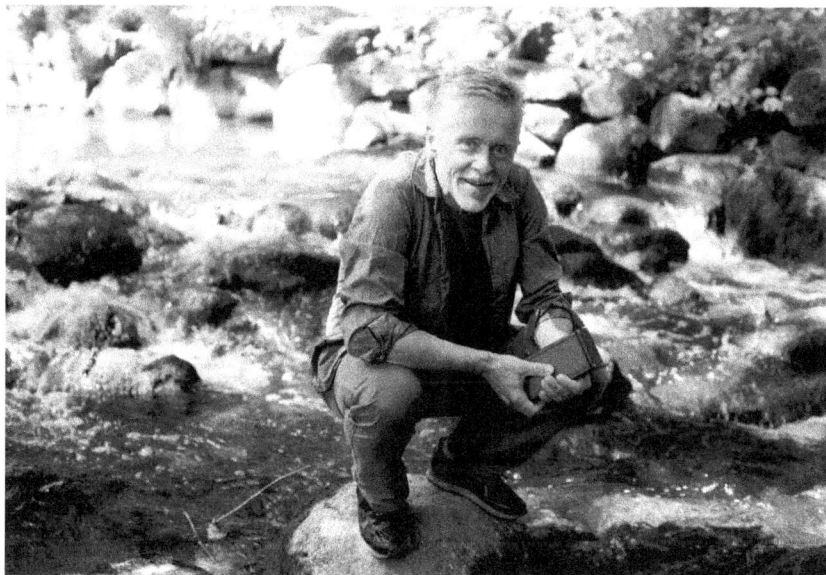

REFERENCES

A More Excellent Way – Spiritual Roots of Disease Pathways to Wholeness – Henry W. Wright – 2005

A Race for Madmen – The Extraordinary History of the Tour De France – Chris Sidwells – 2010

Allergies and Candida – Steven Rochlitz, MD, PhD

Better Bones, Better Body – Susan E. Brown, PhD – 1996

Better Health with (Mostly) Chinese Herbs & Foods – Dr Albert Y. Leung – 1995

Biological Ionization as applied to Farming & Soil Management – DR. A. J. Beddoe, DDS – 1986

Born to Run – Christopher McDougall – 2009

Cell-Level Healing, The Bridge from Soul to Cell – Joyce Whiteley Hawkes, PhD – 2006

Chemtrails Confirmed – William Thomas – 2004

Chronic Fatigue Syndrome, A natural way to treat ME – Professor Basant K. Puri – 2005

Coconut Cures, Preventing and Treating Common Health Problems with Coconut – Bruce Fife, ND – 2005

Confessions of a Medical Heretic – Robert S. Mendelsohn, MD – 1979

Curing the Incurable – Thomas E. Levy, MD, JD – 2009

Dancing with Water, The New Science of Water – MJ Pangman MS & Melanie Evans – The Sauna Cookbook, Food for Body and Soul – Tuula A. Kaitila & Edey E. Saarinen – 2004

Dead Doctors Don't Lie – Dr Joel D. Wallach & Dr Ma Lan – 1999

Detoxification & Healing – Sidney MacDonald Baker, MD – 1997

Don't Drink the Water – Lono Kahuna Kupua Ho'ala – 1998

Earthing, The Most Important Health Discovery Ever? – Clinton Over & Stephen T. Sinatra, MD & Martin Zucker – 2010

Emerging Viruses, AIDS & Ebola, Nature< Accident or Intentional? – Leonard G. Horowitz, MA, MPH – 1996

Excitotoxins, The Taste that Kills – Russell L. Blaylock, MD – 1997

Exuberance, The Passion for Life – Kay Redfield Jamison – 2004

Fats that Heal, Fats that Kill – Udo Erasmus – 1986

Fighting Body Pollution, Staying Healthy in an Unhealthy World – Paul Kramer, RCN – 2003

Fire in the Belly – Keith Scott-Mumby, MD, MB, ChB, PhD – 2012

Food in History – Reay Tannahill – 2007

Fresh Air for Life, Indoor Air Pollution – Allen C. Somersall, Ph.D. MD – 2006

Guds Egen Signatur – Grant R. Jeffrey – 1996

Gym Free and Ripped, Weight Free Workouts That Build and Sculpt – Nathan Jendrick – 2011

Healing Celebrations – Dr Leonard G. Horowitz – 2000

Healing is Voltage, Healing Eye Diseases – Jerry Tennant, MD(H), MD(P), FAAO – 2011

Healthy Recipes for Your Nutritional Type – Dr Joseph Mercola & Dr Kendra Degen Pearsall – 2007

Herbal Antibiotics, Natural Alternatives for Treating Drug-Resistant Bacteria – Stephen Harrod Buhner – 2012

Hormone Replacement Therapy, Yes or No? – Betty Kamen, PhD – 1993

How to Swap Asthma for Life – Michael Clark – 2007

How We Heal, Understanding the Mind-Body-Spirit Connection – Douglas W. Morrison – 2001

Hydrogen Peroxide, Medical Miracle – William Campell Douglass, MD – 1990

In the Mind of a Master – Susan Anderson with Sim Spurling – 2012

Introduction to Structured Water with Clayton Nolte – 2011

Invisible Killers – Rik j. Deitsch & Stewart Lonky MD – 2007

Life's Operating Manual – Tom Shadyac – 2013

Living Clay, Nature's Own Miracle Cure, Calcium Bentonite Clay – Perry A. – 2006

Medical Intuition – C. Norman Shealy, M.D. PhD – 2010

Mind Over Medicine, Scientific Proof that you Can Heal Yourself – Lissa Rankin, MD – 2013

Miracle Food Cures from The Bible – Reese Dubin – 1999

Natural Progesterone, The Multiple Roles of Remarkable Hormone – John R. Lee, MD – 1993

Naturlig Progesteron – Dr John R. Lee, MD – 1996

Nourishing Traditions – Sally Fallon – 1999

Nutrition and Physical Degeneration – Weston A. Price, DDS – 1939

On The Track of Water's Secret – Hans Kronberger – 1998, 2011

Optimal Health Guidelines, Second Edition – John R. Lee, MD – 1993

Ormus, Modern Day Alchemy – Chris Emmons RPH – 2009

Pemf, The 5th Element of Health – Bryant A Meyers – 2013

PEO Solution – Brian Scott Peskin, BSEE-MIT & Robert Jay Rowen, MD – 2014

Pity the Nation – Lebanon at War – Robert Fisk – 1990

Porphyria, The Ultimate Cause of Common, Chronic & Environmental Illness – Steven Rochlitz, PhD – 2010

Power Up Your Brain, The Neuroscience of Enlightenment – Dr David Perlmutter, FACN & Albert Villoldo, PhD – 2011

Rare Earths – Forbidden Cures – Joel D. Wallach, BS, DVM, ND & Ma Lan, MD, MS – 1994

Rip It Up – Richard Wiseman – 2012

Secrets of Your Cells – Sondra Barrett, PhD – 2013

Seeds of Deception – Jeffrey M. Smith – 2003

Solved: The Riddle of Illness – Stephen E. Langer, MD & James F. Scheer – 1984

Spark – John J. Ratey, MD – 2008

Spirit Filled Life Bible – New King James Version

Sweet Deceptions – Dr. Joseph Mercola & Dr Kendra Degen Pearsall – 2006

Take Control of Your Health, and Escape the Sickness Industry – Elaine Hollingsworth – 2003

Textbook or Orthopaedic Medicine, Volume 1, Fifth Edition – James Cyriax – 1947

The 4-Hour Body – Timothy Ferriss – 2010

The 4-Hour Workweek – Timothy Ferriss – 2007

The Art of Fermentation – Sandor Ellix Katz – 2012

The Art of Healing – Bernie S. Siegel, MD – 2013

The Blood and its Third Element – Antoine Bechamp – 2002

The Body Electric – Robert O. Becker, MD & Gary Selden – 1985

The Cancer Industry, Ralph W. Moss, PhD – 1999

The China Study – T. Colin Campbell, PhD & Thomas M. Campbell – 2004

The Clinical Science of Mineral Therapy – Leslie Fisher – 1991

The Complete Book of Running for Women – Claire Kowalchik – 1999

The Concept of Water – R. D. V. Glasgow – 2009

The Cure for All Diseases – Hulda Regehr Clark PhD, ND – 1995

The Doctor Who Cures Cancer – William Kelley Eidem – 1997

The Extracellular Matrix and Ground Regulation – Alfred Pischinger – 2007

The Field – Lynne McTaggart – 2001

The Fluoride Deception – Christopher Bryson – 2004

The Fourth Phase of Water, Beyond Solid Liquid Vapour – Gerald H. Pollack – 2013

The Genie in your Genes – Dawson Church, PhD – 1956

The Great Cholesterol Myth, Why Lowering your Cholesterol Won't Prevent Heart Disease – and the Statin-Free Plan that Will – Jonny Bowden, PhD, CNS & Stephen Sinatra, MD, FACC – 2012

The Hidden Messages in Water – Masaru Emoto – 2001

The Hidden Story of Cancer – Brain Scott Peskin, BSEE, MIT – 2006

The Homeopathic Treatment of Emotional Illness, A self-help guide to remedies which can restore calm and happiness – Dr Trevor Smith – 1983

The Honeymoon Effect – Bruce H. Lipton, PhD – 2013

The Immortal Edge – Michael Fossel, MD, PhD & Greta Blackburn & Dave Woynarowski, MD – 2011

The Maker's Diet – Jordan S. Rubin – 2003

The Medical Mafia – Suylaine Lanctot – 1999

The Miraculous Properties of Ionized Water, The Definitive Guide to the World's Healthiest Substance – Bob McCauley – 2006

The Prophet – Kahlil Gibran – 1926

The Rife Handbook of Frequency Therapy with a Holistic Health Primer – Nenah Sylver, PhD – 2009

The River Why – David James Duncan – 1983

The Science of Water, Concepts and Applications – Frank R. Spellman – 2008

The Secret of Quantum Living – Frank J. Kinslow – 2010

The Seven Pillars of Health – Dr Don Colbert – 2006

The Snowflake, Winter's Secret Beauty – Kenneth Libbrecht – 2003

The Sports Gene, What Makes the Perfect Athlete – David Epstein, 2013

The Tension Network of the Human Body – Robert Schleip & Thomas W Findley & Leon Chaitow & Peter A Huijing – 2012

The Truth About Air, Electricity & Health, A guide on the use of air ionization & other natural approaches for the 21st Century health issues – Rosalind Tan – 2013

The Untold Story of Milk – Ron Schmid, ND – 2003

The Virus and the Vaccine – Debbie Bookchin & Jim Schumacher – 2004

The Warrior Diet – Ori Hofmekler – 2003

The Whole Soy Story – Kaayla T. Daniel, PhD – 1999

The Wound and the Doctor – Glin Bennet – 1987

Transdermal Magnesium Therapy – Dr. Mark Sircus, Ac, OMD – 2011

Vaccination and Immunisation: Danger, Delusions and Alternatives – Leon Chaitow – 1987

Van Gogh and The Colours of the Night – 2008

Vibrational Medicine – Richard Gerber, MD – 1988

Walk on Water – Dr. Leonard G. Horowitz – 2006

Water – A Natural History – Alice Outwater – 1996

What Doctors Don't Tell You – Lynne McTaggart – 1996

What Your Doctor May NOT Tell You About Premenopause – John R. Lee, MD – 1999

When Healing Becomes a Crime – Kenny Ausubel – 2000

You Are Your Own Gym – Mark Lauren with Joshua Clark – 2010

Your Body's Many Cries for Water – F. Batmanghelidj, MD – 1992

Your Hands Can Heal You – Stephen Co & Eric B. Robbins, MD, with John Merryman – 2002

Your Own Perfect Medicine – Martha M. Christy – 1994

INDEX

Butyl-Ether 110

K

L

M

Microbes 77
Microbial 77, 196
Migraine 185
Milieu 148, 149, 384
Mindfulness 55
Mitochondria 66, 126, 145, 303, 478, 508
Monosodium Glutamate 95, 128, 140
Monoterpene 455
Moses 300, 388, 469
MRSA 125, 179
MSM 366
MTBE (Methyl—T- Butyl-Ether)   110
Mycotoxins 366
Myth 69, 96, 259
Mythology 39, 453
N
N-Acetyl Cysteine (NAC) 366
NAC (N-Acetyl Cysteine) 366
Naproxen 90
NASA 141, 188, 225, 234, 248, 249
Naturopath 117, 167, 168, 235, 319
Nausea 78, 99, 107, 108, 110, 114, 115
Nebuchadnezzar 328
Nella Fantasia 292
Neuralgia 443, 454, 469
Neurology 233
Neuron-Toxin 107, 356
Neuroscience 405, 514
Neurotransmitter330
Newton's Apple 57
Niacin 265, 466
Nickel 31, 115, 368
Nicola Salvi 284
Niels Bohr 97
Niesen 39
Nigella Sativa 444
Nigellone 444
Nikoline Broccolini 450
Nitric 471
Nitrogen 76, 108, 109, 110, 112, 287, 373, 377, 394
Nitrosamine 366
Noble Herb 465
Nose 110, 184, 189, 200, 206, 214, 220, 234, 315, 405
NRK (Norwegian Broadcasting) 165
Nucleotide 80, 155
Nuts 269, 278, 298, 323, 403, 410, 411, 415

www.ingramcontent.com/pod-product-compliance
Lightning Source LLC
Chambersburg PA
CBHW072104270326
41931CB00010B/1450